An Introduction to Neurophysiology

An Introduction to Neurophysiology

J.F.STEIN
MA, BSc, BM, BCh, MRCP
Lecturer in Physiology
University of Oxford and
Fellow of Magdalen College
Oxford

Blackwell Scientific Publications

OXFORD LONDON
EDINBURGH BOSTON MELBOURNE

First published 1982

Photoset by Enset Ltd,
Midsomer Norton, Bath, Avon
Printed and Bound in Great Britain
at the Alden Press, Oxford.

DISTRIBUTORS

USA
  Blackwell Mosby Book Distributors
  11830 Westline Industrial Drive
  St Louis, Missouri 63141

Canada
  Blackwell Mosby Book Distributors
  120 Melford Drive, Scarborough
  Ontario M1B 2X4

Australia
  Blackwell Scientific Book Distributors
  214 Berkeley Street, Carlton
  Victoria 3053

British Library
  Cataloguing in Publication Data

Stein, J.F.
  An introduction to neurophysiology.
  1. Neurophysiology
  I. Title
  612'.8   QP361

ISBN 0-632-00582-3

Contents

Preface

This book arose out of disappointment with most existing accounts of neurophysiology. Over ten years of tutoring and lecturing to medical and psychology students, neurologists, psychiatrists and even anaesthetists in training, I have come across very few texts which have managed in the least to convey the fascination and excitement of neurophysiology. Most fail rather dismally to overcome a central problem which neurophysiology faces: its techniques generate a wealth of results yet these often contribute rather little to our understanding of how the brain actually works. Indeed there are many who believe that the subject is regressing because it is incapable of interpreting its own data. This schism between results and their explanation is a particular problem of multi-authored books in which individual specialists cautiously under-interpret their contributions and carefully eschew speculation, presumably because they feel that textbooks should always stick to 'established facts'—as if there were such things. The result is that they succeed in producing rather dry and fact-filled texts which fail to capture the excitement of the subject.

Immodestly, therefore, I have tried to cover the whole of neurophysiology, adopting the same style and approach throughout. I have attempted to include only results which help to explain how particular neurophysiological mechanisms work, and have avoided those that do not contribute to such understanding. I fear the reader will find that this impudent aim has far exceeded the modest capacities of the author. It has certainly led to far more speculation than one would normally expect to find in a textbook. This is particularly true of the second half of the book, which deals with motor systems, because these are so much more difficult to study or understand. I am confident that most of these speculations, and I fear that also many of the 'facts' presented, will turn out to be wrong. But I crave the reader's indulgence and bid him remember the words of Lord Bacon: 'Truth is more likely to come out of error if this is clear and definite, than out of confusion.'

I am very much indebted to Geoffrey Walsh's *Physiology of the Nervous System* (Longman, London), which is a shining example of how neurophysiology can be made interesting and exciting. Naturally, I am also indebted to current texts in neurophysiology, such as those written by V. Mountcastle, T. Ruch & H.D. Patton,

S.W. Kuffler & J.G. Nichols and B. Katz, whose ideas for presenting material have, of course, influenced my own. I am grateful to my colleagues in the University Laboratory of Physiology, Oxford, many of whom, unwittingly or not, have helped with the writing of this book. I am grateful also to Blackwell Scientific Publications for their editorial help, and to Clare Little of Oxford Illustrators for converting my appalling scrawls into the delightful illustrations you see before you. I thank my wife, Clare, for putting up with the long gestation of this book, but above all I appreciated the company of my daughter, Lucy, each morning. Watching her 'doin' some drawin'' generated more ideas about how sensory and motor systems work than I would ever have believed possible.

Magdalen College,
Oxford

Chapter 1
Basic Structure of the CNS—
Neuroanatomy and
Neuroanatomical Methods

The foundation of neurophysiology is neuroanatomy. Without a thorough knowledge of the 'wiring diagram' of the brain we would be quite powerless to understand it. Without details of the microscopic structure of nerve cells and particularly of their contacts with each other we would be equally lost.

CELLS IN THE NERVOUS SYSTEM

The nervous system of most animals consists of separate nerve cells or *neurones*. These communicate with each other at specialized contact areas called *synapses* (a term coined by Sir Charles Sherrington from the Greek word for 'to clasp'). In the human nervous system there are perhaps 10^{15} neurones, and even these are outnumbered by their supporting cells, known as *glia* (Fig. 1.1), which include: *oligodendrocytes* which supply the myelin sheaths for central nervous fibres; *Schwann cells* which do the same for peripheral nerves; *astrocytes* which surround blood vessels, filling the role of fibrous tissue in other tissues; *microglia* which are the central-nervous scavengers, analogous to the macrophages found in the rest of the body; and *ependymal* cells which line the spinal canal and cerebral ventricles.

A 'typical' neurone consists, like most other cells, of a nucleus surrounded by cytoplasm which contains organelles such as mitochondria, ribosomes, vesicles, microtubules, etc., and is bounded by a cell membrane. It is bathed by a small amount of extracellular fluid (e.c.f.) which is doubly protected from the vagaries of the blood itself by the *blood–brain barrier*.

Nerve fibres

What distinguish nerve cells from other cells morphologically are their extended processes—branched *dendrites* often bearing thousands of 'spines', upon which other neurones synapse. These dendrites lead signals towards the cell body or soma, and usually a single *axon* leads away from the cell (Fig. 1.2). In some sensory neurones, e.g. those carrying cutaneous signals from the foot, the dendrites and axon together may be as long as 2 m. By contrast, small *interneurones* within the central nervous system may possess axons which are only a few microns in length. Many axons are ensheathed, by oligodendrocytes within the CNS or by Schwann cells peripherally; these provide a layer of thick insulating material, *myelin*, for the larger, rapidly conducting axons.

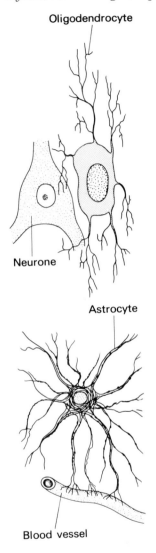

Oligodendrocyte

Neurone

Astrocyte

Blood vessel

Fig. 1.1. Glial cells.

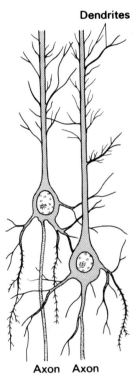

Dendrites

Axon   Axon

Fig. 1.2. Pyramidal neurones in cerebral cortex.

Reflex arc

The basic organization of the CNS is surprisingly simple (Fig. 1.3). Receptors in the periphery (skin, eyes, ears, etc.) connect with sensory nerve fibres. These are the long processes of nerve cells whose cell bodies lie close to, or within, the CNS. In the case of spinal sensory nerve fibres, the cell bodies are found in the *dorsal root ganglia* which lie near the dorsolateral surface of the spinal cord. The central processes of these neurones pass into the spinal cord via the *dorsal roots* and either (1) pass immediately upwards towards the head; or (2) make contact in the *dorsal horn* of *grey matter* of the spinal cord with second-order, relay neurones which then pass information upwards towards the brain; or (3) make contact with *interneurones* (none of whose processes extends further than a few millimetres locally); or (4) make contact directly with *motoneurones* situated within the ventral part of the grey matter, the *ventral horn*. The axons of ventral horn cells (which constitute the *motor nerves*) are directed back via the *ventral roots* to the motor apparatus of the body, the skeletal muscles. Thus the basic organizational unit of the

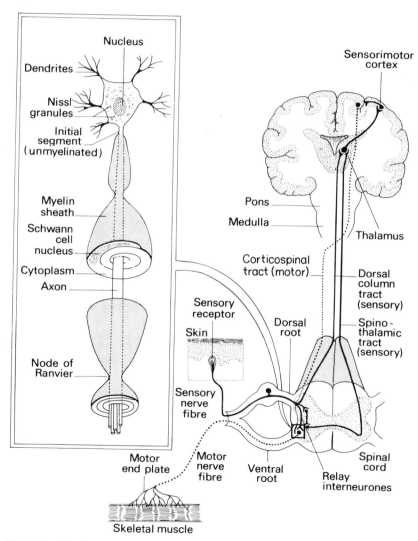

Fig. 1.3. Basic circuits in the CNS.

spinal cord (a *reflex* arc) consists of sensory nerve fibres passing via dorsal roots to the dorsal horn to connect with mononeurones in the ventral horn whose axons leave for the muscles via the ventral roots. The unidirectional flow of signals into the spinal cord via the dorsal roots and out of it via the ventral roots is known as the Bell–Magendie 'law'; unfortunately it is now known to be an over-simplification, and therefore cannot be considered a law.

Spinal segments

The spinal cord derives many of its features from the segmental organization of the lower animals from which we have evolved. It consists of 31 segments, each giving rise to a pair of spinal nerves which contain both dorsal (sensory) and ventral (motor) root fibres. These 31 pairs are distributed as follows: eight cervical, twelve thoracic, five lumbar, five sacral and one coccygeal. Because inner-vation of the upper and lower limbs demands more neuronal machinery than the rest of the trunk, the spinal cord is enlarged at the point where the cervical and lumbar roots emerge. The sensory innervation of the skin of the trunk (the dermatomes) is very orderly, but because the basic innervation of the body segments occurs early in embryonic life, before the limb buds have developed, the migration of the portions of embryonic segments which form the limbs confuses the pattern of cutaneous innervation. Similarly, the sensory and motor supply to the muscles of the trunk is simple, but the segmental nerve roots supplying the different muscles of the limbs intermingle in the cervical, brachial, lumbar and sacral plexuses, so that it is often difficult to determine from the site of a muscle which spinal cord segments innervate it.

General structure of the brain

Like the spinal cord, the brain develops from the hollow dorsal neural tube of the embryo. Quite early in development, the anterior end of this tube shows three clearly identifiable enlargements: the forebrain, midbrain and hindbrain. The remnants of the interior of the tube are the hollow lateral and third ventricles of the forebrain, the midbrain 'aqueduct of silvius', the hindbrain fourth ventricle and the spinal canal. During development these cerebral enlarge-ments subdivide further. The forebrain gives rise to the telen-cephalon (which later forms the cerebral hemispheres and basal ganglia) and the diencephalon (which develops into the thalamus and hypothalamus); the midbrain develops into the mesencephalon which forms the tectal region (superior and inferior colliculi), midbrain reticular formation and cerebral peduncles; whilst the hindbrain gives rise to the pons, cerebellum and medulla.

The entire brain is contained in, and suspended and protected by, three membranes, the meninges, known as the dura mater, arachnoid mater and pia mater. The innermost, the pia mater, envelops neural elements themselves. The arachnoid mater lies outside the pia, enclosing the subarachnoid space which contains cerebrospinal fluid (c.s.f.). This fluid, whose composition is controlled more closely than that of blood as a result of the blood–brain barrier, is secreted by *choroid plexuses* in the ventricular system of the brain, flows from there into the subarachnoid space surrounding the brain and spinal cord, and is reabsorbed into the venous sinuses by the arachnoid villi. The blood–brain barrier (Fig. 1.4) is not a single anatomical entity but refers to the protection afforded by the combined effect of the cerebrospinal fluid (c.s.f.) and extra layers of arachnoid and pial membrane interposed between the blood capillaries and nerve cells in the brain. Thus the brain floats in c.s.f. and is chemically and mechanically protected by it. Furthermore, wherever blood vessels enter the brain, continuations of the pial and arachnoid membranes accompany them, forming an important part of the blood–brain barrier. The outer meninx is the dura mater, which lies immediately underneath the cranium and spinal canal. Within the layers of dura are formed the venous sinuses, which drain blood from the brain and reabsorb c.s.f. through the arachnoid villi.

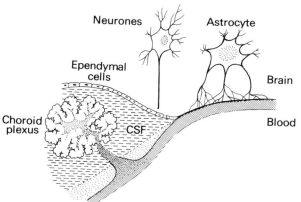

Fig. 1.4. The blood–brain barrier. Neurones are separated from blood by c.s.f., ependymal cells and astrocyte processes surrounding blood vessels.

The cerebral hemispheres (Fig. 1.5)

The left and right cerebral hemispheres are the most conspicuous structures in the human nervous system. It is their complexity and size which provides us with consciousness and our superior ability to adapt and react to changing circumstances, and to profit from the previous experiences not only of ourselves, but also of others with whom we can communicate complex ideas by speech and writing.

The hemispheres are separated from each other by the longitudinal (or sagittal) fissure. This deep cleft is crossed by the corpus callosum, which is a large band of fibres connecting the two hemispheres. Within the hemispheres lie the lateral and third ventricles and the basal ganglia, thalamus and hypothalamus. The cerebral cortex is greatly increased in area by folding into convolutions (gyri), which are separated by fissures (sulci). The lateral sulcus (Sylvian fissure) is the most prominent of these and separates the temporal lobe from the frontal, parietal and occipital lobes above it. The second largest is the central or Rolandic fissure which passes downwards, laterally and slightly forwards from a point about a third of the way between the frontal and occipital poles. It delineates the frontal lobe from the parietal lobe posterior to it. The parietal lobe is separated from the occipital lobe behind it by the parieto-occipital sulcus.

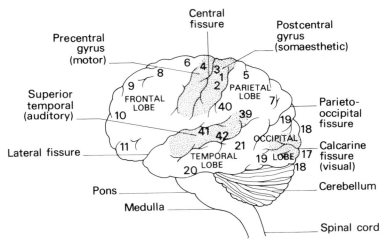

Fig. 1.5. External view of brain showing Brodmann's cytoarchitectonic numbers.

The precentral gyrus, just in front of the central fissure, is also called the motor cortex, because stimulation here causes movements of different parts of the body. In general the frontal lobe is most active during movement and may be considered the motor part of the cerebral cortex. Behind the central sulcus in the postcentral gyrus, lies the primary somaesthetic sensory area; in the superior temporal gyrus lies the primary auditory receiving area; whilst at the very back of the occipital lobe, surrounding the calcarine fissure, lies the primary visual cortex. Between these specialized sensory regions lie large areas of 'association' cortex. Thus areas behind the central sulcus are mostly devoted to sensation rather than movement.

Basal ganglia (Fig. 1.6)

The basal ganglia or deep cerebral nuclei (cf. deep cerebellar nuclei) are paired masses of grey matter lying within the cerebral hemispheres. The most prominent of these is the corpus striatum which consists of the caudate nucleus and putamen, separated from each other by the internal capsule. These project to the globus pallidus which lies medial to them, and this in turn mainly projects medially to the thalamus.

Thalamus (Fig. 1.6)

The thalamus is a large, oval structure lying above the hypothalamus and medial to the basal ganglia, beside the lateral and third ventricles. It develops from the diencephalic division of the forebrain, and almost all fibres passing to the cerebral hemispheres relay in one of its many nuclei (as shown in Fig. 8.8). These include nuclei relaying specific sensory information [the lateral geniculate (vision), the medial geniculate (hearing), the ventroposterolateral (somaesthesia)]; motor afferent nuclei (the ventrolateral and ventroanterior); nuclei supplying association cortex (the pulvinar, dorsomedial and anterior); and non-specific nuclei which project to other thalamic nuclei and to the basal ganglia (the intralaminar and reticular).

Hypothalamus (Fig. 1.6)

The hypothalamus is a small portion of the diencephalon forming the floor and lower part of the wall of the third ventricle. Like the thalamus, it consists of many small nuclei. These are responsible for many of the homeostatic functions of the body by regulating the autonomic nervous system and the hormone orchestra, and by influencing drives and emotions, such as eating, drinking, defence, sexual behaviour and sleep.

Midbrain (Fig. 1.7)

The midbrain or mesencephalon extends from the upper pons to the lower border of the hypothalamus. The most conspicuous features of its ventral part are two huge fibre bundles, the cerebral peduncles, which carry motor fibres away from the cerebral cortex and sensory fibres towards the thalamus. On the dorsal surface of the midbrain (also called the tectum or tegmentum) lie the superior (visual) and inferior (auditory) colliculi, together called the corpora quadrigemina. Within the substance of the midbrain lie two motor nuclei, the red nucleus and substantia nigra (black nucleus), and the

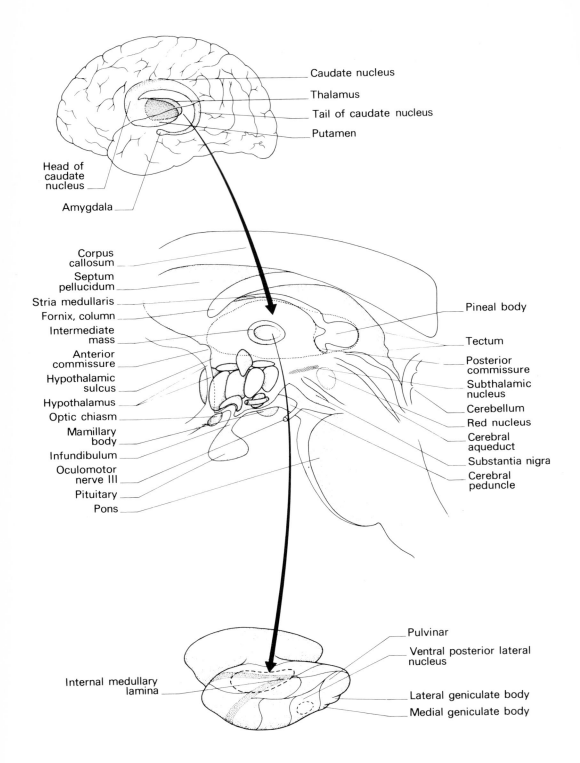

Caudate nucleus

Thalamus

Tail of caudate nucleus

Putamen

Head of
caudate
nucleus

Amygdala

Corpus
callosum

Septum
pellucidum

Stria medullaris

Fornix, column

Intermediate
mass

Anterior
commissure

Hypothalamic
sulcus

Hypothalamus

Optic chiasm

Mamillary
body

Infundibulum

Oculomotor
nerve III

Pituitary

Pons

Pineal body

Tectum

Posterior
commissure

Subthalamic
nucleus

Cerebellum

Red nucleus

Cerebral
aqueduct

Substantia nigra

Cerebral
peduncle

Pulvinar

Ventral posterior lateral
nucleus

Internal medullary
lamina

Lateral geniculate body

Medial geniculate body

Fig. 1.6. Basal ganglia, thalamus and hypothalamus.

nuclei of the third and fourth cranial nerves, which supply extrinsic and intrinsic muscles of the eyes.

Pons varioli (Fig. 1.7)

The pons appears to form a bridge between the two halves of the cerebellum, hence its name. Its most obvious feature is the band of fibres on the ventral surface connecting the pontine nuclei within it to the cerebellar hemispheres via the middle cerebellar peduncles. The pontine nuclei receive signals from the cerebral cortex destined for the cerebellum. Through the pons pass the motor and sensory fibres which form the cerebral peduncles in the midbrain. It also contains nuclei of the Vth, VIth, VIIth and VIIIth cranial nerves and motor nuclei in the pontine reticular formation which participate in postural, cardiovascular and respiratory control.

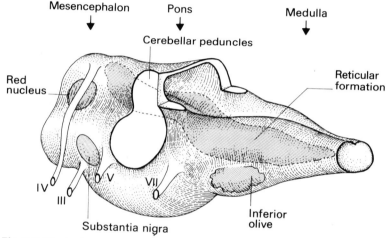

Fig. 1.7. The brainstem.

Medulla oblongata (Fig. 1.7)

The medulla is continuous with the pons above and the spinal cord below and therefore carries all the ascending and descending tracts which communicate between the spinal cord and brain. On its ventral surface lie two roughly pyramid-shaped structures, the 'medullary pyramids', which are the 10% of corticofugal fibres remaining after the rest of those passing through the cerebral peduncles have left the pons to supply the cerebellum and other brainstem motor structures. Just above the junction of the medulla with the spinal cord, at the pyramidal decussation, most of the left-hand-side pyramidal tract fibres cross over to the right and vice versa. They then form the lateral corticospinal tract in the lateral column of the spinal cord. Above this decussation, somaesthetic fibres relaying in the dorsal column nuclei also decussate to form the medial lemniscus, which passes upwards towards the thalamus. Thus these sensory fibres come to lie on top of the medullary pyramids.

In addition, the medulla contains nuclei of the Vth, IXth, Xth, XIth and XIIth cranial nerves, another large relay of signals destined for the cerebellum (the inferior olive) and further dispersed collections of cell bodies separated by a network of fibres, which participate in respiratory, cardiovascular and postural control (the medullary reticular formation).

NEUROANATOMICAL METHODS

Study of the intact or coarsely sliced brain has now revealed most of what it can. However, examination of the brain's intimate structure by light and electron microscopy remains extremely fruitful.

Golgi technique

Because there are perhaps a thousand million million (10^{15}) neurones in the brain, dyes which stain every neurone are not much help in elucidating the structure of any individual neurone as each would be overlaid by thousands of others. However, the technique introduced by Golgi enables a single neurone to be stained. For some reason still unknown, this technique stains 'capriciously', particularly in neonatal animals, impregnating only about one cell in a hundred with silver. But those few cells which are stained are outlined in their entirety, so that all their processes can be seen. Golgi's technique has revealed more information about the structure of individual neurones than any other. It is ironic that Golgi used it to try to support his belief that the CNS consists of a continuous network of fibres with a continuous cytoplasm (a 'syncytium'), rather than many thousands of discrete but contiguous neurones as suggested by Schwann's *cell theory*.

Neurone doctrine

Ramon y Cajal, who laid the foundations of much of our knowledge of the structure of the nervous system, exploited Golgi's technique to demolish the nerve net theory and to substantiate in its place the 'neurone doctrine'—the cell theory applied to the nervous system. He realized that the Golgi method stained whole individual neurones but not their neighbours, and therefore that all neurones must be separate from one another. He was able to demonstrate that each neurone receives signals from others via its dendrites, transfers them to its cell body or *soma* and dispatches the signals onwards, sometimes great distances, via its axon (Fig. 1.3) which then makes synaptic contacts with the next neurone's dendrites. Neurones are thus 'contiguous not continuous'. Seldom can a duo with such antagonistic beliefs as Golgi and Cajal have shared a Nobel prize!

Anterograde degeneration

The next important advance in neuroanatomy was the discovery that chemical changes in damaged neurones could be detected using special stains. When an axon is cut off from its parent cell it begins to degenerate within 12 hours, and dies within a week. The degenerating material binds silver stains particularly well. Thus if a nerve tract of interest is cut in an operation under anaesthetic and the animal killed after about six days (the optimum time to observe degeneration), the normal course of the tract can be traced in microscopic sections by looking for the places where stained degeneration products may be seen. Early variations of this technique, such as the Marchi method, suffered from the disadvantage that an axon's terminals were not stained. This is a serious drawback since, if one cannot visualize the actual nerve endings, one cannot be sure whether a pathway under study actually terminates in a particular structure or simply passes through it. In the hands of Nauta, Fink and Heimer, however, methods have been perfected for staining degenerating axon terminals and visualizing them using the electron microscope.

Autoradiography

Degeneration techniques were the major tools used by neuroanatomists until very recently, but now more direct methods for outlining neurones and their processes are available. Radioactive amino acids injected in the vicinity of nerve cell bodies are taken up and transported right out to the peripheral terminations of their axons. The site of radioactivity in sections of the brain cut a few hours later can then be detected by its effect on a photographic emulsion (autoradiography). Thus the course of fibres originating in the injected nucleus can be determined, without having to make lesions. Also, using microelectrodes inserted into nerve cells it is now possible, although difficult, to inject dyes such as 'procion yellow' into nerve cells identified electrophysiologically, and thus visualize them afterwards in their entirety.

Retrograde degeneration

It is often useful to be able to detect not only where a fibre goes but also where it comes from. Loss of its axon causes compensatory changes in a nerve cell body. Such 'retrograde' effects of lesions can be detected with suitable stains. However, retrograde degeneration only occurs if a substantial proportion of the terminal branches of a neurone are destroyed. Consequently, if axons branch to two quite different areas the technique will not usually work.

HRP

Curiously, however, a large molecule totally unconnected with the nervous system, horseradish peroxidase (HRP), is taken up by nerve terminals and transported back to their parent cell bodies. Thus, if HRP is injected into a region, the origin of fibres terminating there can be determined by looking for the cell bodies in which HRP reaction products are found. It does not matter whether the axon has one or many branches, as the HRP will still be transported back to the parent cell body. It is even possible using two substances of this sort staining or fluorescing different colours to label the same cell body from two different sites and thus show that its axons branch to both of them.

Transneuronal degeneration

If a large proportion of the terminals normally impinging on a neurone are removed, the receiving neurone may also show changes which can be detected with suitable stains (*transneuronal degeneration*). A classic instance of this is the effect upon the lateral geniculate nucleus of removing one eye. The main input to three of its six layers is removed by this means, so the neurones in these layers degenerate even though they themselves, projecting on-wards to the visual cortex, have not been touched.

Electroanatomy

At this point we should consider a technique not strictly neuro-anatomical which will be considered in greater detail later, namely electrical stimulation and recording in anaesthetized animals. This is often somewhat disparagingly called 'electroanatomy', since in many ways it is analogous to the neuroanatomical techniques we have considered already. In brief, sites in the nervous system are stimulated electrically and activity evoked elsewhere is recorded by means of suitable electrodes. With this technique both *orthograde* (normal direction of flow of signals) and *retrograde (antidromic)* activity can be detected, so that it can be used to supplement neuroanatomical delineation of pathways between structures.

Chapter 2
Physiological Techniques

Although a knowledge of the connections between regions, the 'wiring diagram', is essential background for studying the functions of the nervous system, by itself neuroanatomy can never show us how a neural network really works. Neuroanatomists, of course, often suggest how structures they see might work, usually by comparing them with similar structures whose functions are well known; but eventually the only way to reveal mechanisms is to watch them at work by recording electrical changes, by observing the effect of 'fraudulent' messages introduced by electrical stimulation, or by observing what goes wrong when bits of the system are removed or ablated; in short the neurophysiologist's trusted triad of techniques: ablation, stimulation and recording. To these we must now add pharmacological counterparts: pharmacological inhibition, stimulation by chemical transmitter *agonists,* and recording transmitter release.

Ablation

Ablation is what nature unfortunately achieves when disease destroys parts of the brain. However, because most pathological processes do not abide by neuroanatomical boundaries, it is often very difficult to interpret a patient's symptoms in terms of particular structures damaged. If they are sufficiently skilful, neuroscientists can make discrete lesions with a greater certainty of hitting a particular region. Nevertheless, the results are still difficult to interpret. However well placed a lesion is, it is almost certain to interrupt fibres which may have nothing to do with the region being studied but simply pass nearby. The consequences of severing these fibres may easily be mistaken for the functions of the target area. For some systems this problem can be partly overcome by using drugs which selectively poison certain types of neurones only— pharmacological ablation. For instance, 6-hydroxydopamine (6-OHDA) is taken up predominantly by those neurones which employ dopamine in the synthesis of their transmitters. The drug cannot be metabolized further and quickly kills the cell. For example, when 6-OHDA is injected into a nucleus containing dopaminergic cells, such as the substantia nigra, it kills only the dopaminergic neurones, not neurones employing other transmitters or fibres of passage. Likewise, another poison, kainic acid (a glutamate analogue), is thought to be absorbed only by cell bodies, and thus kills only neurones originating at the site of injection.

Neural plasticity

A second major problem in interpretation of the results of lesions in the CNS is that when one part is damaged other parts can often take over many of its functions. This capacity of the brain for lasting self-modification is known as *plasticity*, and its mechanism is far from understood. The process often occurs rapidly; within a few hours of making a lesion many of the initial symptoms may have disappeared, so it is impossible to be sure whether defects seen in the early period are actually a result of the lesion itself or were just due to temporary disturbances consequent upon the trauma of surgery, anaesthesia, etc. Assessment of lasting deficits requires sophisticated testing. Usually, the animal must be trained beforehand to perform a task designed to reveal the expected deficit. Even if a disability does become apparent upon behavioural testing, this only tells us about that part of the total set of functions of the ablated area which other parts of the brain cannot take over, rather than about important roles the area might perform under normal circumstances. For example, if a lesion is made in the motor cortex of a monkey, the animal is initially paralysed on the opposite side of the body. Quite quickly, however, it recovers almost complete use of these limbs and eventually the only demonstrable deficit is its inability to move the fingers separately, so it uses the hand as a single unit like a spatula. It would be a mistake to deduce from this that the only normal function of the motor cortex is to move the fingers independently; this is just the only function of the motor cortex which other structures cannot take over.

Reversible inactivation

New techniques which may help to overcome these problems are local cooling and the local administration of short-term drugs. Using these methods one can temporarily inactivate a defined region of the brain in unanaesthetized animals, and observe changes in behaviour. Thus one can investigate the immediate effects of such temporary disruption and compare these with performance before and after treatment. This goes some way towards defeating the brain's plasticity because the normal functions of a region may be revealed before other parts of the brain have time to take over. Furthermore, by varying the degree of cooling or the amount of drug administered one can produce greater or lesser degrees of impairment at will.

A further problem with ablation techniques is that the result of a lesion may not be the loss of some function (negative symptom), but the release of activity normally kept under inhibitory control by the ablated area (positive symptoms). Such effects are predictable from the important part that inhibition plays in controlling the operations of the central nervous system, but they serve to confuse the unwary experimenter. The classic examples of positive release symptoms (disinhibitions) are found in the involuntary movements of basal ganglia disease—tremor, chorea (dance-like movements) and hemiballismus (uncontrolled throwing about of a limb); these are essentially normal sequences of movements released inappropriately and repeatedly.

Stimulation

The second class of technique employed by neurophysiologists is electrical stimulation. The great advantage of this approach is that the timing and magnitude of the stimulus can be clearly defined. It is therefore easy to see whether any neural response is related in time to the stimulus and hence likely to be 'driven' by it. The delay between the stimulus and response (the *latency*) can give much useful information about the pathways between the sites of stimulation and response. Further important data can be derived from changing the magnitude of the stimulating current and its frequency.

For example, the pontine nucleus lies in the midbrain and is known to project axons to the opposite cerebellar cortex, a distance of about 20 mm in the cat. Stimulation of the nucleus gives rise to single unit responses which may be recorded from the granule cell layer of cerebellum about 5 ms later (Fig. 2.1a). These responses disappear if the stimulating current is dropped below a *threshold* of about 15 μA, and they fail even at high stimulus intensities if the frequency of stimulation is greater than about 20 pulses per second (p.p.s.). These facts may be interpreted as follows: the 5 ms latency of this 20 mm pathway indicates a conduction velocity for these fibres of about $20 \times 10^{-3} \div 5 \times 10^{-3} = 4 \ \mathrm{ms^{-1}}$; axons with a diameter of about 0.7 μm have this conduction velocity and their cell bodies would be *c.* 40 μm in diameter. Neuroanatomical studies of the pontine nucleus confirm that these deductions are correct.

The fact that the responses begin to drop out when the stimulating frequency is raised above 20 p.p.s. suggests that there is a *synapse* between recording and stimulating electrodes which cannot faithfully follow higher frequencies. The recording electrode is not actually recording from the fibre which left the pontine

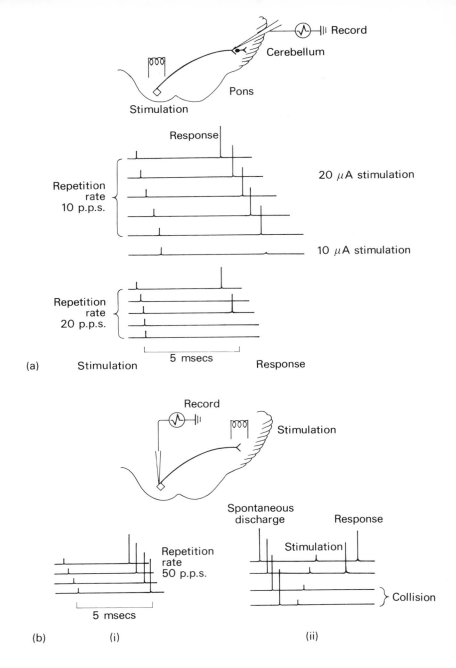

Fig. 2.1. (a) Stimulation in pontine nucleus; recording trans-synaptically from second neurone in cerebellar cortex. A 20 μA stimulus causes a regular response in a cerebellar neurone when repeated 10 times per second, but the neurone fails to follow at 20 pulses per second or if the intensity is halved to 10 μA. (b) Stimulating pontine neurone terminals in cerebellar cortex excites them antidromically. Since there is no synapse they follow a much higher frequency of stimulation (50 p.p.s.) (i). If an antidromic stimulus follows shortly after a spontaneous discharge of the neurone, orthodromic and antidromic impulses meet each other's refactory periods (collide) and the antidromic signal drops out (ii).

nucleus—a difficult feat anyway—but from the next neurone in this particular pathway, a cerebellar granule cell. The axon from the pontine nucleus makes synaptic contacts with the dendrites of granule cell. These contacts transfer the impulse but have a lower security of transmission than the axon itself, so they fail to conduct at higher frequencies. Had we been recording from the axon itself we would expect it to follow at frequencies of up to about a hundred p.p.s.

If we reverse the recording and stimulating electrodes, and now stimulate the axon terminals in the cerebellar cortex, recording from the neuronal cell bodies in the pontine nucleus (Fig. 2.1b), we can activate the pontine cells by 'backfiring' them *antidromically*. (Axons, unlike synapses, will transmit messages in either direction.) When this is done, the latency from stimulus to antidromic activation of the pontine neurone is slightly shorter than before, since we now avoid perhaps 0.5 ms of synaptic delay in the cerebellum, so we should recalculate the conduction velocity (this gives a figure of 4.4 ms^{-1}). We now find that the axon will follow stimulating frequencies up to perhaps 100 p.p.s. Furthermore, if we can arrange things in such a way that the stimulation of the cerebellum follows shortly after a spontaneous discharge of the pontine neurone (Fig. 2.1bii), then the orthodromic impulse passing towards the cerebellum collides with the antidromic impulse coming back from the cerebellum and the two cancel out. This collision technique is the only sure way of knowing that stimulating and recording electrodes were at the two ends of the same neurone. Conveniently, unlike the recording electrode, the stimulating electrode does not have to be particularly close to the axon terminal, as current will spread to it from some distance away.

A major disadvantage of electrical stimulation is that it is most unnatural. The nervous system does not normally encounter large electrical shocks causing many thousands of neurones to discharge synchronously. Rather, natural stimuli set up complex patterns of activity, distributed in both space and time, which are transformed and redirected during the normal operations of the nervous system; so electrical stimulation is essentially a crude artifice. However, it is especially useful in the study of electroanatomy, as we have seen. Also it may provide qualitative information about whether a pathway is excitatory or inhibitory and quantitative information about how effective it is. Lacking any knowledge of electrophysiology, Cajal never entertained the possibility of inhibition, and therefore made limited functional sense of the structures he discovered. However, Sherrington, using electrical as well as natural stimuli, was able to deduce the existence of inhibition and with it lay the foundations of much of our understanding of how the nervous system works.

Natural stimulation

One might think that light shone in the eye, touch on the skin, or sound at the ear (natural stimulation) would overcome many of the disadvantages of electrical stimulation. However, natural stimuli also have several disadvantages. Their timing is usually much more difficult to define precisely. Sensory energy must be transferred to sensory receptors and transformed into nervous impulses. This all takes time, and the length of time often varies. After a bright light is shone onto the retina it takes perhaps 10 ms for the first impulses to reach the optic nerve leaving the eye, but with a dim light it may take up to 100 ms. When the skin is pressed it takes an amount of time, which varies with temperature, local circulation, etc., for the full pressure to be transferred to nerve terminals within the dermis.

Moreover, it is often difficult to decide what is the appropriate natural stimulus to apply. It was not until Hubel and Wiesel started using slits rather than spots of light that the sensitivity of neurones in the visual cortex to the orientation of lines and edges in the environment was appreciated (Chapter 6). It is still an open question as to which is the best sort of stimulus to use for auditory cortical neurones and many others. One has to be very careful what is meant by the word 'best' in this context. The relatively simple criteria used by neurophysiologists, such as a neurone's peak discharge frequency or total number of impulses per stimulus, may not be at all significant to the brain. The CNS as a whole may be interested in much more complex and sophisticated patterns of discharge than we yet comprehend.

Pharmacological stimulation

A new twist to the study of stimulation has arisen from pharmacological techniques. Many of the chemicals responsible for transmitting messages between the synapses of neurones have now been identified and synthesized. These, or their analogues (agonists), can be introduced artificially into the CNS with the aim of selectively stimulating the neurones which normally employ them as transmitters. Thus, for example, the transmitter acetylcholine (ACh) injected near to motoneurones in the spinal cord selectively excites small interneurones there known as Renshaw cells, whose effects on the motoneurones may thus be studied.

Pharmacological inhibitors

Similarly, pharmacological agents which block the action of transmitter systems are useful. Strychnine has long been employed in this way, though the rationale for its efficacy has only recently become clear. It seems to block postsynaptic inhibition by suppressing the action of a normally inhibitory transmitter (gamma-aminobutyric acid (GABA)). The consequence is that neurones normally kept under tight control by the action of GABA are disinhibited by strychnine and discharge continuously. Thus strychnine turns out to be rather a convenient way of stimulating the nervous system. Because the CNS usually has a very efficient means of disposing of its own excitatory transmitters in order that they will not continue their excitatory effects for too long, they themselves are not the most useful experimental tools. However, the CNS is not used to strychnine and has no efficient means for disposing of it, so it remains active for much longer to exert continuing stimulation.

Electrical recording

Probably the most informative neurophysiological technique is to record from neural structures while they are in action. (Galvani was the first to suggest that the nervous system might operate by means of electricity.) Modern developments in electronics make it quite a simple matter to record and amplify the relatively small potentials produced by nerve cells (Fig. 2.2). This has become the technique of choice, because it offers a way of 'spying' on neurones going about their normal business. The most recent development—recording from fully awake, moving animals—is even more promising as it disposes of the need for anaesthetics which depress and alter normal neuronal activity.

When recording from the CNS one can either measure, using relatively large electrodes, the potentials produced by large groups

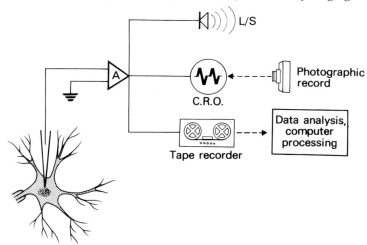

Fig. 2.2. Basic intracellular recording set up. The microelectrode is connected to a very high impedance amplifier. Discharges are heard on a loudspeaker, inspected on a cathode-ray oscilloscope (C.R.O.) and recorded for subsequent analysis on a tape recorder.

of cells (these are known as *gross potentials* for obvious reasons) or, using very small microelectrodes, record from just a single neurone either extracellularly by placing the electrode close to the neurone or, with greater difficulty, intracellularly by piercing the cell and recording from inside it.

Gross potentials

Gross potential records are difficult to interpret. This is because in most areas of the brain there are large numbers of different sorts of neurones distributed with different geometric relationships to one another and to a recording electrode. What it records, therefore, is a composite potential from all these neurones, weighted according to their distances from, and the attitude of their electrical axes to, the electrode. Thus, even if it were possible, by suitable stimulation, to make every neurone of a particular sort fire synchronously (and it usually is not), the potential recorded by a gross electrode would still be complicated by the different distances and axis angles of the cells relative to the electrode. Furthermore, neurones stimulated first excite then inhibit other cells in turn, so the recorded potential is quickly affected by secondary activity.

In short, gross potential recording is very frustrating. Nevertheless, it can help to give a general impression of the activity occurring after a stimulus. Gross potentials evoked by a stimulus confined to different parts of the visual field have been used to map the projection of the retina on to the visual cortex in a far more precise way than is possible neuroanatomically. This still remains the quickest and most convenient way of determining where on the cortical representation of the visual fields an electrode happens to lie. Furthermore, computerized methods now allow us to record gross potentials through the human scalp or vertebral column and offer exciting prospects for the application of electrophysiological techniques to the study of neurological disease.

In certain favourable areas gross potential recordings can be used more analytically. In the retina, cerebellum and hippocampus, for example, cell types are segregated in different layers and are arranged in well-defined geometric relationships to one another. The effects of stimulating a particular afferent can therefore be related to the cell type receiving the input by advancing a gross electrode through the layers of cells and noting the timing and amplitude of the potential fields set up by the stimulus at different depths. This technique is called *laminar field analysis*.

Microelectrode recording

It is now possible to record from single neurones intracellularly. A very fine microelectrode (tip diameter less than 1 μm) is made to penetrate the cell membrane, which then seals around it. Intracellular recording is technically very demanding as neither the neurone or the electrode can be permitted to move so much as a micron or the cell is lost. This is very difficult to achieve *in vivo*, since the brain and spinal cord tend to move small distances each time the heart beats or the animal breathes and these movements clearly cannot be stopped altogether! It is the only technique, however, that can give direct information about the electrical state of the membrane, the *membrane potential*; such knowledge is essential for determining the precise nature of *synaptic inputs* to a cell. Furthermore, only by penetrating a cell can one inject dyes to identify the neurone from which one has been recording.

Extracellular recording from single neurones

Extracellular recording is rather easier. A microelectrode made of glass or insulated wire (commonly tungsten) etched to a fine point is brought sufficiently close to a cell or fibre to record the small extracellular currents which flow when it discharges an *action potential*. The electrode is advanced towards the neurone with a suitable microdrive; proximity is usually judged by listening to the amplified crack of the neurone's discharge heard over a loudspeaker.

One has no choice which particular neurone in an area of interest is approached, although one may be able to identify it histologically afterwards. It is widely suspected that electrodes tend to record from the largest neurones in an area but, for unknown reasons, different types of electrode record from different sorts of neurone. The experimenter tries to record from as many neurones as possible in a region and thus derive general principles about the properties of the whole population of neurones from this small sample. However, he cannot easily allow for the bias introduced by the electrode's properties.

Furthermore, the activity of any single neurone is probably relatively unimportant by itself. (We can happily lose a very large number of cells as a result of disease, neurosurgery or an excessive affection for alcohol and not notice any obvious changes until late in life.) What is important is the overall activity of a whole population of neurones, all doing approximately the same thing. It may be impossible to judge from the behaviour of one cell that happens to be at the end of one's electrode what the emergent properties of the whole population would be. Nevertheless, extracellular recording from single neurones is one of the best techniques we have at the moment, and much of what follows in this book has depended on it.

Local blood flow

Very recently, promising techniques have been introduced for visualizing which cerebral regions become active under different circumstances. When neurones are activated their consumption of glucose increases, and if there is enough regional activity local blood flow will also increase. Radioactive deoxyglucose can enter the cell in place of glucose but since it cannot be metabolized it accumulates in the cell and may therefore be used as a very precise indicator of which individual cells were active just before an animal is killed and its brain fixed. This technique has been used, for example, to confirm that all the cells in a 'column' of the visual cortex respond to only one orientation of a bar of light.

In conscious animals, including man, local increases in blood flow may be detected using radioactive isotopes circulating in the blood. Counters sited around the head are used to determine where the isotope has concentrated, and so the regions in which blood flow has increased. This technique has been used to confirm that an area just in front of the 'mouth' region of the left motor cortex (Broca's speech area) increases its activity during speech, and that when we conceive an action but do not execute it an area medial to the motor cortex, the supplementary motor area, increases its activity although the motor cortex does not.

Chapter 3
The Electrical Properties
of Neurones

Our present understanding of the nervous system was certainly not achieved in a logical order. The history of neurophysiology has been marked by a series of fits, starts, blind allies and prejudices. Nevertheless, it is clear that if we are to compress what actually took 500 years of faltering progress to understand into the few months the average student can afford to spend upon neurophysiology, we will have to approach it in a much more orderly way—with the logic of hindsight.

Nerve membrane

What distinguishes nerve cells from most other cells functionally is their property of electrical excitability, which is highly developed. This is afforded by the special characteristics of their cell membrane. This membrane is thought to consist of a double layer of fatty acid (lipid). Lipid molecules are made up of two carbohydrate chains with one end relatively highly charged, or polar, and the other nonpolar. The polar ends of the two chains are situated on the surfaces of the membrane facing outwards towards the e.c.f. and inwards towards the interior of the cell. A layer of protein is probably adsorbed onto each of these surfaces. Lipid-soluble substances pass through such a membrane fairly easily, whilst water-soluble (polar) substances should not. Yet water and ions do pass into nerve cells, though relatively slowly. It is likely that there are discontinuities in the structure of the membrane where the lipid molecules are rearranged to form 'channels' lined with protein through which water and selected ions can pass. The size of ions surrounded by their hydration shells varies, as does their charge density. Thus the channels can exhibit *ionic selectivity* and *voltage sensitivity*. Some also show sensitivity to particular chemical triggers. This is known as chemical gating. These properties confer upon nerve cells their excitability. At present we have no technique to visualize these channels directly and their structure must be deduced from their electrical and other properties.

RESTING POTENTIAL

Although it was Galvani who first suggested that muscles can produce their own electricity, it was Julius Bernstein who, in 1902, found the first vital clue as to how the electrical charge is produced. Bernstein discovered that the interior of nerve and muscle cells is rich in potassium and organic ions (charged proteins which cannot escape from the cell) whilst poor in sodium and chloride, unlike the extracellular fluid which has much Na^+ and Cl^- but little K^+. He proposed therefore that the electrical charge on excitable membranes is *electrochemical*, consequent upon unequal distribution of ions.

Electrochemical gradients

If two solutions containing the same ion at different concentrations are brought together at an interface permeable to that ion, two forces determine its movements (Fig. 3.1). On the one hand, concentration gradients tend to cause ions to flow from the stronger to the weaker solution. On the other hand, each ion which does migrate carries a charge which tends to increase the potential in the weaker solution and decrease it in the stronger. At equilibrium the fluxes in the two directions are equal; the potential difference tending to attract ions back exactly balances the concentration difference tending to make them migrate.

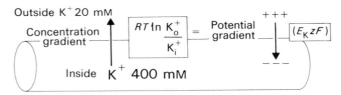

Fig. 3.1. K^+ concentration gradient tends to move K^+ ions out of axon. The resulting accumulation of positive charge outside tends to move K^+ ions in again. At equilibrium, the Nernst equation applies.

Nernst equation

This situation was described mathematically by Nernst. The potential gradient for K^+ ions is equal to $E_K.zF$, where E_K is the equilibrium potential for K^+ ions, z is their valency (1), and F is Faraday's constant—96 500 coulombs—the quantity of electricity conveyed when one mole of a univalent ion passes from one solution to another. At equilibrium, we can equate this with the kinetic energy ratio of the two solutions—$RT \ln[K_o]/[K_i]$ (where K_o is the external K^+ concentration, K_i is the internal K^+ concentration, R is the gas constant and T is the absolute temperature). Thus at equilibrium:

$$E_K zF = RT \ln[K_o]/[K_i]$$

or

$$E_K = RT/zF . \ln[K_o]/[K_i].$$

The latter is the usual form of the Nernst equation.

Bernstein proposed therefore that the charge across an excitable cell membrane is the result of the *potassium concentration difference* between the inside and the outside of the cell. In 1902 however, it was only possible to guess at the exact value of these concentrations and impossible to measure the resting membrane potential. Since the introduction of microelectrodes which can be inserted inside axons without damaging them, and of amplifiers and cathode ray oscilloscopes capable of recording the tiny potentials and currents involved, Bernstein's hypothesis for the resting potential has been largely confirmed. Perhaps the most important step was made by J. Z. Young, a zoologist, who drew the attention of physiologists to the 'giant' motor nerve trunk supplying the mantle of the squid. This consists of two axons each about 1 mm in diameter. Fairly large electrodes can be inserted into these without causing any serious damage to their electrical properties.

Intracellular recording

When a microelectrode is inserted into the squid giant axon, the potential recorded between it and the extracellular fluid drops to about −65 mV, the resting potential (Fig. 3.2). This is quite similar, though not identical, to the Nernst equilibrium potential for potassium (−75 mV). The resting membrane is thus permanently charged or *polarized*. If the concentration of K$^+$ in the fluid bathing the axon is changed, the resting potential recorded changes by 58 mV ($= RT/zF$ at 20°C) for each tenfold change in [K$^+$] (Fig. 3.2). This logarithmic relationship is what we should predict from the Nernst equation if the resting potential is the result of potassium

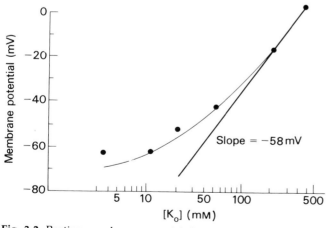

Fig. 3.2. Resting membrane potential changes by 58 mV for each tenfold change in external K$^+$ concentration. At low [K$_o^+$] the effect of permeability to other ions is apparent.

concentration differences between the inside and outside of the membrane.

Selective permeability

However some awkward problems remain. First, the resting potential is not precisely equal to the potassium equilibrium potential but more positive, which suggests that perhaps other ions are involved. Secondly, radioactive tracer studies have shown that the membrane is in fact not only permeable to K^+, but also to Cl^- and slightly to Na^+. The concentration and potential gradients for Na^+ should combine to force Na^+ into the cell at a high rate; yet the resting membrane potential remains at -65 mV. The explanation is that although the resting membrane is slightly permeable to Na^+, it is about 80 times more so to K^+. Despite a lower atomic weight, Na^+ ions surrounded by their hydration shells are considerably larger than K^+ ions. Thus the contribution of Na^+ influx to the resting membrane potential is only 0.125 (the ratio of Na^+/K^+ permeabilities) times that of K^+. This serves to raise the resting potential from the K^+ equilibrium potential of -75 mV to its normal level of -65 mV.

THE SODIUM PUMP

As the cell membrane is permeable to both K^+ and Na^+, we must explain how the observed concentration differences of these ions across the membrane are preserved; why Na^+ and K^+ ions do not run down their concentration gradients and eventually eliminate the membrane potential as their concentrations equalize. If an axon is poisoned with a metabolic inhibitor, such as dinitrophenol (DNP),

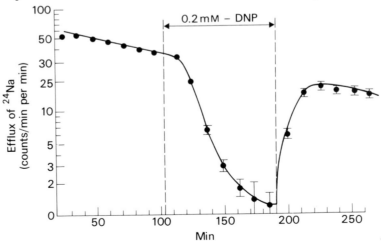

Fig. 3.3. When the sodium pump is stopped by DNP, the efflux of Na^+ ions is reduced to zero.

this is exactly what does happen (Fig. 3.3). Over the course of a few minutes or hours (depending on the degree of activity of the neurone), the electrochemical 'battery' runs down and the resting potential disappears. This suggests that in the unpoisoned axon Na^+ ions which pass into the cell and K^+ ions which pass out are actively pumped back again by a process requiring metabolic energy (Fig. 3.4).

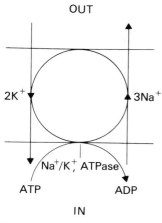

OUT

$2K^+$ $3Na^+$

Na^+/K^+ ATPase

ATP ADP

IN

Fig. 3.4. The sodium pump.

The exact mechanics of the *sodium pump* are still not fully understood. They are known to involve the splitting of the ubiquitous energy store ATP by an enzyme whose activity is dependent upon the presence of Na^+ and K^+ ions. This Na^+ and K^+-dependent ATPase is probably situated on the inside of the membrane (Fig. 3.4). Activation of the pump is favoured by a high concentration of Na^+ inside the cell, but it also requires the presence of K^+ ions outside. If a higher than usual concentration of K^+ ions is placed inside the cell, a high concentration of Na^+ maintained outside and no ATP provided, the pump can actually be made to work backwards, i.e. Na^+ and K^+ run down their concentration gradients and ATP is resynthesized from ADP. It seems likely that pumping involves either the physical shuttling of some energy-rich intermediate carrier binding K^+ on the outside and Na^+ on the inside (unlikely), or (currently favoured) a 'conformational' change in the shape of a specialized protein running from one side of the membrane to the other, in such a way that it locally reverses the electrochemical forces on the ions. Such a protein has now been isolated; it is a dimer (two molecules joined together) and each part consists of a heavy and a light chain.

The pump is blocked by the glycoside *ouabain*; this is similar to digitalis, an extract of foxgloves introduced in the seventeenth century by William Withering for the treatment of heart failure.

Ouabain binds to the pump protein; using radioactive ouabain one can therefore mark and count the actual number of pumping sites.

Electrogenic action of sodium pump

Accurate measurements of the amounts of Na^+ and K^+ pumped suggest that the transport of ions in each direction is not symmetrical. Three Na^+ ions are usually extruded for every two K^+ ions pumped in (Fig. 3.4). Hence, when the pump is highly active it can have a direct (*electrogenic*) effect on the membrane potential. Since more Na^+ is pumped outwards than K^+ is moved inwards, the resting potential becomes more negative (*hyperpolarized*) when the pump is activated, e.g. after a train of impulses, or when the internal Na^+ concentration is increased in other ways. The hyper-polarization caused by increased pumping is most easily observed in small neurones since the number of pumping sites per unit surface area is approximately constant and smaller neurones have a higher surface to volume ratio.

ACTION POTENTIALS

The resting potential of a nerve membrane is only the background to the story of how neurones transmit signals to each other. Trans-mission of information down axons and some long dendrites takes place by means of trains of electrical impulses known as *action potentials* or 'spikes' (named thus from the way in which they appear on an oscilloscope screen showing change in potential with time; Fig. 3.5).

All-or-none law

If an action potential is generated at all it achieves a standard size and shape (the all-or-none 'law'), constant for each neurone. In-formation is not carried in the shape or size of the impulse, which is a function of the responding axon, but is *coded* in the timing of these standard impulses and the number and type of fibres activated. We shall have much more to say later about this largely unsolved problem of coding.

Na^+ current

Although Bernstein's hypothesis explained the resting membrane potential quite satisfactorily, he could not account for the action potential. He suggested that when a neurone is excited the negative internal potential is simply shorted out, so that the internal resting level is temporarily reduced to zero. This did not explain Overton's observation that no action potential occurs unless Na+ ions are present in the external fluid, which had prompted him to suggest that Na+ ions normally pass into the cell during an action potential.

The use of intracellular microelectrodes allowed Cole & Curtis and Hodgkin & Huxley, in 1939, to show that at the peak of an action potential the membrane potential does not merely reduce to zero, but actually reverses to reach a value of about +40 mV (the *positive overshoot;* Fig. 3.5). That overshoot is quite close to the value of the sodium equilibrium potential (+55 mV) derived from the Nernst equation applied to Na+ concentration differences across the membrane, so maybe the sodium permeability of the membrane somehow increases during an action potential, Na+ ions cascading into the cell for a brief period and sweeping the membrane potential towards the Na+ equilibrium potential. However, this was difficult to prove. Hodgkin and Katz showed that the size of the positive overshoot varies with the external Na+ concentration, which is consistent with the hypothesis. Cole and Curtis showed that the overall conductance of the membrane is increased markedly during the action potentials—again consistent with the idea that Na+ permeability increased.

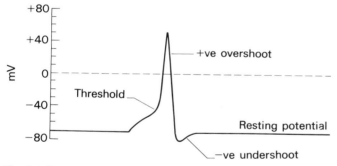

Fig. 3.5. Intracellularly recorded resting and action potentials.

Voltage clamp

Direct proof required a technique for measuring the Na+ current and its time course—almost watching the Na+ ions flow in. Membrane currents vary both with the level of the membrane potential and with the time which has elapsed since they started—they are both voltage- and time-dependent. Some means of 'freezing' the membrane potential during different stages of development of an action potential was required, so that the time course of ionic flows could be examined without the complications of changing membrane potential. The voltage clamp technique introduced by Cole and Curtis in 1939 provided just this. Their idea was to clamp the membrane at a fixed potential and measure the currents which flowed. The reason why the potential across a membrane changes is that ionic currents flow across it; so if equal and opposite currents are applied to the membrane by the experimenter, no potential changes can occur. The amount of current necessary to keep the membrane potential at a chosen level is then equal to the current carried by the ions which would otherwise change the potential.

The voltage clamp technique was made possible by the development of negative feedback amplifiers. The clamp potential chosen by the experimenter is compared by the amplifier with the actual membrane potential measured by means of an intracellular recording microelectrode; the difference between them is used to calculate and generate a current sufficient to prevent the two diverging, which is then delivered via the current electrode (Fig. 3.6). The current generated by the voltage clamp amplifier is then equal and opposite to any underlying ionic flows.

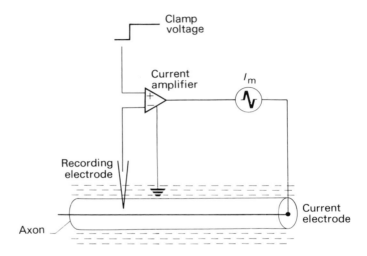

Fig. 3.6. Voltage clamp.

It was then necessary to determine which ions are responsible for the membrane currents which flow during the action potential. The concentration of Na^+ and K^+ in the bath fluid can be varied; and in the squid giant axon, whose axoplasm can be squeezed out rather like toothpaste, the concentration inside the axon can also be controlled. If a change in concentration of an ion leads to a change in a membrane current under study, that ion is implicated in the mechanism of that current.

Capacitative current

When the membrane potential is stepped from its resting level to zero (a depolarizing step) the membrane capacitance is first discharged, causing a momentary outward 'capacitative' current (Fig.

3.7). Fortunately this stage is over long before the ionic currents become significant (though, as we shall see later, it may mask small 'gating' currents which cause the alterations in membrane structure underlying ionic permeability changes).

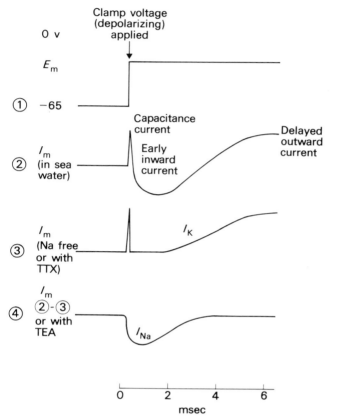

Fig. 3.7. Voltage clamp records. The membrane is clamped at a depolarizing voltage E_m (1). Rapid membrane current is = I_{m} (2)(3) and (4). Rapid capacitance current gives way to an early inward current carried by Na$^+$ ions (4), followed by a delayed outward current carried by K$^+$ ions (3).

Na$^+$ inward current

There follows a large inward current lasting 1 ms or so (Fig. 3.7(2)). This is later replaced by a slow outward current over the next 3–4 ms. The inward current is carried by Na$^+$ ions. It is abolished by removing external Na$^+$ (Fig. 3.7(3)) and returns on replacing the Na$^+$ or substituting lithium. It is also abolished by treating the axon with a powerful poison, tetrodotoxin (TTX), derived from the puffer fish (a Japanese culinary delicacy). The immense potency of this poison, which attests the importance of inward Na$^+$ currents to the well-being of our nervous systems, makes the consumption of this fish an exciting, if anxious, experience for neurophysiologists.

Current reversal

If the membrane potential is not clamped at zero but at $+55$ mV (i.e. the equilibrium potential for Na^+) then the early inward current disappears. This is to be expected if the inward current is carried by Na^+ ions, because when the membrane potential is raised to the Na^+ equilibrium potential there is no longer any force acting to push Na^+ ions into the cell. The electrical gradient now prevents their entry, as it exactly balances the chemical gradient pushing them in. If the membrane potential is made still more positive than this *reversal potential* the small number of Na^+ ions inside the axon and other ions which can use the same channel are actually forced outwards.

All these observations support Overton's original hypothesis that Na^+ ions rush into the axon during the upstroke of the action potential. The axon's normal, low Na^+ permeability is temporarily increased and so the membrane sweeps towards the Na^+ equilibrium potential. In fact the action potential never reaches this level because the Na^+ permeability channels begin to 'inactivate' at positive membrane potentials. Also, the delayed outward current referred to earlier begins to build up to limit the depolarization of the membrane potential.

K^+ outward current

The magnitude of the outward current diminishes on raising external, or lowering internal, K^+ concentration. Its reversal potential lies at the K^+ equilibrium potential (-75 mV); so it is probably carried by K^+ ions. It too can be blocked using a poison (tetraethyl ammonium—TEA) (Fig. 3.7④) which is therefore a useful tool for further analysis of membrane phenomena. This delayed outward current, together with Na^+ channel inactivation, bring the membrane potential back towards the resting potential. The membrane actually undershoots its normal resting level (the *negative undershoot*) as the K^+ equilibrium potential is below the normal resting potential, and the K^+ conductance of the membrane remains higher, while the Na^+ conductance is temporarily lower, than normal.

Hodgkin–Huxley equations

The quantitative detail furnished by the voltage clamp technique enabled Hodgkin and Huxley to model the action potential mathematically using a system of differential equations which describe the voltage and time dependence of ionic conductances. The theoretical purposes of such a mathematical model are to pinpoint deficiencies in our knowledge about a system, to predict properties

of the system which would not have emerged without the abstract
model, and to deduce from the form of the mathematical equations
clues to the native of the physical mechanisms underlying them.
Thus Hodgkin and Huxley found that the voltage dependence
of their variable 'm', which describes the activation of Na^+
conductance, can be modelled by a cubic equation. The simplest
hypothesis to account for this is to suppose that three charged
particles must all interact before a local modification of the membrane structure will allow Na^+ ions to pass through.

Membrane channels

The most recent observations suggest that activation of three
charged sites on a helical protein chain causes a conformational
change—the helix twists—and this probably lowers energy barriers
to free passage of Na^+ ions. Artificial membranes consisting of lipid
bilayers 'doped' with quite simple helical polypeptide chains have
been constructed which mimic the ionic selectivity and voltage-
dependent conductances of natural membrane channels to a quite
remarkable degree.

The fact that the Na^+ and K^+ currents can be independently
blocked, by TTX and TEA respectively, strongly suggests that these
two currents travel through different channels in the membrane.
These two channels must therefore have different physical dimensions and charge profiles, since on activation they show different
selectivities for different sized ions surrounded by their hydration
shells.

Gates

It is convenient to postulate that these ionic channels in the
membrane contain *gates* which can be either open or shut according
to their degree of activation. These gates are presumably charged,
since they are voltage sensitive, i.e. they change state when the
electric field across the membrane changes. Their movement must
therefore consume electrical energy, which should be detectable as
a *gating current*, at the beginning of membrane excitation. Unfortunately, this current is usually masked by capacitance current
occurring at the same time; nevertheless gating currents have now
been identified experimentally by subtracting from each other the
currents following equal and opposite voltage steps from the resting
potential. The Na^+ gates open following a positive voltage step, so
gating current flows in addition to the current discharging the
membrane capacitance. However, a negative voltage step from the
resting potential cannot close the Na^+ gates, which are already shut
at the resting potential; it only charges up the membrane capaci-

tance further. The difference between the currents flowing in the two directions must therefore be equal to the current required to open the Na$^+$ gates, as the symmetrical capacitance currents cancel one another out (Fig. 3.8). More detailed analysis of these gating currents under various conditions will contribute further to our understanding of the molecular mechanisms underlying membrane permeability.

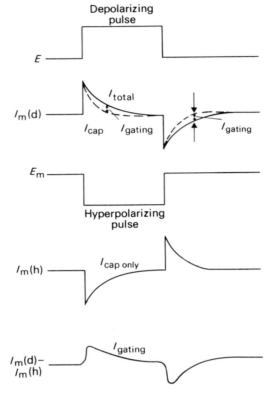

Fig. 3.8. Gating current. Depolarizing voltage pulse (E_m) causes capacitance current and gating current to flow through the membrane. A hyperpolarizing pulse causes capacitance current only, as closed gates cannot close further. The difference between the two [I_m(d)–I_m(h)] equals current consumed in opening the Na$^+$ gates.

Threshold

An action potential does not develop unless the membrane potential is brought to a certain *threshold* rate of depolarization. At this level, inward current resulting from increase in Na$^+$ conductance brought about by depolarization exceeds the outward current of K$^+$ ions, which is also encouraged by the depolarization but more slowly. Above threshold therefore the membrane becomes more depolarized and Na$^+$ conductance increases still further, which in turn causes greater membrane depolarization. This is an example of *positive feedback*, where a stimulus enhances, rather than reduces, itself. Such systems are inherently unstable; hence there is a self-amplifying cascade of increasing depolarization and increasing Na^+ conductance, leading to the peak of the action potential. As the number of Na^+ channels involved is quite small, and the actual quantity of ions transferred is modest, the overall 'bulk' concentrations of K^+ and Na^+ inside and outside the neurone may not change much during nervous activity. Hence the maximum point (Na^+ equilibrium potential) and the minimum point (K^+ equilibrium potential) of the action potential are fixed by the bulk concentrations of these ions on either side of the membrane. This is why, if an action potential is triggered at all, it is of a standard 'all-or-none' size.

Refractory period

Immediately after an action potential it is impossible to elicit another one for a short period of time (about 1 ms), known as the *absolute refractory period*. This is because during this time Na^+ channels are fully inactivated and K^+ channels are fully activated. Therefore no amount of depolarization can trigger an action potential. For a longer period after this (about 4 ms), known as the *relative refractory period*, it becomes progressively less difficult to excite an action potential as the inactivated Na^+ conductance, the activated K^+ conductance, and hence the negative undershoot, revert to normal.

LOCAL CURRENT SPREAD

So far, we have considered the generation of action potentials without considering what can raise the membrane potential to threshold in the first place. Experimenters apply electrical currents, but in the intact nervous system local currents generated by receptor, synaptic or action potentials in adjacent parts of the membrane are the causes of excitation.

When depolarization occurs at a point on the membrane it acts as a 'sink' of current, attracting positive charges from neighbouring regions of the outside of the membrane and neutralizing negative charges on the inside of the membrane (Fig. 3.9). Hence adjacent parts of the membrane become depolarized. It is important to realize that these local or *electrotonic* currents are not carried by the relatively slow migration of ions which underlies the transmembrane currents causing the action potential. Instead, charge is transferred from one ion to the next at the speed of light, rather as a row of marbles transfers a knock quickly from one end to the other without much movement of any individual marble. Local currents are therefore extremely rapid, like the flow of electricity in a conductor, but they *attenuate* as a result of losses across the membrane. The membrane is not a perfect insulator, of course, because of its ionic conductances. One of the penalties for evolving the action potential mechanism, which maintains nervous impulses at a standard size, is the attenuation of local currents.

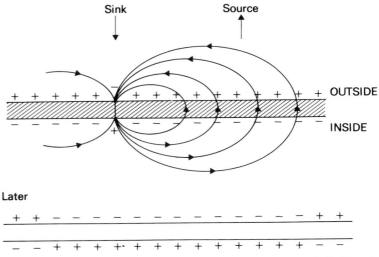

Fig. 3.9. Local currents. Local depolarization acts as a current sink. Positive charges are attracted from neighbouring regions on outside of membrane. Negative charges on the inside are neutralized. Hence depolarization spreads outwards, attenuating with distance and time.

Cable equation

The way in which local currents diminish can be modelled mathematically using the *cable equation*, first developed in order to understand electrical losses from submarine telephone cables. Essentially, each section of the membrane is modelled by an equivalent electrical network consisting of membrane resistance and capacitance in parallel (Fig. 3.10 ①), connected to the next sections (②, ③, etc.) by the internal resistance of the axon (R_i) and the external resistance of the e.c.f. (R_o). The magnitude of the currents set up by a potential occurring at any point on the membrane can then be calculated as a function of the distance from the point and the time elapsed.

Length and time constants

The solutions of the cable equation (see Fig. 3.10) give rise to two important constants: the length constant ($\lambda = \sqrt{R_m/R_i}$), which describes the distance along the membrane over which the potential passively falls to $1/e$ (about ⅓) of its original value; and the membrane time constant ($\tau = R_m \times C_m$), which defines the amount of time it takes for the local potential to fall to $1/e$ of its initial value. So these two constants together define, for any particular axon, the decrement of a potential as a function of the time elapsed and the distance along the fibre.

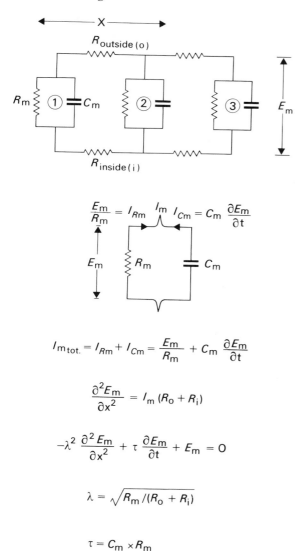

$$\frac{E_m}{R_m} = I_{Rm} \quad I_{Cm} = C_m \frac{\partial E_m}{\partial t}$$

$$I_{m\,tot.} = I_{Rm} + I_{Cm} = \frac{E_m}{R_m} + C_m \frac{\partial E_m}{\partial t}$$

$$\frac{\partial^2 E_m}{\partial x^2} = I_m (R_o + R_i)$$

$$-\lambda^2 \frac{\partial^2 E_m}{\partial x^2} + \tau \frac{\partial E_m}{\partial t} + E_m = 0$$

$$\lambda = \sqrt{R_m / (R_o + R_i)}$$

$$\tau = C_m \times R_m$$

Fig. 3.10. Model of local current spread. The cable equation.

Conduction velocity

The speed of conduction of action potentials can be calculated as a function of membrane resistance and capacitance, and of the internal resistance of the axon. Since these three all vary with diameter of the axon, they give rise to the important property that conduction velocity increases with fibre diameter. In unmyelinated fibres, conduction velocity increases as the square root of the diameter. Thus the squid giant axon is 1000 μm in diameter and in seawater at 20°C conducts at c. 25 ms^{-1}. Small unmyelinated fibres of 0.1 μm diameter conduct at c. 0.25 ms^{-1}.

Saltatory conduction

Ia fibres are in fact enveloped by an insulating myelin sheath provided by Schwann cells. Action potentials are not generated in every part of such a fibre, only at the *nodes of Ranvier* where the sheath is interrupted at the junctions between Schwann cells so that action currents can take place. Furthermore, repolarization after the action potential occur only by Na$^+$ current inactivation. Myelinated fibres have disposed with the need for additional outward K$^+$ current—another economy.

One can think of the nodes of Ranvier as analogous to the amplifiers situated every few miles along a sub-Atlantic telephone cable. The signals decrease in size because of leakage across the insulation, but are boosted every few miles by the amplifiers. Similarly, local currents set up by an action potential diminish as they spread over the myelin sheath (although not as quickly as if the myelin were not there), and they are boosted by the generation of an action potential at the next node of Ranvier. In a sense, therefore, the action potential can be said to jump from node to node, and the conduction in myelinated fibres is termed *saltatory*—from the Latin *saltare*, to jump (nothing to do with table salt).

The advantages of this system are twofold. In the first place, the myelin insulation gives much higher capacitance and resistance, so that its length and time constants are increased and conduction velocity is also increased. The conduction velocity of myelinated fibres increases approximately linearly with axon diameter, so that the velocity of conduction in ms^{-1} is roughly six times the axon diameter in microns.

Secondly, utilizing only Na$^+$ channels and confining the generation of action potentials to only a small portion of the membrane reduces the transfer of ions across it. Since all ions so transferred have to be pumped back again and this pumping accounts for much of the energy expended by the CNS, ATP supplies are conserved.

RECEPTORS

The majority of signals dealt with by the nervous system commence with the activity of sensory receptors. There are two broad classes of sensory receptor: *mechanoreceptors* and *chemoreceptors*. (Thermo-receptors and photoreceptors are probably specialized forms of chemoreceptor, making use of thermo- and photochemical effects.) Most is known about mechanoreceptors and photoreceptors, and we will be dealing with some of them in greater detail later. However it is worth introducing a few basic ideas here.

The task which receptors have to perform is to convert the form of sensory energy to which they are sensitive into the currency which the nervous system uses, trains of action potentials. This process is known as transduction. One can split it into three steps.

(1) Delivering the stimulus energy to the sensory nerve terminal (*translocation* of the stimulus).

(2) Transforming the sensory energy into a *receptor potential* in the nerve terminal (*transduction* proper).

(3) Coding the receptor potential as a train of nerve impulses (*action potential generation*).

Each of these processes probably takes place at a separate site.

Translocation

The first step, translocation, is often ignored but is in fact very important. For example, mechanoreceptors in the skin sit well below the surface, yet one is able to feel the slightest touch. Mechanical conduction from skin surface to nerve endings must therefore be very efficient. How it is accomplished by a variety of mechanisms such as skin hairs, dermal ridges, strategically sited sweat drops and so on, we will examine in Chapter 8. But the point to be emphasized here is that these mechanisms themselves confer on the receptors some of their functional properties. Hairs bend, so that only a proportion of the force impinging on them is transferred to the nerve endings at their roots; skin tissues are *viscous*, so that if they are indented rapidly they deform underlying nerve terminals maximally, but if they are deformed slowly they may be able to absorb much of the energy without passing all of it on. Thus in Fig. 3.11 the 'step' displacement of the probe is converted into a peak followed by a lower plateau. This is known as *mechanical adaptation* and is a result of the mechanical filtering properties of the receptor. These can often be modelled by relatively simple mechanical analogues such as Voigt elements (Fig. 3.11). For chemoreceptors, other than photoreceptors, very little is known about translocation or indeed about the subsequent steps of transduction and action potential generation. The translocation of light by the optics of the eye is, of course, a subject in its own right, and we will leave it for a later chapter.

Transduction

The exact mechanisms of transduction, by which mechanical force or chemical change is converted into membrane currents followed by *receptor potentials,* are unknown. As in the case of the action potential, it is likely that an increase in membrane permeability to sodium is involved since removing external sodium abolishes receptor potentials; moreover, their reversal potential lies close to the Na^+ equilibrium potential. But TTX does not affect the receptor potential, implying that it uses a different mechanism to the Na^+ channels used by the action potential; furthermore, the channel concerned shows less ionic selectivity than the classical Na^+ channel. Precisely how permeability changes are effected is still a mystery. Presumably, mechanical deformation of the membrane causes a distortion in some critical protein, which leads to conductance changes. However, its precise nature is unknown.

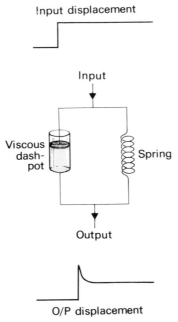

Fig. 3.11. Voigt element. Dashpot and spring in parallel convert step input into pulse followed by step. Pulse magnitude is proportional to rate of change of input.

Action potential generation

It is probable that the part of the terminal membrane specialized to respond to mechanical deformation cannot itself generate action potentials. This is not surprising since, as noted earlier, Na^+ channels for receptor and action potentials are probably separate entities. Ionic currents activated by the permeability changes in a receptor terminal set up local electrotonic currents which spread passively, as elsewhere, decreasing with time and distance. Many sensory receptors are supplied by myelinated nerve fibres but lose their myelin at the receptor terminals. It appears that the first site on these fibres able to generate action potentials is the initial node of Ranvier. Thus, as long as the size and rate of change of the potential reaching the first node by electrotonic spread exceed threshold, an action potential will occur there. While receptor currents continue, action potentials will be generated. It is easy to see qualitatively that their frequency will depend upon the size of the receptor potential, though the details of this relationship are a great deal more complicated than this.

In particular, almost all sensory receptors show the phenomenon of *adaptation*—their response to a constant stimulus is not constant, but is greatest when the stimulus is first applied and then diminishes. This can be the result of the mechanical filtering effects mentioned earlier, or of adaptation of the receptor potential itself, or of adaptation at the spike generator site. The mechanisms underlying these last two include a slow K^+ channel activation, Na^+ and Ca^{2+} channel inactivation sodium pump stimulation, depending on the particular receptor studied.

Chapter 4
Synaptic Transmission

The most important source of local currents generating and modulating the frequency of action potentials in a neurone is synaptic activity. To start with we will consider transmission not within the central nervous system at all, but at the *neuromuscular junction* (NMJ)—the synapse between somatic motor nerves and skeletal muscles. This is not because it is in any way typical (indeed in many ways it is highly specialized), but more is known about the neuromuscular junction than any other, because it is so easy to isolate and visualize. We hope that knowledge gained about its properties will give us reliable insights into the behaviour of CNS synapses, which are so much more difficult to study.

Neuromuscular junction

On entering a muscle, a motor nerve splits into separate *motor endings*. The number of endings derived from one nerve depends on the degree of precision with which the muscle can be used. A large antigravity muscle, such as gastrocnemius, has a small number of motor nerve fibres supplying a large number of muscle fibres; each fibre has a large number of branches, which together with the muscle fibres it innervates is known as a *motor unit*. A fine muscle such as an eye muscle is comprised of a large number of smaller motor units, each supplying just a few muscle fibres. The motor ending synapses with a specialized region of the muscle known as an *end plate* (Fig. 4.1).

At the end plate the muscle membrane is thrown into a large number of junctional folds. The distance between nerve and muscle membranes is reduced to about 20 nm (20×10^{-9} m), but this is still too great for local currents to traverse the gap by direct electrical transmission and necessitates some kind of amplifier mechanism. This is not, in fact, primarily because the gap is too large, but because the pre- and postsynaptic membranes interpose a very large resistance to electrotonic current spread. Since the normal membrane resistance is about 100 ohms m^{-2}, the resistance to current flow over the 5 μm of synaptic contact is about 3000 megohms. Any postsynaptic voltage change would be reduced to less than one per cent of the presynaptic value. Therefore some sort of amplification is needed; transmission across the neuromuscular

synapse must occur by some mechanism other than simple
electrotonic current spread.

Most synapses cause a delay in conduction ranging from a few
hundred microseconds at the neuromuscular junction to several
tens of milliseconds at autonomic synapses. No such delay would be
expected with electrical transmission. Furthermore, most synapses
only conduct in one direction, whereas electrical conduction can
usually occur in both directions. Nevertheless until the 1930s many
physiologists believed that synaptic transmission was electrical.
They were finally convinced of the reality of *chemical transmission*
only by the brilliant experiments and the authority of Sir Henry
Dale.

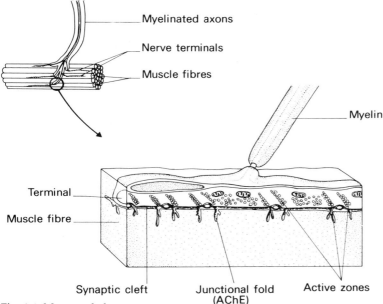

Fig. 4.1. Motor end plate.

CHEMICAL TRANSMISSION

Elliot (1904) noticed that extracts made from the adrenal gland
mimicked the effects on the circulation of stimulating the sympathetic division of the autonomic nervous system; he suggested
that perhaps these nerves normally worked by releasing chemicals
similar to those found in the adrenal gland. However, this unlikely
tale appeared so preposterous to his colleagues that he was dis-
couraged from even publishing it.

Loewi's experiment

In 1924 Otto Loewi performed his famous experiment, which put
the idea of chemical transmission firmly on the map. Loewi had a

curious dream about frog hearts, which he wrote down in the middle of the night. His writing the next day proved indecipherable. Fortunately the following night, the dream, like the ghost in *Hamlet*, returned; wanting no mistakes this time, Loewi rushed to his laboratory and performed the experiment there and then, at dead of night. Many of us wish we had such fruitful visions!

Loewi took a frog's heart and stimulated the vagus nerve which, when activated, slows the heart. He collected the fluid bathing the slowed heart, perfused a second frog's heart, deprived of its vagus nerve, with this fluid, and observed a dramatic slowing of the second heart's beat. Something released into the perfusate on stimulating the vagus nerve of the first heart had slowed down the second.

Loewi was extraordinarily lucky. The slowing agent, which he called 'vagusstoff', would have been produced locally in minute amounts, and should have been immediately destroyed. But fortunately frog heart lacks the hydrolytic enzyme *acetylcholinesterase (AChE)*, which normally breaks down vagusstoff (now known to be *acetylcholine (ACh)*); so acetylcholine released from the vagus nerve terminal was free to flow into the bath to inhibit the second heart, thus providing the first sound evidence for chemical transmission.

Criteria for chemical transmission

The evidence that ACh is also released at skeletal neuromuscular junctions depended upon the use of drugs such as eserine which block the acetylcholinesterase which is found in large quantities bound to the muscle membrane at the end plates. Then a Loewi-type experiment could be performed to demonstrate two of the

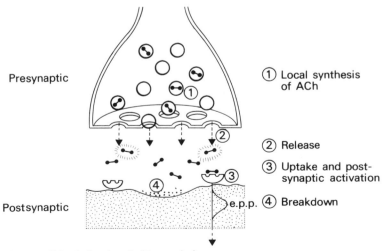

Presynaptic

Postsynaptic

① Local synthesis of ACh

② Release

③ Uptake and post-synaptic activation

④ Breakdown

e.p.p.

Fig. 4.2. Criteria for chemical transmission.

phenomena essential to prove chemical transmission—first, that the postulated transmitter is in fact released during presynaptic activity of a nerve (②) in Fig. 4.2) and secondly that this same substance will mimic the normal action of the nerve on the postsynaptic membrane ③.

It is necessary to satisfy three further criteria, namely: evidence that the enzymatic machinery necessary to synthesize the substance is present locally ①; evidence that there exists a local mechanism for breaking it down or otherwise removing it ④; and since chemical processes are involved, demonstration that there are other chemical substances (drugs) with similar structures which are able to block transmission at each of its stages: synthesis ①, release ②, postsynaptic action ③ and breakdown or removal ④.

Chemical transmission at the NMJ

In the case of the neuromuscular junction all these criteria have been met. (1) Hemicholinium blocks the synthesis of acetylcholine from choline and acetyl coenzyme A by the enzyme choline acetyl transferase, which has been shown to be situated in the presynaptic terminal. (2) Botulinum toxin is the immensely potent poison produced by *Clostridium botulinum* in inadequately sterilized canned produce. It has such a powerful effect because it prevents any release of ACh from presynaptic nerves. (3) Curare, used from prehistoric times by South American Indians for incapacitating hunted animals and unwanted humans, paralyses by occupying the postsynaptic sites normally employed by ACh. (4) Eserine blocks the active sites of acetylcholinesterase, so that the life of ACh is prolonged.

Similarly, Dale's criteria for identifying chemical transmitters have been satisfied for ACh at sympathetic and parasympathetic ganglia and at parasympathetic terminals, and for noradrenaline at sympathetic nerve endings. But nowhere in the central nervous system has such strong evidence been achieved, as synapses there cannot be physically isolated and studied.

Presynaptic mechanisms

Vesicles

If presynaptic terminals from the neuromuscular junction are examined using the electron microscope, they are seen to contain large numbers of vesicles loaded with acetylcholine (Fig. 4.3a). This discovery was linked with the electrophysiological observation that random fluctuations occur in intracellular records of the postsynaptic *end plate potential* (Fig. 4.3b). These were called *miniature*

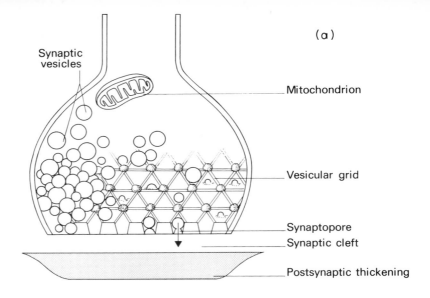

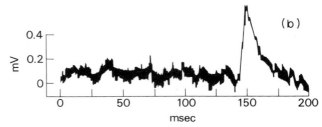

Fig. 4.3. (a) Presynaptic vesicles. (b) Spontaneous miniature end plate potential (m.e.p.p.) superimposed on synaptic noise.

end plate potentials (m.e.p.p.s) by Katz. They occur spontaneously, independently of any pre- or postsynaptic action potential, and they are all the same size (*c.* ½mV). It seemed possible that each m.e.p.p. was the result of the spontaneous release by exocytosis of the contents of one vesicle containing a standard-sized packet (known as a *quantum*) of the transmitter acetylcholine. It was proposed that a presynaptic action potential markedly enhances the probability of release of vesicles, so that 50–100 empty their contents into the synaptic cleft simultaneously, and thus ensure a postsynaptic end plate potential sufficiently large to trigger the muscle's action potential.

The vesicle hypothesis still remains only a hypothesis however, even though it is supported by a wealth of circumstantial evidence, because no-one has yet managed to show that vesicles are the sole source of ACh appearing in the cleft. Questions also remain about how each vesicle is filled with such a high concentration of ACh (about 10^4 molecules); about how the vesicular membrane is formed; about what happens to a vesicle after it has emptied its contents; and most importantly, about what propels vesicles towards the presynaptic membrane and dissolves away both vesicular and presynaptic membrane for exocytosis to occur.

Intracellular calcium release

These exocytotic events certainly involve calcium ions since they are sensitive to the level of external Ca^{2+} and can be triggered by micro-injections of Ca^{2+} into the terminal. Ca^{2+} channels confined to the terminal are activated following an action potential, so that Ca^{2+} enters the presynaptic terminal during its action potential. It may activate a system of contractile microfilaments, analogous to the sliding filaments of muscle, containing proteins known as neurin and stenin which are similar to actin and myosin; however, only the barest outline of this process is yet understood. Another function of Ca^{2+} may be to neutralize negative charges on vesicle and terminal membranes, enabling them to coalesce and exocytosis to ensue.

The size of an action potential is a very sensitive determinant of the amount of Ca^{2+} which flows into the presynaptic terminal. This Ca^{2+} current varies as the fourth power of external Ca^{2+} concentration. Internal Ca^{2+} is removed by a mechanism which involves Na^+ flowing down its concentration gradient into the terminal, in exchange for Ca^{2+} extrusion. Ultimately, therefore, the sodium pump provides the power to pump out Na^+ which enters the terminal as a result not only of the action potential but also of the Na^+/Ca^{2+} exchange mechanism—the *calcium pump*.

Postsynaptic mechanisms

Once released, acetylcholine diffuses across the synaptic cleft to exert its postsynaptic effects. The easiest way to monitor these is by inserting a micropipette electrode into the muscle fibre close to the end plate in order to measure the end plate potential. The spontaneous release of quanta of ACh is signalled by the m.e.p.p.s, as we have seen, whilst large end plate potentials, culminating in muscle action potentials, occur after each presynaptic nerve impulse.

ACh receptors

The detailed mechanisms underlying end plate potential changes have been dissected using the same techniques as for nerve membrane potentials, i.e. manipulating ion concentrations, application of specific drugs and use of the voltage clamp technique.

After its release, each molecule of ACh binds to a *receptor* protein situated on the muscle membrane; this event triggers a train of processes leading to muscle membrane permeability changes— 'chemical gating'. The concept of a receptor was introduced in order to explain the specificity of the postsynaptic membrane for ACh and other substances with similar chemical structures. It was necessary to postulate some sort of chemical 'lock' to take the ACh 'key'.

Despite their similarity to ACh most substances which bind to the ACh receptor, such as curare and succinylcholine, have the effect of *blocking* neuromuscular transmission. Although they fit the lock they cannot open it. Recently, using a snake venom, bungarotoxin, which binds specifically and irreversibly to acetylcholine receptors, it has become possible to isolate the receptor protein, and hence to begin to characterize its chemical and physical properties.

Postsynaptic permeability changes

The important function of the acetylcholine receptor when activated is to effect changes in postsynaptic membrane permeability leading to end plate potential changes. An unselective increase in both Na^+ and K^+ conductances seems to occur, as though ACh punches a hole in the muscle membrane. In voltage clamp experiments, Takeuchi showed that current reversal through the activated end plate lay neither at the Na^+ nor the K^+ equilibrium potential, but at a point half-way between. Furthermore, changing either Na^+ or K^+ concentration changes the magnitude of the end plate potential; so both Na^+ and K^+ fluxes are probably involved.

Many unsolved problems still remain. How does the activation of ACh receptors actually effect the change in the membrane channels? Does the binding of ACh to its receptor trigger a conformational charge in an ACh channel protein, which then relaxes automatically to its initial state? Or does the channel remain open until ACh is broken down by acetylcholinesterase? ACh probably only acts as a trigger. The channel then opens and closes automatically, whether or not ACh remains *in situ*. Are separate Na^+ and K^+ channels involved? Probably not. Do several ACh molecules cooperate to open up an end plate conductance channel? Many of these questions should be amenable to investigation now that the receptor protein itself has been isolated.

The contribution to the end plate noise of a single ACh-gated channel may now be estimated, either by analysis of synaptic noise, or by sucking a very small patch of end plate membrane containing a single channel onto the end of a micropipette. This 'micro' end plate potential is *c.* 0.1 μV. i.e. 1/5000th of an m.e.p.p. generated by a quantum of 2×5000 ACh molecules, or $1/(5000 \times 50)$ of a full e.p.p. set up by the release of 50–100 vesicles following an action potential.

ACh appears to be the chemical transmitter employed by all large neurones whose axons leave the central nervous system, including their branches known as *collaterals*. Thus skeletal muscle is excited by ACh released from the axons of spinal cord motoneurones, and spinal cord *Renshaw cells* are excited by ACh released from their collaterals. The neurones of the *sympathetic ganglia* lying alongside the vertebral column are also excited by ACh released from the axons of *lateral horn cells* in the thoracic part of the spinal cord. The preganglionic terminals of the *parasympathetic* system (found in the walls of the organ they supply) similarly release ACh; these arise from motoneurones in the brainstem and sacral portion of the spinal cord. ACh is also released from the postganglionic fibres of the parasympathetic system, but not from those of the sympathetic system.

At each of these sites, the action of ACh can be mimicked or blocked by appropriate drugs (known as *agonists* and *antagonists*, respectively). At the neuromuscular junction choline, carbachol and nicotine act as agonists, whilst curare, succinylcholine and gallamine are antagonists. At sympathetic ganglia, the lateral horn axons are blocked by hexamethonium and decamethonium (very similar to succinylcholine but with a longer C-chain backbone), whilst their action is again mimicked by nicotine. At parasympathetic ganglia, preganglionic fibres are blocked by atropine and ACh is mimicked by muscarine. At postganglionic parasympathetic endings muscarine is an agonist and atropine, an antagonist. The agonistic properties of muscarine at parasympathetic pre- and postganglionic sites, and of nicotine at sympathetic ganglia and the neuromuscular junction, enable the synaptic effects of ACh to be classified as *muscarinic* or *nicotinic*; this division is carried over into the central nervous system, though muscarinic receptors seem to be much commoner in the CNS.

Noradrenaline (NA)

A conspicuous gap in this picture of peripheral synaptic transmission is the identity of the agent released by postganglionic sympathetic nerve endings. This is *noradrenaline* (also known as norepinephrine in the USA). Though much is known about its biochemistry, less is known about its electrophysiology, as noradrenergic synapses are not easy to study using recording techniques. Each axon contains numerous varicosities, which make multiple *'en passant'* synapses with target cells (Fig. 4.4), either smooth muscle or glandular cells. These cells have their own inherent electrical activity and do not necessarily produce action potentials at all. Thus, the function of their innervation is not necessarily to trigger contractions, etc., as is the case with skeletal muscle, but rather to modulate activity which is taking place anyway. Hence, deprived of clear-cut electrical signs of synaptic activity, electrophysiologists have, to a large extent, yielded noradrenergic synapses to the biochemists.

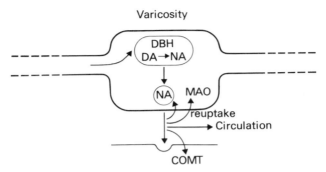

Varicosity

Fig. 4.4. *En-passant* noradrenergic synapse. Dopamine is converted into noradrenaline within presynaptic vesicles. After release it is removed either by the circulation or be re-uptake pre- or postsynaptically, where it is either re-used or broken down by monoamine oxidase (presynaptic) or catechol-o-methyl transferase (postsynaptic).

Noradrenergic vesicles

Biochemistry has provided compelling evidence of the exocytosis of sympathetic transmitters from vesicles. When sympathetic nerve terminals are activated, all the contents of their 'dense-cored' vesicles seen under the electron microscope are emptied into the synaptic cleft. These include not only noradrenaline itself but small quantities dopamine (its precursor), DOPA β-hydroxylase (which is responsible for converting dopamine to noradrenaline) and a pigment, chromogranin, whose function is probably to bind the noradrenaline within the vesicle. All these substances are found in intact vesicles in presynaptic noradrenergic endings, before exocytosis. It looks as though all the contents of a vesicle are unceremoniously dumped into the synaptic cleft.

TRANSMISSION IN THE CNS

Although the identification of transmitter substances in the CNS has proved difficult, electrical recording from CNS neurones has revealed much about what they do. Motoneurones in the ventral part of the grey matter of the spinal cord are large and reasonably easy to penetrate with an intracellular microelectrode. Hence, without knowing precisely which synapses or transmitters are responsible, one can examine central synaptic phenomena; these have turned out to be reassuringly similar to those in the periphery.

Excitatory synaptic potentials

On stimulating fibres known to be excitatory to motoneurones, such as the large sensory fibres from muscle spindles (Ia afferents), excitatory postsynaptic potentials (*e.p.s.p.s*) occur in the motoneurone a short time afterwards (Fig. 4.5). These are positive local potentials diminishing with time and distance from the site of the synapse. If there is sufficient excitatory synaptic action, the motoneurone membrane potential is brought to the threshold of an action potential at the *axon hillock*, where the action potential threshold is lowest (Fig. 4.5). The reversal potential of the e.p.s.p. (about − 15 mV) and the qualitative results of attempts at ionic substitution (which can only be performed rather crudely in CNS neurones, by injecting ions intracellularly) are consistent with increased permeability to both Na^+ and K^+ underlying the e.p.s.p. However, the transmitter responsible is probably not ACh, as this, choline acetylase and acetylcholinesterase are not found in appropriate positions pre- and postsynaptically. One of the likely candidates for excitatory transmission is an amino acid—glutamate.

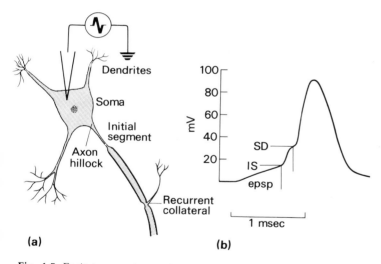

(a) (b)

Fig. 4.5. Excitatory postsynaptic events. Initial segment has lowest threshold. Full somadendritic (SD) spike follows.

Another important difference from chemical transmission at the neuromuscular junction is that a presynaptic action potential at the NMJ always results in a muscle action potential immediately afterwards, whereas transmission at the motoneurone is much less secure. Some hundreds of terminals probably have to discharge excitatory transmitter before there is a certainty of a motoneuronal action potential.

Postsynaptic inhibition

The motoneurone acts as the 'final common path', in Sherrington's phrase, for all muscle contractions called for, and controlled by, the CNS. As such, it receives not only excitatory inputs but also inhibitory ones derived from sensory receptors, interneurones in the spinal cord, and fibres descending from higher centres. Just as excitatory synapses cause excitation by depolarizing the membrane, inhibitory synapses may cause inhibition by *hyperpolarizing* it, i.e. increasing its normal negative potential, thus making it more difficult for excitatory inputs to reach threshold (Fig. 4.6). This process can be studied in the motoneurone by stimulating an inhibitory

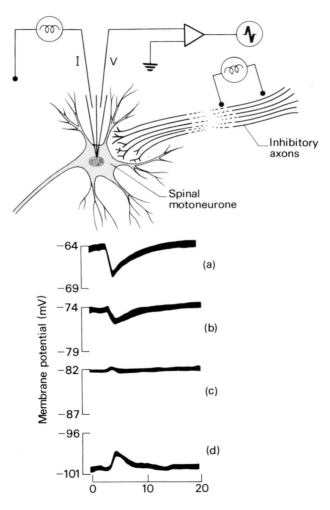

Fig. 4.6. (a) Hyperpolarization follows stimulation of inhibitory axons if the motoneurone is already depolarized. If motoneurone is hyperpolarized by injecting current (I), the hyperpolarizing effect of inhibitory input is reduced (b), then reversed (c), becoming depolarizing (d).

input, for example from the muscle spindle afferents of an antagonistic muscle.

Crayfish muscle inhibitory synapse

A much more convenient preparation to study is the inhibitory
neuromuscular synapse of the crayfish. No such thing is found in
vertebrates, but one trusts that the mechanisms found in the crayfish are shared by the mammalian central nervous system. The
inhibitory transmitter employed at the crayfish neuromuscular
synapse is gamma-amino-butyric acid (GABA). This was discovered by analysing the contents of inhibitory and excitatory
axons separately, as they can easily be distinguished under the
microscope. Inhibitory axons contain about 100 times more GABA
than excitatory ones. Furthermore, inhibitory axons release GABA
on stimulation. Takeuchi clinched the argument by showing that
artificially applied GABA mimics the hyperpolarizing effects of
stimulating inhibitory axons.

Ionic basic of postsynaptic inhibition

Hyperpolarization is probably not brought about, as one might have
expected, through increasing K^+ conductance, which would make
the membrane potential more negative, dragging it towards the K^+
equilibrium potential. Rather, GABA appears to cause an increase in
Cl^- conductance. This only causes a hyperpolarization if the
membrane is already partly depolarized (Fig. 4.6), as the Cl^- equilibrium potential is close to the normal resting membrane potential.
Nevertheless, it is true inhibition, as the membrane potential is
thereby pegged at the Cl^- equilibrium potential. This makes it much
more difficult for any subsequent excitatory synaptic currents to
depolarize the membrane. In effect, an increase in Cl^- conductance
lowers membrane resistance so that, by Ohm's Law, a larger
synaptic current is required to shift the neurone's membrane
potential to threshold. Of course the inward transfer of Cl^- pro-
moted by GABA must be compensated for by yet another pump, the
chloride pump, about which we know very little as yet.

It is known that in spinal motoneurones, postsynaptic inhibitory
effects are also brought about by increased Cl^- conductance.
Here, since the membrane is usually partially depolarized, hyperpolarization is usually seen, but can be reversed if the resting
potential is made more negative beforehand (Fig. 4.6 c,d). It is
unlikely that the transmitter responsible in the spinal cord is GABA.
Another amino acid, glycine, may be involved. In the cerebellum,
basal ganglia and cerebral cortex however, it is very likely that
GABA is the usual inhibitory transmitter.

Presynaptic inhibition

In 1961, Eccles and his colleagues noted that inhibition of spinal motoneurones could occur without any change in membrane potential or membrane conductance. They concluded that the inhibition was due to a reduction of the amount of transmitter released by the presynaptic nerve terminals. It has subsequently been shown that some synapses end upon afferent terminals rather than upon cell bodies (these are termed 'axo-axonic' synapses) (Fig. 4.7). They can cause slight depolarization of presynaptic terminals (*primary afferent depolarization*). This causes a reduction in the size of any subsequent action potential in the presynaptic terminal as it starts from a higher initial level; whilst its peak, determined by the Na^+ equilibrium potential, is fixed. Therefore the voltage swing of the presynaptic potential is reduced. This reduces the amount of Ca^{2+} entering the terminal, hence the amount of transmitter released is diminished.

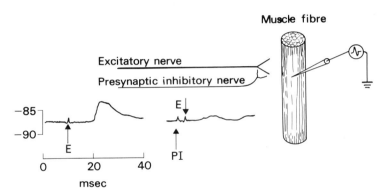

Fig. 4.7. Presynaptic inhibition in crayfish. Stimulation of excitatory nerve (E) causes depolarization. Prior stimulation of the presynaptic inhibitory (PI) nerve depolarizes the excitatory nerve, so that the excitatory nerve subsequently has no effect on the muscle.

The time course of presynaptic inhibition in the spinal cord is much longer than postsynaptic inhibition, lasting for some hundreds of milleseconds. This corresponds to the duration of a negative potential which can be recorded from dorsal roots entering the spinal cord following stimulation of a sensory nerve—the negative *dorsal root potential* (Fig. 4.8). It is likely, therefore, that the negative dorsal root potential represents the sum of presynaptic depolarizations occurring in the terminals supplied by a particular dorsal root, spreading back down the afferent fibres electro-tonically. Paradoxically, at the same time as reducing the amount of transmitter released, this subthreshold depolarization of presynaptic terminals makes them more excitable, since they are brought closer to their thresholds. Therefore, another way of detecting

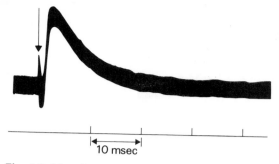

Fig. 4.8. Negative extracellular potential (corresponding to positive, depolarizing intraterminal potential) recorded from dorsal roots of mammalian spinal cord.

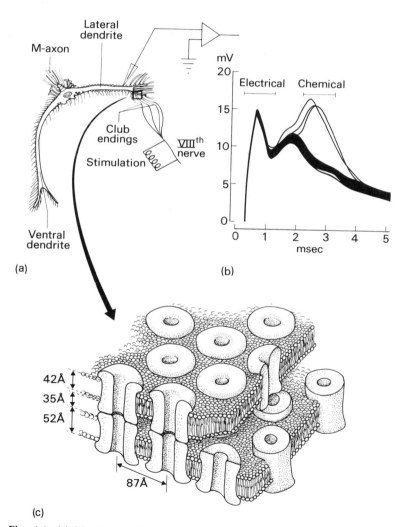

Fig. 4.9. (a) Mauthner cell (present in teleosts). (b) Early response of electrical synapse then later response of chemical synapse following stimulation of VIIIth nerve. (c) Gap junction.

presynaptic inhibition is to test for this increase in the excitability of afferent fibres (Wall's technique).

ELECTRICAL TRANSMISSION

Recently, it has emerged that chemical transmission is not universal. Electrical transmission does indeed take place at some sites, where there are specialized tight *gap junctions* no more than 2 nm wide traversed by membrane cross-bridges offering low-resistance pathways to current spread (Fig. 4.9c). The most closely studied of these is in the Mauthner cell of teleost fishes. The lateral dendrite of this large cell in the medulla oblongata forms gap junctions with club endings of the VIIIth (vestibular) nerve. Presynaptic currents pass directly across the junctions with little or no synaptic delay (Fig. 4.9b). Currents injected postsynaptically will pass just as easily back into the presynaptic terminal. Other sites where electrical transmission of this sort probably occurs are: between the neurones of the inferior olive, which give rise to the climbing fibres projecting to the cerebellum of vertebrates; in the heart, where the separate muscle cells are joined together electrically by gap junctions; in the retina between neighbouring receptors and between horizontal cells; and most interestingly of all, between the cells which make up the very primitive embryo, before their differentiation into organs. This last observation has given rise to the speculation that electrical transmission across these tight junctions is no more than a coincidence. What they are really for is to transmit regulating substances, rather than electricity, from cell to cell. So electrical synapses may be no more than primitive chemical ones after all!

Chapter 5
Introduction to Sensory
Neurophysiology

Although Descartes (1596–1650) was confident enough to explain the whole of perception in terms of a system of pneumatic tubes, pulleys and levers, more cautious minds in later centuries have contented themselves with trying to explain sensation only—a rather more modest aim. Though these two words, perception and sensation, are sometimes used interchangeably, they should really be used of two rather different concepts. Sensation is the neural mechanism by which data about the physical world are brought to the sensorium—the sensory part of consciousness; whereas perception is what the mind does with the information—comparing it with previous experiences stored in the memory, adding emotional connotations, etc. So sensation is the physical process of information transmission from the outside world, common to everyone, whilst perception is a person's private experience dependent to some extent upon his past encounters and his own personality, as well as on what is happening in the outside world. Of course the interface between the two will remain ill-defined whilst we have to use words such as 'mind', which cannot be defined clearly in physiological terms.

Traditionally, sensation has been the province of physiologists whilst perception has been studied by psychologists and philosophers. However, sensory physiology has recently begun to provide clues to the processes of perception itself; for example, the predilection of neurones in the visual cortex for lines and edges orientated at particular angles begins to explain how we can recognize the shape of an object, say a chair. A unique array of orientation detectors is stimulated by a chair. This pattern is presumably compared with patterns previously experienced and found to correspond most closely with that class known as chairs. This matching process may thus be the physiological substrate of perception. Attaining more detailed knowledge of sensory processes enables us to specify more precisely what perceptual processes must do, though we still know very little about how they do it.

To begin to understand how a sensory system works we must first be familiar with its anatomy—the connections between *sensory receptors* and *relay stations* within the central nervous system and the topographical organization of these connections. To what extent is there a correspondence between the location of a receptor, the location of fibres within the array leaving the receptive surface and the site of their terminations at relay stations and within the cerebral cortex? As we shall see, topographical organization of neurones is of the utmost importance to localization and spatial resolution in sensory systems.

After considering its neuroanatomy, we need to examine the capabilities of each sensory system in order to see what degree of precision humans can actually achieve. We can thus gain a clearer idea of what physiological attributes of the nervous system we should search for. For each sense we need to know the limits and powers of resolution (the largest and smallest intensities it can cope with); the range of qualities (also known as modalities, colours or tones) it can distinguish; and its capacity to resolve these with respect to magnitude, position and timing.

The four fundamental properties of a stimulus

In fact, complete information about four basic variables is all that is necessary for the CNS to be able to reconstruct a complete picture of the outside world. These variables are the *modality* of a stimulus, its *intensity, position* and *timing*. More complex characteristics of an object can then be deduced using appropriate combinations of these variables, e.g. the movement of an object can be judged from the rate of change of its position with respect to time; and its shape may be discovered by following its edges and contours, which are discontinuities in the intensity (or modality) of stimulation at different points on a receptive surface. For example, if you feel a 50p piece it has seven edges along which the intensity of stimulation of touch receptors abruptly diminishes, and seven vertices where the orientation of the edges changes through about 50 degrees. Putting all this information together enables you with very little difficulty to identify a 50p piece by touch alone.

Neural signalling

One of the major difficulties for sensory physiologists is that these four basic variables—the modality, intensity, position and timing of a stimulus—cannot be signalled by fully independent mechanisms within the nervous system. There are only two fundamentally different ways in which the CNS can transmit information: by the frequency of impulses in single fibres (which usually signals the intensity and timing of a stimulus) and by the choice of which particular fibre of an array is activated (which helps to indicate its location and modality (Fig. 5.1)). These two ways of signalling are sometimes known as *frequency* coding and *labelled line* coding respectively.

It follows from the necessity of transmitting four variables of a stimulus using only two fundamentally distinct means of coding that there will be a certain degree of ambiguity. In fact, the CNS itself is sometimes confused. For example, when the intensity of a monochromatic light is increased, its apparent colour sometimes changes. It is not at all surprising that neurophysiologists too are often very confused!

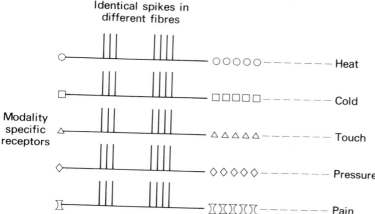

Fig. 5.1. Labelled-line coding. Modality-specific receptors connect to specific areas of the CNS. Their modality is reconstructed from their site in the periphery and the regions in the CNS to which they project, rather than from the spike trains which they generate.

Modality

It is worth examining the four essential properties of a stimulus and their coding a little further. First, the nature of the stimulus—its modality. What is it? Humans are often said to possess only five senses: touch, vision, hearing, taste and smell (whilst the sixth sense is 'extrasensory': premonition, clairvoyance and so on), but to these we should add at least temperature, pain, position and visceral sensations; and remember that different qualities, or 'sub-modalities', exist within each sense.

Muller's doctrine

Johannes Muller was the first to suggest that the modality of a stimulus is not signalled by any special characteristic of the message transmitted by a single nerve fibre, but by which type of nerve fibre is stimulated. This was enshrined in his famous doctrine of 'specific nerve energies' in which he stated his belief that no matter how a sensory nerve is stimulated, when it discharges it is interpreted by the sensorium as signalling the stimulus to which it normally responds: 'Sensation consists in the communication to the sensorium, not of the quality or state of the external body, but of the condition of the nerves themselves, excited by whatever external cause'. He deduced this from such familiar phenomena as the flash of light experienced when the eyeball is hit and, during the operation of 'couching' for cataract, the flash experienced by the patient when the retina is pierced by a needle. Volta connected a large battery to metal rods inserted into the ears, and when he closed the switch, heard a noise like 'the boiling of thick soup'. Weber persuaded his brother (!) to place electrodes over his eyes; when current was applied, the brother experienced a light that passed right through his head. Such observations all supported the idea that however a sensory nerve is activated, its discharge is interpreted according to the type of receptor to which it is attached, rather than the type of sensory energy exciting it.

The basic truth of Muller's doctrine has withstood the test of time; in general we can say that the nature of a stimulus is signalled to the CNS by 'private labelled lines' for each modality. The stimulus to which a particular receptor responds preferentially is called the *adequate stimulus* for that receptor. Receptors are connected to a series of 'relay' neurones, termed 'first-order', 'second-order', etc., which carry the information towards the cerebrum. Although Muller's doctrine implies that all such connections are specifically designated to carry one particular modality, it turns out that only a proportion of receptors and nerve fibres are *modality-specific* in this way. However, as we shall see, so long as even a proportion of fibres are modality-specific, the modality of the original stimulus can usually be reconstructed.

Types of receptor

The major sensations then are served by *modality-specific receptors*, situated at different anatomical sites. These may be broadly divided into *mechanoreceptors* (responding to stretch, pressure or other types of mechanical deformation) and *chemoreceptors* (visual, thermal, taste, pH, PO_2, etc.). Receptors are also classified according to their site and function: *teleceptors* (distance receptors) in the head, found in eyes, ears, nose and throat; *exteroceptors* in the skin; *proprioceptors* in muscles, joints and deep connective tissues; and *interoceptors* in the visceral, respiratory and cardiovascular systems.

Within each broad category of sensation there are many qualitative differences. These are also sometimes known, confusingly, as modalities, submodalities or qualities. Within the sense of touch there are hair touch, light touch, deep pressure, flutter and vibration senses; there are sharp, burning and aching qualities of pain; kinaesthesia and stataesthesia (the sensations of limb movement and limb position); warm and cold temperature senses; we distinguish tone, timbre and quality of sound and colour of light; sweet, sour, bitter and salt tastes; and so on. A comprehensive list is impossible (where would tickle and itch come?). It is unlikely, despite Muller's doctrine, that all of the more subtle, qualitative distinctions within a sensation can be entirely explained by the existence of different receptors and pathways for each. Only the major categories can be accounted for in this simple way. Submodalities and qualities of sensation are probably the result of the way in which information from different receptors is put together, dependent on the overall pattern of discharge in the whole array of fibres leaving a sensory surface.

Intensity

A second important characteristic of a stimulus is its intensity. How much of it is there? Adrian showed that the all-or-none law applies to sensory nerve fibres as much as to motor ones. Thus the only way in which a single fibre can transmit information must be by altering the number of impulses it generates per unit time. In 1932, he showed that the degree of extension of a muscle stretch receptor is signalled by the impulse frequency in the nerve fibres leaving it. This basic *frequency code* is used to signal intensity by all sense organs that have been studied, and also by their relay neurones in the pathways leading to the cerebral cortex.

For many sensory neurones it is very difficult to decide what we should consider the correct measure of frequency of discharge. The frequency of action potentials in a nerve is their number per unit time, but what time period should we choose? From the point of view of the synapse made with the next neurone in a sensory chain, the important variable is the time between successive impulses, each of which causes transmitter release, compared with the rate of decay of the postsynaptic potentials which they produce, since this determines the degree to which the next neurone's membrane potential is affected by the input. Perhaps, therefore, we should measure inter-pulse intervals rather than average firing frequencies. If the neurone is firing regularly, the only advantage of expressing the pulse interval as a frequency is that increased frequency of stimulation is associated with an increased frequency of discharge, as opposed to decreased inter-spike interval. A measure which increases with increased stimulation strength is easier for experimenters to handle.

However, there are all sorts of possible codes other than frequency, such as *probability of discharge, phase* encoding and *burst duration* coding, which may be employed by the nervous system particularly if discharge is not regular; their subtleties are entirely lost when discharge frequency is simply averaged over a longer period. But unless one has some clue as to which other form of coding might be employed one has no choice but to use the average frequency of discharge. One should always remember however that this parameter is arbitrary; it may be particularly misleading in the case of those neurones which discharge irregularly, and may therefore be using a more complex code.

Psychophysics of intensity discrimination

The correlation of subjective estimates of the magnitude of a stimulus with objective measures of its actual physical intensity (psychophysics) has exercised a continuing fascination. In the nineteenth century it even seemed possible to 'quantify the mind' in this way. With the mind measured it was hoped that maybe its mysteries would unfold; for had not measuring matter by physicists opened up the physical sciences? Although the secrets of mental processing have failed to yield to psychophysical methods, nevertheless, quantification of the relationship between the amount of sensory energy applied and resultant subjective experiences has proved to be an immensely useful technique. This assessment of the overall treatment of a stimulus by the CNS can then be compared with what is known from experiments on animals about the behaviour of neurones in sensory pathways, and many of the operations of the intact sensorium thus explained.

One of the most important principles to emerge from psychophysics is the Weber–Fechner law. In 1850, Weber found that the smallest difference which could be detected between two weights (the just noticeable difference—j.n.d.) was directly proportional to their actual weights. So the j.n.d. appeared to be a constant fraction of the level of sensory stimulation with which it was being compared (mathematically $\Delta S/S = K$). Fechner confirmed these observations and extended them to other sensations (he claimed that his mathematical expression of them was the law which related body and mind). Fechner's modification of Weber's principle implied that the physical intensity of a stimulus has to change geometrically to produce an arithmetic change in its perceived strength ($S = K \log I$). Thus the intensity of a light must increase ten times for it to appear twice as bright, and sound pressure must increase by ten times for it to seem twice as loud.

Actually the Weber–Fechner logarithmic equation fails to describe the relationship between sensation and stimulus completely accurately, particularly at low intensities. It appears that perceived magnitude of sensation also increases geometrically rather than arithmetically; thus it is the perceived ratio of magnitudes rather than the perceived difference which remains constant. Stevens showed that plotting the data from such psychophysical experiments yields an S-shaped curve, better fitted by a power function ($S = K.I.^n$) or $\log S = \log K + n \log I$. Thus a plot of log S against log I gives a straight line (e.g. for estimating a wide variety of stimuli (Fig. 5.2)).

$$\text{Log } S = \log K + n \log I$$

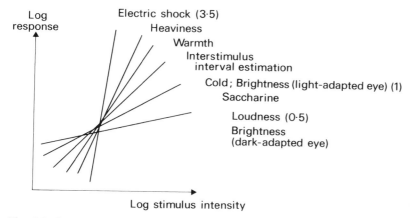

Fig. 5.2. Stevens' power law holds true for the psychophysical response to many stimuli.

Stimulus position

A third characteristic of a sensory stimulus which must be signalled to the CNS is its *location*. Where is it? In general this information is transmitted as a result of *point-to-point correspondence* between loci on sensory surfaces and loci within the central nervous system. An orderly arrangement of the spatial relationships of sensory neurones within the CNS preserves the spatial relationships of stimuli right through to the primary receiving areas in the cerebral cortex (Fig. 5.3). This is known as *topographical mapping*. Of course things are not as simple as this when examined more closely. The maps are always distorted. The density of receptors in different regions varies according to the use to which they are put; for example, the fingers have more receptors than the back of the hand; and the part of the retina which serves the optical axis of the eye, called the *fovea*, has more receptors than the periphery. Hence the number of fibres leaving the fingers or fovea is higher than elsewhere, and they take up more room. Further, more neurones are employed centrally in analysing the information they bring. Thus, when the cortex is finally reached, a greater cortical area is devoted to the fingers and fovea than to the back of the hand and periphery of the visual field. The maps of the skin and retina on the cerebral cortex are thus very distorted.

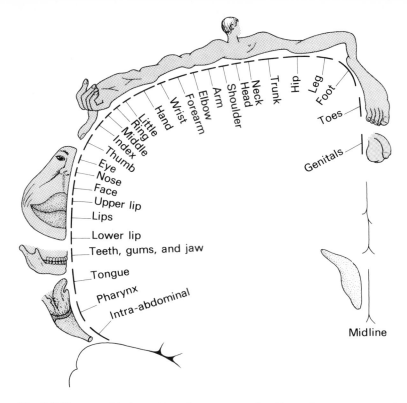

Midline

Fig. 5.3. Topographical mapping of receptors on the skin surface on to somaesthetic cortex (postcentral gyrus). The area of cortex employed by each receptor is uniform; hence the higher the density of receptors in a region, the more cortex is employed in analysing its signals.

Receptive fields

A further complication is that there are *'lateral'* interactions between neighbouring receptors and first-, second- and third-order neurones. These interactions are both excitatory and inhibitory, and are crucially important to spatial resolution of a stimulus, as we shall see. They mean that the *receptive field (RF)* (i.e. the area of sensory surface which will influence firing of a neurone under study) is much bigger than the individual receptor endings contributing to it. However, the resolution which the system can ultimately achieve is much finer than the size of even the smallest receptive field. This is because sensory neurones are organized in a way which enables them to respond most actively to *spatial discontinuities* in the environment.

Changes in stimulation with time are perhaps the most obvious discontinuities in the environment which are of potential importance for survival. In many ways, however, spatial discontinuities—lines, edges and contours—carry more information. As we have noted, the shape of an object is discovered by following its edges. Edges are changes in light intensity, colour, skin impression, etc. with respect to position. Just as adaptation enables receptors to respond exclusively to stimuli which change with time, so there is a neural procedure for enhancing differences which are a function of position. This mechanism is known as *surround inhibition* or *lateral inhibition*; it is probably the most important analytical process in the CNS that we understand as yet.

Lateral inhibition

The best-known examples of lateral inhibition occur in ganglion cells of the retina and in neurones in the dorsal column nuclei receiving from cutaneous nerves. The receptive fields of these neurones are circular. Stimulation in the central region of the receptive field causes excitation of the cell, whereas stimulation in the periphery causes inhibition. Because many receptive fields overlap, the inhibitory surround of one receptive field is the excitatory centre for many of its neighbours. Each neurone has laterally orientated inhibitory connections with surrounding neurones.

   This arrangement has the important effect of enhancing spatial discontinuities in the environment, and thus improving spatial resolution. If an edge falls upon an array of receptive fields as shown in simplified form in Fig. 5.4, then receptive fields situated wholly to the left of the edge are stimulated in both their excitatory centres and inhibitory surrounds. Thus, excitation of their centre is counteracted by inhibition exerted by their surround, and the neurones discharge weakly. Receptive fields situated wholly to the right of the edge are not stimulated at all, so their firing rate lies at a low

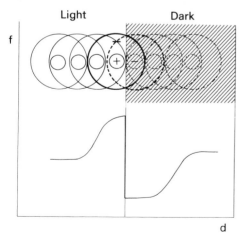

Fig. 5.4. Frequency of discharge of an array of overlapping centre–surround receptive fields at a light/dark interface. Peak discharge within array represents the place where light intensity changes most, i.e. the edge.

'spontaneous' level. However, for neurones whose receptive fields are situated along the edge, the state of affairs is more complicated. Part of their inhibitory surround is stimulated and part is not. The excitatory centres of those to the left of the edge are activated, and those to the right are not. Hence the excitation of neurones with the centres of their receptive fields situated just to the left of the border is offset only by partial inhibition from their surround, whilst those with centres to the right are not excited at all but still receive inhibition from the region of their surround situated to the left of the edge. So, at an edge, lateral inhibition ensures an abrupt change from neurones whose discharge is enhanced to those in which it is diminished, as shown in the figure.

The resolving power of the system is thus determined not by the size of individual receptive fields, but by the degree of overlap between neighbouring ones; for it is the difference in position of one receptive field with respect to its neighbours which determines whether one excitatory centre or the next is excited. This distance can actually be less than the size of one receptor if the receptor contributes inputs to neighbouring excitatory centres. A line falling across the middle of a receptor then contributes equal inputs to both receptive fields and can, in principle, be assigned its correct position by splitting the difference between the two.

Receptor arrays

Furthermore, receptors are not arranged in neat rows but in random patterns, so a unique array of receptors, and hence a unique set of relay neurones, is stimulated by a line falling on the receptive surface. The width of the line can be reconstructed from information about which particular neurones were stimulated (see Fig. 5.5). Again, the minimum width detectable is not determined by the size of individual receptive fields but by the amount by which they overlap. Maximum resolution can only be achieved by considering the output of the whole array of neurones together.

There is ample evidence that a large number of receptive fields

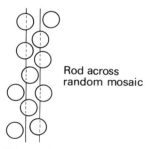

Rod across
random mosaic

Fig. 5.5. Rod width may be reconstructed from knowing which particular receptors were stimulated, even if it is narrower than the smallest receptive field.

must be activated to achieve the finest resolving power of the visual system. For example, the minimum interval between two lights on a black background which can be detected subtends about 30'' of arc at the retina; this is approximately equal to the diameter of the smallest cones. But vernier acuity (the detection of horizontal separation between two vertical lines) of about 10'' of arc can be achieved, and binocular disparities of only a few seconds of arc can be used to indicate the distance of an object from the observer. In the latter two cases, the visual system is able to pool the outputs from a much larger number of neurones (over the length of the vertical lines and over the entire contour of the object at a distance) and hence achieve better resolution.

Statistical operations

These examples illustrate another important generalization: sensory systems perform their feats of analysis statistically. The outputs from many hundreds of first-order neurones converge ultimately on one cortical cell. The probability of this neurone responding depends on the proportion of its particular set of inputs which are excited. Slightly different sets of first-order neurones converge upon neighbouring cortical neurones. At the same time, any individual first-order output diverges to hundreds of different cortical neurones. The important thing is that the set of first-order receptive fields projecting onto one cortical cell is different from that projecting to its neighbour. Thus, further stages of inhibition in the cortex can detect the cortical neurone in which the highest proportion of its input set of receptive fields is maximally active, and reject those with slightly less afferent input. As we shall see, further analysis in the cortex does not usually take the form of simple surround inhibition yielding concentric fields, but is more complex. In the striate visual cortex, fields are 'polarized'; so that they are cigar shaped, responding best to lines and edges orientated in the plane of their polarization. Thus these cells can 'look' for peaks of activity corresponding to lines or edges in the environment having a particular orientation, and thus begin the analysis of shape and contour.

Adaptation and surround inhibition are the operations in the sensory periphery of which we have the greatest understanding. As a result of adaptation, the signals which pass centrally are not proportional to the intensity of a stimulus alone, but also to the rate of change of intensity (dI/dt). Similarly, surround inhibition transforms the signal in an array of fibres from a simple record of the intensity of the stimulus at a particular position to a differential—the rate of change of stimulus intensity with respect to its position on the receptive surface (dI/dx).

Cross-modality inhibition

We may be encouraged to look for analogous operations involving modality, another of our four vital properties of a sensory stimulus. We will see that changes in neuronal discharge occur when the colour of a retinal stimulus changes, as a function of its position ('opponent-colour' coding). This we may call 'cross-modality' inhibition. Cross-modality inhibition also occurs in the cutaneous system. Cutaneous touch receptors can inhibit the transfer of pain signals to second-order neurones in the spinal cord; this underlies the 'gate' theory of pain control. In the central nervous system, inputs from totally different sense organs can converge and inhibit each other. For example, properly timed auditory stimuli can inhibit visual input in the cerebellum (Fig. 5.6); and proprioceptive inputs from eye muscles can inhibit visual signals in the superior colliculus. We might call this 'cross-sensory' inhibition. Thus operations analogous to lateral inhibition, which enhances discontinuities in the spatial domain, also occur between modalities and sensations; they presumably serve a similar function in emphasizing transitions from one form of sensory energy to another.

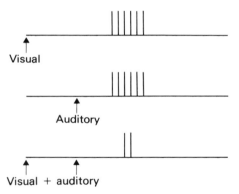

Fig. 5.6. Cross-modality inhibition. A cerebellar Purkinje cell responding to visual and auditory stimuli. If stimuli are applied one after the other with appropriate timing, they inhibit one another.

Timing

The fourth characteristic of a sensory stimulus which is needed to assemble a complete reconstruction of the outside world is its timing; when it starts, when it stops and how its intensity, colour, tone or position change with time. In general, these things are signalled by the temporal characteristics of the impulses elicited by the stimulus.

The start and finish of a pulse train signal the start and finish of the stimulus. A change in frequency within a train can signal a change in stimulus intensity. However, this arrangement could easily allow misinterpretation of signals. First, the speed of transduction at different receptors and the conduction velocities of different fibres vary widely. So the start of a stimulus may give rise not to a synchronous volley arriving at the cerebral cortex, but to a ragged array of bursts arriving at different times. Furthermore, most receptors *adapt,* lowering their discharge frequency to a constant stimulus, as discussed in Chapter 3, so a change in the frequency of discharge may signify either a change in the stimulus intensity or merely adaptation of the receptors. However, the CNS is presumably programmed to expect receptor adaptation in certain pathways, i.e. it is a 'constant' in the interpretation of signals. Hence any unexpected changes are likely to result from changes in the stimulus. A corollary of this is that, since the majority of receptors do adapt, if a stimulus does not alter with time more and more receptors stop discharging altogether and a constant stimulus begins to fade. This is one of the reasons why we rarely feel the clothes on our body or the hardness of our seat, and why retinal images fade away completely if movements of the eye are entirely prevented.

Dynamic sensitivity

The greater responsiveness of sensory systems to changes than to steady states is of great survival value, since discontinuities in the environment provide important information. The rate of adaptation of a receptor determines its sensitivity to the rate of change of a stimulus with time (sometimes called its *velocity sensitivity* or *dynamic sensitivity*). A receptor, such as a Pacinian corpuscle, which adapts quickly will respond very weakly to a slowly changing stimulus but vigorously to a rapidly applied one; whilst a slowly adapting receptor will signal the final 'static' intensity of the stimulus, rather than its rate of application.

Oscillatory activity

Even more complicated inhibitory interactions than lateral inhibition and cross-modality inhibition take place in the temporal domain. Following the arrival of an excitatory sensory volley in the CNS there is almost always a period of reduced activity followed by a rebound of excitation, giving rise to oscillations which may continue for several seconds (Fig. 5.7). The role of these oscillations in sensory processing is something of a mystery, but one can speculate that the interruption of a pattern of oscillations by a further sensory stimulus is in itself a way of emphasizing a new event in the periphery, rather as throwing a second stone into a

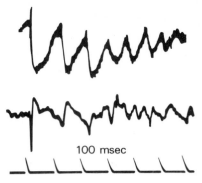

100 msec

Fig. 5.7. Long-lasting oscillatory response in thalamus (VPL) (upper trace) and postcentral gyrus (lower trace) following a single cutaneous stimulus.

pond complicates the pattern of ripples caused by the first, by an order of magnitude.

Reverberating circuits

Another possible explanation is that these oscillations represent the activation of 'reverberating circuits' which are set up when chains of interneurones excite each other. They may underly phenomena such as: long-lasting 'central excitatory and inhibitory states'; reflex activity which well outlasts the original stimulus; 'habituation'—the tendency of sensory systems to react to regularly repeated stimuli with smaller and smaller responses; and even short-term memory which, as we shall see, is probably an 'electrical' phenomenon.

Function of dynamic responses

One might ask why it is necessary for receptors and sensory systems in general to signal rates of change (velocities) as well as the changes themselves, since the former can in principle be derived simply by dividing the difference before and after the change by the time taken to achieve it. Surely the nervous system must be capable of such a simple calculation.

The disadvantage of deriving rates of change in this way is that the calculation can only be performed after the change to which it refers has taken place. It is easier to see that this could be a profound drawback if we consider a specific example—the spinal stretch reflex—but the argument can be extended to cover all sensory receptors and sensation in general.

Instability in the stretch reflex

Stretching a muscle excites length receptors (muscle spindles) within it. These cause the muscle's motoneurones to discharge, opposing the stretch, as if in an attempt to keep the muscle at a constant length. The resultant reflex contraction takes place with a minimum latency of about 10 ms and a maximum power at about 50 ms. Suppose the muscle were alternately extended and shortened every 50 ms by some external agency (Fig. 5.8a); then the main reflex response to the extension would take place after a delay of about 50 ms (Fig. 5.8b). By this time however, the muscle would already be shortening; the reflex would add to this and actually reinforce it (Fig. 5.8c). This would tend to cause extreme instability of the muscle, as negative feedback would be converted into positive feedback because of the phasing of the lengthening and shortening of the muscle in relation to the loop time of the reflex. Of course, regular extension and flexion of a muscle every 50 ms seldom occurs in real life; but it is often the case that afferent signals fluctuate greatly over this sort of time scale, so the circumstances of negative feedback being converted to positive feedback can often arise. Indeed, everybody is found to possess a normal 'physiological' tremor of about 10 c.p.s. (half period = 50 ms). In some people it is much more noticeable than others. It is highly likely that this tremor is the result of just the process outlined above—namely fluctuating length feedback interacting with varying muscle activity giving a half-cycle time of about 50 ms.

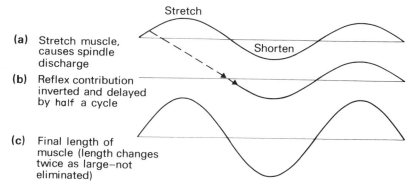

(a) Stretch muscle, causes spindle discharge

(b) Reflex contribution inverted and delayed by half a cycle

(c) Final length of muscle (length changes twice as large—not eliminated)

Fig. 5.8. Effect of stretch reflex delay converting negative length feedback to unstable positive feedback.

Velocity signals—prediction and damping

The role of velocity feedback from muscle spindles is to help prevent oscillations and instability—to 'damp' and smoothen body movements. This can be seen crudely in Fig. 5.9. In the absence of muscle spindle damping, muscle contraction in response to motocortical stimulation is jerky and ill coordinated, with the unregulated contractions occurring at about 10 c.p.s. (Fig. 5.9B).

It is easy to see that a limb is more likely to overshoot its target if it is moving fast, than if it is moving slowly. However, if the motor control system is provided with an up-to-date signal about how fast the limb is moving (its velocity) it can predict where the limb will have reached at some instant in the future and take appropriate braking action (stronger for fast than for slow movements). This principle, employed routinely by control engineers, allows velocity signals to compensate for delays in negative feedback systems and to contribute to damping.

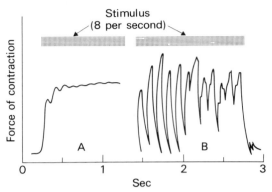

Fig. 5.9. Contraction of soleus following motocortical stimulation before (A) and after (B) section of dorsal roots.

A little thought will show how the same principle may be applied to sensation. For example, the speed of a moving bird can be assessed instantaneously, its future position predicted with a high degree of accuracy and a shotgun fired in front of it with a good chance of bagging a meal.

Centrifugal control of afferent input

It must not be thought that the transformations of sensory information in the CNS by means of temporal modulation, lateral inhibition and so on are passive, fixed and immutable. Almost all sensory relays and some sensory receptors themselves (e.g. muscle spindles, the cochlea in mammals, the retina in birds) receive efferent fibres from higher levels of the nervous system, which can alter the way in which incoming sensory information is treated. This is known as *centrifugal control*. Usually, centrifugal fibres are derived from the same areas of the cerebral cortex as those to which the sensory neurones which they regulate ultimately project. Thus, for example, there is a point-to-point correspondence between afferent and efferent fibres linking the lateral geniculate nucleus with primary visual cortex, and a similar arrangement of those linking dorsal column nuclei with primary sensory somaesthetic cortex. These projections may be both excitatory and inhibitory.

Relay stations also receive modulating inputs from the reticular formation. These probably control overall levels of excitability; they are not topographically organized.

Centrifugal inputs may help to explain the phenomenon of *selective attention*—the mechanism which enables one to enhance sensory acuity to a particular stimulus: a mother to her baby's cry, the particular sound of a favourite person at a cocktail party or the specific feel of a key in one's pocket.

Active filters

Sensory relays are, therefore, far more than passive staging posts on the way to the sensory cortex. They actively transform incoming information under central control and they can redirect information from one receiving area to another. One should therefore think of them not as substations or even telephone exchanges but as *filters* of sensory input, whose properties can be varied from moment to moment. They may enhance certain aspects of a stimulus, in particular its spatial and temporal discontinuities, under central control, and filter this information while diverting or discarding other facets of the stimulus.

Series *v.* parallel processing

Although information about modality, intensity, position and timing is necessary to build up within the CNS a complete picture of the external world, these variables are never signalled independently, but transmitted as 'differentials'—rates of change of one with respect to another. Changes in intensity with time are signalled by alterations in discharge frequency, while change of intensity of stimulation with respect to position (e.g. the edge of an object) is signalled by which neurones in the array leaving a sensory surface are most active.

Although the simplest model of how further analysis proceeds is a *hierarchical* series of processes, gradually specifying the optimum stimulus of sensory neurones in greater and greater detail, it now seems probably that different characteristics of a stimulus are in fact determined simultaneously, in parallel, by different regions of the CNS. Each cortical area is probably designated to abstract a particular characteristic of an object, such as orientation, shape, colour, movement, etc., in a series of operations; but many such series are arranged in parallel and are active simultaneously. Thus, in the visual system contours and shapes are registered by the neural apparatus in occipital lobe area 17; stereoscopic depth, which is derived from a comparison of the inputs from the two eyes, is dealt with in area 18; and movement and colour are analysed in different parts of the superior temporal sulcus.

The idea that different aspects of a stimulus are abstracted by specialized serial systems of neurones working in parallel with each other was first introduced to explain some results of psychophysical experiments. These showed clearly that some features of a stimulus are analysed independently of others. For instance, an illusion of movement may be obtained by changing the intensity of illumination or the position of contours in a random dot pattern. Changing colour alone, however, never leads to such an illusion of movement. This implies that colour and movement are analysed entirely separately from one another in the visual system. These and many similar observations suggest that separate characteristics of a stimulus are analysed by independent sensory *channels*. This speculation arose long before physiologists had come up with direct electrophysiological evidence for parallel processing.

These channels may often be treated as being entirely independent of each other in psychophysical experiments. One of their most useful characteristics is that they can be selectively fatigued or 'adapted' (not to be confused with receptor adaptation). For example, one way of stimulating the visual system is by the use of a grating of black and white bars in which the intensity of the white bars is made to shade sinusoidally into the black. The advantage of such a stimulus is that a powerful mathematical technique, known as frequency analysis, can be used to quantify experimental results. Fergus Campbell used such gratings with different *spatial frequencies* (number of bars per degree of visual angle) to stimulate the human visual system. Campbell found that if he first exposed a subject to a high-contrast adapting grating of a particular spatial frequency, the subject's threshold for detecting gratings with the same spatial frequency but at lower contrast levels was greatly elevated; but his ability to see other spatial frequencies was normal. Thus the high-contrast adapting grating had selectively fatigued a system of neurones devoted to detecting one spatial frequency, but not those detecting higher or lower frequencies. These systems have come to be known as *spatial frequency channels.*

In order to perform such feats of analysis, these channels probably consist of a series of specialized neurones performing a succession of operations such as temporal, lateral and cross-modality inhibition. One should think of each sensory channel as itself being a hierarchical series of neurones devoted to extracting a particular nugget of information from the environment, and of a large number of such channels operating simultaneously, in parallel, alongside each other. Thus, within each channel, a sequential series of transformations is effected, but the many different features of a stimulus are extracted simultaneously.

Cortical columns (Fig. 5.10)

Some of the physiological mechanisms underlying these parallel sensory channels, each specialized to look for a specific property of a sensation, have now been identified. At the macroscopic level, the analysis of broad classes of characteristics, such as colour, movement, etc., by separate areas of cortex has been conclusively demonstrated. On the microscopic scale, a similar arrangement of parallel processing units can be seen in the organization of cortical cells in columns. The majority of connections between neurones in the cerebral cortex are radial, so that columns of cells normal (at right angles) to the cortical surface are joined together. Each column receives a 'specific' sensory fibre from the appropriate thalamic nucleus to layer 4 of its cortex and 'non-specific' inputs to its superficial layers. Its main 'corticocortical' outputs (to other parts of the cerebral cortex) leave from layer 3 and its 'corticofugal' projections leave the cerebral cortex altogether, for other parts of the CNS, from layer 5.

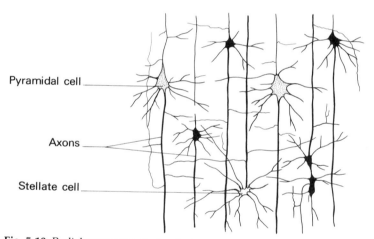

Pyramidal cell

Axons

Stellate cell

Fig. 5.10. Radial arrangement of cortical neurones in 'columns'.

Each sensory column receives information from a particular region of the sensory surface projecting to it. This follows from the topographical organization of primary sensory pathways. What is more remarkable, however, is that each column responds to only a narrow range of properties within the category analysed by the area in which it is situated. Thus, single columns in the visual striate cortex (V1) respond to only one orientation of a line or edge stimulus; those in V4 respond only to a single colour; and those in the second somatosensory area, only to cutaneous stimuli moving in a particular direction. The column appears to be the smallest abstracting unit of a sensory system. Many such columns serve each local area in the outside world, covering all possible orientations, colours, etc. Together they make up cortical areas devoted to broader categories of sensation such as colour or movement; and many cortical areas work together simultaneously to perform the complete analysis of every characteristic of a perceived object.

'Second' sensory systems

A further variation on the theme of parallel processing is the existence of 'second' sensory pathways in addition to the classical primary ones. For cutaneous sensation, parallel projections via the spinothalamic and dorsal column routes have long been recognized though, over-simplistically, they were thought to carry entirely different modalities—pain and temperature as opposed to touch and proprioception, respectively. It is now clear that hearing and vision also employ separate, second, sensory routes which parallel the well-known primary ones. All sensory systems project via dual pathways, sometimes known as 'lemniscal line' (primary) and 'lemniscal adjunct' (secondary) pathways. Like the spinothalamic pathway for somaesthesia, the secondary routes are, in fact, phylogenetically older; only under exceptional circumstances can they be shown to reach consciousness. Their chief role may be to control the orientation response of an animal to sensory stimuli, using rapid brainstem connections with motor systems; they may have gained a cortical projection later in evolution. Thus, the second visual route passes from the eyes to the superior colliculus, which is important in controlling eye and head movements. It then projects, via the pulvinar of the thalamus, to prestriate areas in front of the primary visual projection area of striate cortex, and supplies them with further information about the movement of objects in the visual world and that of the eyes and head for the visual control of body movements. Similarly, the second auditory route pathway helps to control movements of the head and ears in response to sounds.

Decoding

We have made many references to 'sensory coding' in this chapter. Normally, coding in one place implies decoding in another. Some people seem to think that 'a little man' sits somewhere in our brains (Descartes would have suggested the pineal gland) putting together incoming sensory messages and decoding them for the benefit of consciousness. This is an entirely unnecessary complication. The cipher experts at Bletchley in the Second World War intercepted coded messages, but merely translated them into another code—the English language—which generals and admirals could understand and act upon. In the CNS, the cipher experts are the sensory parts of the cortex which transform signals coming from the periphery into other signals which the motor, memory and visceral systems can use to do things: track a visual target, memorize a telephone number, etc. A little man translating these messages into consciousness is totally unnecessary. Consciousness is probably the sum total of sensory transactions and their interactions with memory and movement. Perhaps it was evolved as the only way of keeping them all under control.

Chapter 6
Visual System

The adequate stimulus for the retina is electromagnetic radiation of wavelength 450–700 nm, which we perceive as light. No doubt honey bees, whose photoreceptors respond to longer wavelengths (up to 800 nm), would consider longer wavelengths as 'light' as well. By photographic or electronic trickery we can transform longer or shorter wavelengths to make them visible too, but clearly there was not enough selective advantage for us to evolve photoreceptors to cover a wider spectrum.

The virtues of the visible spectrum are that: the sun can supply the wavelengths reliably; terrestrial objects absorb and reflect them in patterns sufficiently individual for us to detect; light travels in straight lines; and the wavelengths are sufficiently short for the rays to be focused by suitably shaped interfaces. So, unlike sound waves, the spatial relationships of light waves reflected by objects correspond to the spatial relationships of the parts of the object, and the same spatial relationships may be projected onto the retina by the lens. The detection of spatial relationships is all-important in the visual system.

PSYCHOPHYSICS

Spatial resolution

Acuity

A change of only one per cent in light intensity, marking the edge of an object, can easily be detected at the fovea—the area of retina lying on the optical axis. The acuity of the eye (its capacity to resolve local detail in the visual world) is thus very high indeed. Acuity is usually measured using 'Snellen' standard-sized letters and expressed as the ratio of the smallest letters a subject can see at six metres distance to those that a person with normal vision can see. The normal acuity of '6/6' means that a subject can resolve two lines separated by approximately one minute of arc. The smallest receptors lying on the optical axis of the eye (the fovea centralis) are less than 1 μm across and they subtend less than one minute of arc. Nevertheless, this does not mean that one receptor must remain unstimulated between two lines for them to be resolved. Many people can do much better than 6/6; 6/30 is not uncommon (subtending 12 seconds of arc at the retina). Tests such as that of Vernier acuity (the ability to detect very small horizontal displacements between vertical lines) reveal that the fovea can achieve even higher resolutions, but only 2° away from the fovea acuity falls off dramatically (Fig. 6.1).

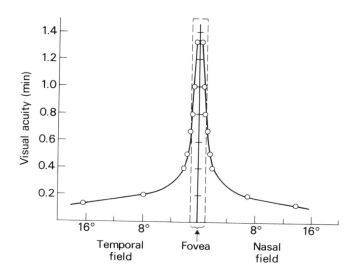

Fig. 6.1. Visual acuity as a function of distance of image from the fovea (i.e. retinal eccentricity).

Direction

The capacity of the visual system to resolve lines, edges and contours in the outside world, to reveal the shape of to whom or what they belong, is obviously of fundamental importance to our survival. Hence, our resolving power for such discontinuities in the environment is extremely high. However, our ability to judge the absolute direction of objects is very much poorer. The complete visual field subtends some 150°. In the centre we can judge the direction of an object to within 1° (a resolution of 0.7%) but in the periphery this falls off to less than 10° (7%).

Distance

Similarly, our absolute judgements of distance are poor, but we can resolve a difference in distance of only a few millimetres between two objects 1 m away. The main cue for distance judgement is the difference between the eyes in the position on the retinae of the two images of an object. This is called the horizontal *disparity*. Disparity is a function of the distance of an object away from the subject and of the distance between the eyes. Hence the distance judgements of a sheep with its wide-set eyes are better than a human's. Our ability to measure absolute disparity (to judge the distance away of a single object) is in fact rather poor; but our computation of comparative disparity is good. The difference in disparity of an object 1 mm in front of another 1 m away is only a few seconds of arc.

Spatial frequency analysis

As described in Chapter 5, a quantitative technique for analysing visual resolution which has turned out to be very useful is *spatial frequency analysis*. Using a grating of black and white bars in which the intensity of a white bar shades sinusoidally into the black bar next to it, one can measure the degree of contrast between black and white bars which can just be detected at each frequency. This gives a picture of a subject's variation of sensitivity across the whole range of gratings from very coarse to very fine—his 'modulation transfer function' (Fig. 6.2). Differences following changes in orientation or colour contrast may also be examined. The former has shown up interesting effects consequent upon, for example, astigmatism in youth, persisting even after the astigmatism has been corrected by

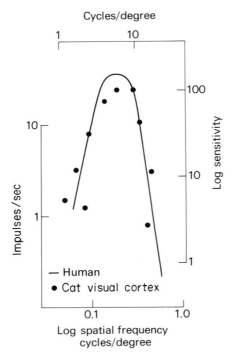

Fig. 6.2. Sensitivity of human observers and neurones in cat visual cortex to different spatial frequencies of a sinusoidal grating.

spectacles. Such people have a residual deficiency in the sensitivity of their whole visual system to gratings orientated in the direction of the plane of their worst astigmatism. This probably reflects the slight inferiority of the image in this plane early in life; in consequence, detectors responding to tht orientation were insufficiently stimulated at a crucial stage in their development, leaving a permanent deficiency of their resolution of lines and edges orientated in that direction.

The neuronal systems dealing with particular bar sizes can be selectively fatigued or adapted. If a subject is first exposed to a high-contrast adapting stimulus of a particular spatial frequency and orientation, his sensitivity for detecting that spatial frequency if it is presented at low contrast is greatly diminished. Neighbouring spatial frequencies and neighbouring orientations are unaffected, however.

Intensity

The range of light intensities over which the human eye can operate is immense. About 10^{10} photons flood the eye when we look directly at the sun yet, when it is fully adapted to the dark, $1/10^9$ of that number, only ten photons, will give rise to a sensation of light. Hecht, Schlaer and Pirenne found that in fully dark-adapted eyes, five of these ten photons are lost *en route* through the rather murky optical media of the eye; and five retinal rods excited by just one photon apiece are sufficient to yield a visual sensation. Over the whole range of light intensities the eye is rather insensitive to changes in overall brightness, although exquisitely sensitive to local changes, as we have seen. A tenfold increase in the physical intensity of a light source is perceived as only doubling its apparent brightness. As noted by Weber and Fechner (Chapter 5), subjective brightness is therefore proportional not to actual light intensity, but to its logarithm.

Dark adaptation

The print on a newspaper viewed in daylight reflects more light than its white background in twilight, yet the contrast appears the same to us. The sensitivity of the visual system must therefore somehow be varied to suit prevailing light conditions.

If a subject is suddenly removed from bright light into complete darkness, over the next half hour or so his threshold for seeing a faint flash of light shows two phases. In the first 10 minutes there is a rapid reduction in threshold, followed by a further, slower reduction over the next 20 minutes (Fig. 6.3).

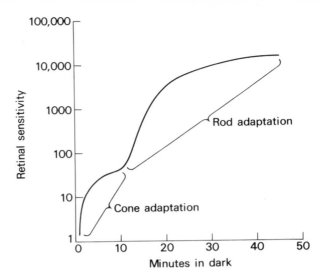

Fig. 6.3. Time course of dark adaptation.

Duplicity theory

These two phases are important evidence for the 'duplicity theory': in daylight, vision is mediated by one type of retinal receptor, the cone, which effects colour vision; whereas in the dark, vision is implemented by rods. Completely colour-blind 'rod mono- chromats', who develop no cones at all, do not show the first phase of dark adaptation. Those who lack rods can see colours but suffer from night blindness; in such subjects the later phase of dark adaptation does not occur. As rods predominate in the periphery of the retina, the first phase of dark adaptation is not found for test flashes projected there. Conversely, since the fovea does not contain any rods, one cannot see a dim star if one looks directly at it. The cones in the fovea do not function in dim light, and it is necessary to look away from the star in order for the rods to see it.

Purkinje shift

In daylight, a wavelength of 570 nm is most efficiently absorbed, so the weakest flash which one can detect is towards the red end of the spectrum. This wavelength represents the average of the absorption peaks of the three pigments found in cones. However, after adapting to the dark, peak sensitivity of the eye shifts to around 500 nm, which is the absorption maximum for rhodopsin—the rod pigment. This change is known as the Purkinje shift (Fig. 6.4), after Johannes Evangelista Purkinje, who discovered the phenomenon as a medical student and went on to lend his name to the chief neurone in the cerebellum and to the conducting tissue of the heart.

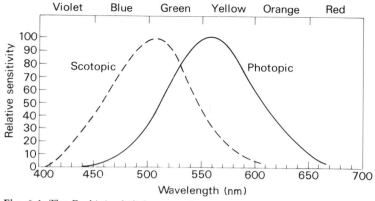

Fig. 6.4. The Purkinje shift from maximum sensitivity at 570 nm (red) in daylight (photopic range) to 500 nm (green) at night.

Colour

The next important characteristic of a visually perceived object with which we have to deal is its colour. In bright light (the so-called *photopic* range of human vision), the eye can distinguish something like 170 different hues. These correspond to the different wavelengths of the light reflected from an object and not absorbed by it. The wavelengths which we can distinguish are not evenly spaced over the visible spectrum; in our most sensitive range, differences of only 1 nm can be detected (Fig. 6.5), whereas all the wavelengths below 300 nm look violet and all those above 650 nm look red. Also, most objects reflect not just one wavelength but several; their colour is thus the result of a mixture of wavelengths reaching the eye. Furthermore, wavelength is not the only parameter which makes colours look different. The same wavelength can change its apparent colour if its intensity is increased or if white light is added;

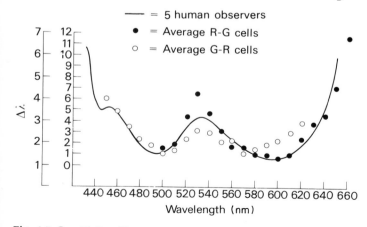

Fig. 6.5. Sensitivity of human observers and monkey lateral-geniculate, red/green, opponent-colour-sensitive neurones to changes in colour (Δλ) at different background wavelengths.

this changes its *saturation*.　Finally, under conditions of very low illumination (the *scotopic* range of vision), when rod vision predominates, perception of colour fails altogether. All wavelengths are perceived as shades of grey.

Young–Helmholtz trichromatic theory

In 1801, Thomas Young demonstrated that any hue which the human eye can detect can be duplicated by mixing suitable amounts of just three primary coloured lights—blue, green and red. This observation was confirmed by Helmholtz, who suggested that a minimum of three different sorts of colour receptor are necessary to signal all the wavelengths we can detect. The shrewdness of this deduction was attested by his successful classification of colour blindness. Sure enough, there turn out to be three types of partial colour blindness: dichromats in which either blue, green or red senses are absent; three types of cone monochromats, in whom pairs of colours are missing; and total (rod monochromat) colour blindness, in which no cones develop at all.

Opponent colour coding

There were many aspects of colour vision which could not be explained by this simple 'trichromatic theory'. The phenomena of *successive* and *simultaneous colour contrast* prompted Hering to introduce a rival theory, that of opponent colour coding. If we stare at a bright red light and then shift our gaze to a white wall, the after-image of the light appears green. Similarly, if we look at a grey square on a red background it takes on a greenish hue. Hering supposed that strong stimulation of red elements in the visual system could fatigue them, and tip the balance in favour of green, with which they were normally in opposition. As we shall see, there is now abundant evidence in favour of Hering's theory of opponent colour processing, for all but the receptor stage in the retina.

McCollough effect

Spatial frequency analysis has also introduced a new dimension to the analysis of colour vision. If an orientated grating is viewed with coloured light, a colour and orientation contingent after-effect may be observed (the McCollough effect). After adaptation to vertical red gratings alternating with horizontal green gratings, a vertical black and white grating looks green, while a horizontal one looks red. Furthermore, after adapting to a red grating tilted clockwise from vertical and a green grating tilted counterclockwise a vertical test grating appears to be tilted counterclockwise when viewed with red light, but clockwise when viewed with green light. The simplest explanation is that the adapting coloured grating fatigues a specific set of orientation- and colour-specific neurones, allowing their opponent-colour counterparts, tuned to the same orientation but not fatigued, to dominate perception. These after-effects are different from the coloured after-images which follow bleaching of visual pigments by bright coloured lights. They are weaker, much slower in onset, last much longer and, unexpectedly, are often stronger half an hour later than immediately after adaptation (reminiscence effect). They exemplify Hering's opponent colour theory; but there is much argument about whether they represent neural adaptation or learning. Perhaps there is no real distinction between the two. Neurophysiologists postulate that learning ultimately involves some form of long-term neural adaptation; the task for the future is to determine its site and mechanism.

Timing

Temporal changes in the visual world take the form either of changes with time of the light intensity at a point (e.g. a winking stationary source of light); or of a change in the position of a light source; or of a change in colour, usually caused by a change in the position of a coloured object. As discussed in Chapter 3 these events are signalled as differentials—changes of intensity or of colour with respect to time.

Critical fusion frequency

The eye is not very good at resolving very rapid changes in intensity or colour, a fact which facilitates film and television technology and A.C. lighting. The threshold for perceiving two bright flashes as being separate, rather than as a single longer flash, is as long as 50 ms, lengthening if light intensity is decreased. The frequency at which bright flashes no longer flicker but fuse together completely, the 'flicker–fusion frequency', is about 30 c.p.s. for bright flashes (equivalent to 33 ms between flashes). The colour signalling system is even slower; the highest frequency at which equal intensity red/green alternations are still seen as colour changes rather than fused to create a new colour (yellow) is as low as 4 c.p.s.

Movement

However, the human visual system is much better at resolving movement, as might be expected of an animal originally adapted for swinging around in trees, avoiding predators and searching for fruit. Changes in the position of objects as slow as $1°\,s^{-1}$ or as fast as $1000°\,s^{-1}$ can be perceived and judged accurately.

THE EYE

Optical media

How does the visual system achieve its resolution of space, colour and time? First, we must consider the equipment with which evolution has provided us to perform these miracles. The optical media of the eye consist of: the cornea, where most of the refraction of light rays take place; the aqueous humour; the lens, whose radius of curvature can be altered to accommodate for objects at different distances; and the vitreous humour filling the posterior chamber.

Lens

The curvature of the lens is adjusted to focus inverted images of objects in the outside world onto the retina. This is effected by circular and radial muscles controlling the tension in suspensory ligaments attached to the circumference of the lens. Contraction of the circular muscle relaxes these ligaments and allows the lens to assume a more spherical shape which refracts light rays more sharply, bringing close objects into focus on the retina. These muscles are under the control of the parasympathetic nervous system and so are inactivated by atropine. Contraction of the radial muscles indirectly tightens the suspensory ligaments; hence they stretch the lens, for focusing on distant objects. They are supplied by sympathetic nerves, so their control is impeded by sympathetic blockers.

Long and short sight

The contraction of the muscles of accommodation is often not properly adjusted to the size of the eyeball, and long or short sight ensues. This seems to be a hereditary problem. Myopia (short sight) is usually considered to be the result of having too long an eyeball, so that light rays converge in front of the retina and distant objects are out of focus; while hypermetropes (those with long sight) are said to have too short an eyeball, so that light rays converge behind it. It can equally well be argued, however, that the circular muscles in the case of hypermetropes, and the radial muscles in the case of myopics, do not contract strongly enough. Thus, although corrective spectacles or contact lenses are the easiest solution to bad eyesight, it is often possible, with the help of a good orthoptist, great patience and self-discipline, to train the erring muscles to do a better job, and thus do without glasses. This does not apply to *presbyopia*—the long sight of older people in whom the lens loses its suppleness and will not bend sufficiently when the circular muscle contracts to accommodate for near objects. Nor, of course, does it apply to *astigmatism*. In this condition the cornea has different horizontal and vertical radii of curvature; so horizontal and vertical elements of an object are brought to a focus in different planes. Hence no single curvature of the lens can achieve a sharp image.

The retina

The retina lies behind all these structures which are, in fact, imperfectly translucent. It is the 'wrong way round', with nerve fibres leaving it on the surface, and receptors lying behind them in the pigment epithelium. This is thought to be an accident of embryology resulting from the fact that the retina is an outgrowth of the forebrain, whose axons lie on the surface. It means that light rays, having traversed the optical media of the eye, must pass through nerve fibres, then ganglion cells, inner plexiform layer, bipolar cell layer, outer plexiform layer, and the inner segment of the receptors, before reaching their outer segments where phototransduction actually takes place (Fig. 6.6).

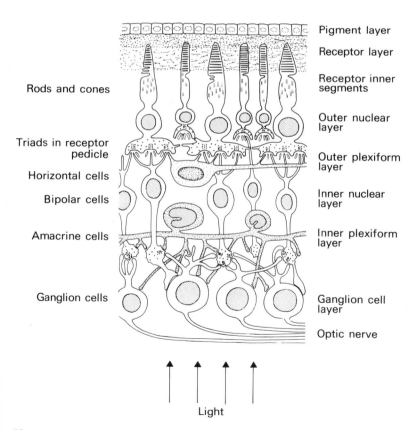

Fig. 6.6. Simplified diagram of retina (after Dowling J.E. & Boycott B.B. (1966) *Proc. Roy. Soc. Lond. B.*, **166**, 339).

Rods and cones

The outer segment of the receptors is buried in a layer of pigment cells containing melanin; these help to cut down stray light, nourish the receptors and remove old receptor membrane. New membrane is under continuous production by the receptor. Photopigment is arranged in an orderly array upon the much-folded outer-segment membrane, which looks like a pile of plates. In cones, the membrane is in free communication with the extracellular space but in rods it is not, perhaps in order to maximize the tiny ionic changes occurring around their membrane in weak light. Rods are responsible for vision in the dark (scotopic vision); they are larger (5 μm across) to optimize their chances of catching quanta of light. Cones are shorter and smaller; the smallest at the fovea being no more than 1 μm across. They are responsible for daylight (photopic) colour vision, where a small quantal catch is not a problem, but resolution of delicate shapes and patterns in the visual scene is. Cones are found in greatest number around the optical axis of the eye. In the fovea, at the very centre of the retina, there are no rods at all. Rods extend right out to the periphery of the eye, where there are no cones (which is why one cannot distinguish colours in the periphery of one's vision).

Photopigments

At the core of visual transduction lie the photopigments: rhodopsin, found in rods, and cyanolabe, erythrolabe and chlorolabe, found in different types of cone. Each rod is thought to contain about 10^9 molecules of rhodopsin; cones contain rather less photopigment. Most is known about rhodopsin, which has been isolated from nocturnal animals with retinae made up entirely of rods; but there is every reason to suppose that the mechanism for capturing photons of light and making use of them is fundamentally similar in all pigments. Each pigment has a different opsin (protein component), while the molecule which captures the photons (retinene) is the same in all of them. Opsins probably determine the spectral sensitivity of the pigments (the wavelength of light that each absorbs most easily) whilst retinene performs the vital role of converting light into electrical potential changes.

Retinene

Retinene can exist in two optical isomers, *cis*- and *trans*-retinene. When primed to absorb a photon, retinene is in the all *cis*- form, tensed like a mousetrap. On absorbing a photon, it springs into the *trans*- form; this triggers a chain of chemical reactions, leading to the bleaching of the rhodopsin. All these reactions are exothermic so that they need no external energy supply. They result in the splitting of rhodopsin into retinal vitamin A and free opsin. In the dark, vitamin A and opsin are joined together and twisted into the *cis-* form; thus rhodopsin is regenerated.

The bleaching of rhodopsin takes a long time (several seconds) to complete, whereas the earliest electrical changes which can be recorded in photoreceptors are almost instantaneous; so bleaching itself probably has little to do with electrical transduction but it is important in light adaptation, as we shall see.

Receptor potentials

The very first potential which can be recorded from receptors (early receptor potential) is probably the electrical sign of the absorption of

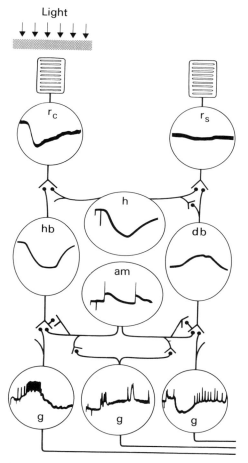

Fig. 6.7. A possible 'wiring diagram' to explain surround inhibition in retinal ganglion cells (after Werblin F.S. & Dowling J.E. (1969) *J. Neurophysiol,* **32,** 339). r_c, receptor in centre; r_s, receptor in surround; hb, hyperpolarizing bipolar; db, depolarizing bipolar; h, horizontal cell; am, amacrine cell; g, ganglion cell.

photons, springing retinene from the *cis-* to *trans-* form. Bortoff first managed to insert electrodes into the outer segments of the giant cones found in *Necturus*, a salamander. He found that their electrical response to a flash of light is not the depolarization that we usually associate with the excitation of neurones, but rather hyperpolarization (Fig. 6.7). In fact, this had already been suspected from studies of the electroretinogram (ERG—the gross potential measured across the whole retina following a flash of light). The hyperpolarizing response of receptors was identified in the ERG by occluding the central retinal artery; this kills all the neural elements in the retina apart from the outer segments of the receptors which are nourished by the pigment epithelium. Subsequent biophysical studies have shown that maintained depolarization of receptor outer segments occurs in the dark, as the result of a continuous sodium current known as the 'dark current'.

The dark current is abruptly halted following a flash of light; hence the receptor hyperpolarizes. It is probable that absorption of one photon, causing photoisomerization of one rhodopsin molecule, leads to the release of perhaps 100 molecules of an 'internal transmitter' (Ca^{2+} and/or cyclic GMP) which are able to plug the same number of sodium channels; this process gives rise to a 'quantal current' of about 1 pA (10^{-12} A) per photoisomerization, causing a potential change of around 50 μV in rods and 25 μV in cones.

Receptor synapses

Neighbouring receptors are often linked together by electrical synapses, so that hyperpolarization of one receptor spreads across a pool of about ten neighbouring receptors. Receptors then communicate with bipolars and horizontal cells by means of a three-way synapse, known as a 'tryad', buried in the receptor pedicle (Fig. 6.6). In addition, chemical transmission in both directions probably occurs here, because there are vesicles beneath receptor, bipolar and horizontal cell membrane surfaces. These are known therefore as reciprocal synapses.

Retinal interneurones

It appears that many *horizontal cells* feed back onto cones. They may show opponent colour coding responses, though some are not differentially sensitive to different wavelengths. *Bipolar cells* project onwards towards the *ganglion cells* which are the output neurones of the retina. However, bipolars can either hyperpolarize (hyperpolarizing bipolars) like the rods and cones supplying them, or they can invert their input and depolarize (depolarizing bipolars).

Amacrine cells which link neighbouring ganglion cells, are the first neurones to exhibit action potentials as well as slow potentials; together with horizontal cells, they probably subserve lateral inhibition. Some feed back upon bipolars, however, whilst others interact with each other. Finally, a new type of retinal neurone has recently been identified. This is the so-called *interplexiform cell,* which is thought to feed back from inner to outer plexiform layer. It could not be clearly separated from the amacrine cell using the Golgi technique, as this does not reliably stain the terminal processes of small neurones; but with the introduction of specific techniques for detecting dopamine in neurones, its true morphology became apparent. It may well play a part in the 'gain control' of the retina, changing its overall sensitivity in light and dark adaptation.

Retinal pharmacology

This most recent information about retinal circuitry has emerged from the combination of classical biophysical with newer pharmacological techniques. It appears that an important excitatory transmitter released from receptors may be aspartic acid, which depolarizes depolarizing bipolars and hyperpolarizes hyperpolarizing bipolars. But the outer layers of the retina also contain dopamine, acetylcholine, large quantities of taurine (which may be converted into another excitatory amino acid, cysteine sulphonic acid) and many peptides such as encephalins, substance P and cholesystokinin. These may also be important in the initial transfer of information from receptors to bipolar and horizontal cells. Dopamine increases the red response and decreases the green responses of colour-type horizontal cells, implying that it is one transmitter employed by the colour system, though details are not yet known. The transmitter released by other, presumably inhibitory, horizontal cells (probably receiving from red cones) is GABA.

The inner plexiform layer contains large quantities of ACh, dopamine, 5HT, GABA and glycine. Snippets of information are now available about some of these. For instance, dopamine-containing amacrines do not make contacts with ganglion cells or bipolars but only with other amacrines; whilst 5HT-containing amacrines feed back predominantly onto bipolars. Many cholinergic amacrine cells appear for some reason to be 'displaced', and are found in the ganglion cell layer. This leaves still other transmitters unaccounted for. These presumably mediate further lateral interactions between ganglion cells which are important for the final construction of the centre–surround organization of ganglion cell receptive fields.

Dark adaptation

Recent advances in our understanding of retinal function have considerably illuminated the mechanisms involved in light and dark adaptation.

Receptor adaptation

A major component of light adaptation, which has only recently been identified, is local desensitization of the processes which release internal transmitter within receptor outer segments. If an adapting light is confined to just the base of a single rod outer segment, it reduces the photocurrent elicited by a dim test light subsequently shone on the same region of the base; but it has no effect on the response to the same light directed at the tip. Hence local adaptation of the receptor occurs under these conditions. This process probably has nothing to do with pigment bleaching, as it has a much quicker time course. It suggests that there may be only a limited local store of internal transmitter molecules, which can be used up quickly.

Bleaching

Photopigment bleaching does, however, account for a major part of light adaptation. There is a logarithmic relationship between rhodopsin concentration and rod sensitivity (Fig. 6.8). Following an adapting light which reduces rhodopsin concentration by only eight

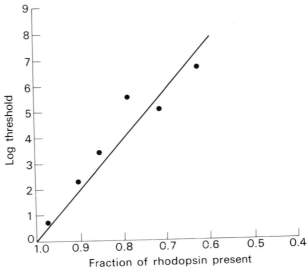

Fig. 6.8. Logarithmic elevation of threshold for seeing is a function of the fraction of rhodopsin remaining unbleached.

per cent, rod sensitivity is decreased by about 100 times; whilst a reduction of 16% reduces it not by 200 times but 1000 times. This proportional relationship is probably the result of the laminar structure of rods. When the first 'plate' of rhodopsin is bleached following the absorption of light, it tends to reflect all wavelengths (which is why it looks white or bleached); hence plates deeper in the rod receive less light than they would if the superficial plates were more translucent. Thus bleaching not only reduces the amount of pigment available to absorb light but increases the proportion of the incident light which is reflected away from receptors altogether.

Neural adaptation

These local processes are by no means the whole explanation for light adaptation however. If they were, adaptation would be confined to the areas of the retina which had received illumination. Yet Rushton showed for rod vision that if a spot of light is used to bleach a small area of the retina, the resultant decrease in light sensitivity is not confined to this area but spreads to the surrounding retina. So probably, in addition, there are 'neural' mechanisms for changing the sensitivity of the retina to light, at least for rods. We know very little about these as yet; though the newly discovered interplexiform cell is probably implicated.

Pupillary changes

We already do know, however, that a mechanism for measuring average light intensity over wide areas of the retina must exist. For although change in pupil size makes a fairly minor contribution to adaptation (its area can only vary by about 20 times), pupillary diameter accurately reflects the average light intensity falling on the eye; this implies that there is a mechanism for measuring it. About 10% of ganglion cells respond not to any of the more esoteric features of a visual stimulus, but simply to the intensity of light falling on their receptive fields. These are sometimes called 'luminosity detectors'. They project both to the LGN and to the *pretectal region*, where pupillary control is organized, and thence to the parasympathetic Edinger–Westphal nucleus. This is responsible for controlling the circular fibres which constrict the pupil.

Like the lens, the pupil also possesses radial muscle which dilates it, supplied by sympathetic nerves. The drug atropine has been known from earliest times as 'belladonna', since it paralyses the circular muscles of the pupil causing it to dilate, thus lending additional beauty to any donna! It is probable that luminosity detectors determine the normal balance of activity of pupillary muscles. They are also involved in dark adaptation.

Ricco's Law

The human capacity to sense changes in overall light intensity varies linearly with the area stimulated (Ricco's Law), up to a maximum plateau. Since the maximum area over which Ricco's Law operates is larger than the receptive-field size of single luminosity detectors, a number of receptive fields must be pooled to complete a sensation of brightness. It is highly likely that luminosity detectors are not alone in joining this pool. During dark adaptation, concentric receptive fields of ganglion cells lose their inhibitory surrounds; they can then contribute to the detection of dim lights over their whole receptive field.

CENTRAL VISUAL PATHWAYS (Fig. 6.9)

The optic nerves which take the axons of ganglion cells from the retinae into the brain pass beneath the frontal lobes towards the brain stem.

Optic chiasm

Just in front of the pituitary stalk, in the *optic chiasm*, the optic nerve fibres coming from the nasal half of the retina of one eye change place with those from the nasal half of the retina of the other eye. The temporal fibres (from the temple-side of the retina) stay where they are. Thus proximal to the optic chiasm (nearer the brain), in the *optic tract* projecting to the *lateral geniculate nucleus* (LGN) of the thalamus, fibres from the temporal half of one retina travel with those from the nasal half of the other. Put another way, fibres leaving the right-hand side of each eye project to the right hemisphere, while those from the left hand side of each eye project to the left hemisphere. In the optic tract, therefore, both sets of fibres deal with the same half of the visual world; thus each half of the brain maps the opposite visual hemifield.

Many fibres divide before they reach the lateral geniculate nucleus. These collaterals pass to the superior colliculus and pretectal region. In both the LGN and superior colliculus therefore, fibres dealing with each half of visual space collect in register to form a 'retinotopic map' of the opposite hemifield.

Lateral geniculate nucleus (LGN)

The LGN has six layers; fibres from the nasal retina of the ipsilateral eye pass to layers 1, 3 and 4, whilst those from the temporal retina of the other eye pass to layers 2, 5 and 6. At this stage, fibres from the two eyes do not interact, although interneurones here receive from both eyes. The significance of the six layers is by no means clear. An early suggestion that the three layers receiving from each eye corresponded to the three types of cones thought to underlying colour vision has not survived; but the layers probably do correspond to some degree of specialization of function. The two deepest layers contain very large neurones which receive and project large fibres onwards to the visual cortex. These are part of the rapidly conducting Y or 'transient' system which we shall consider later. Other visual projection neurones are classified as W (luminosity type) or X (dealing with fine detail and colour). W cells project to the pretectal area, which organizes the pupillary response to light, and also to the superficial layers of the LGN, as do X cells. So the four superficial

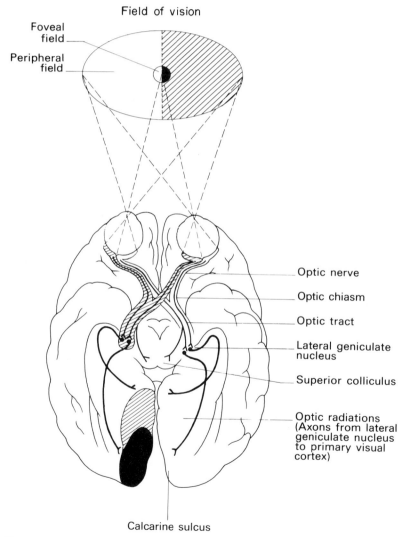

Field of vision

Foveal field

Peripheral field

Optic nerve

Optic chiasm

Optic tract

Lateral geniculate nucleus

Superior colliculus

Optic radiations (Axons from lateral geniculate nucleus to primary visual cortex)

Calcarine sulcus

Fig. 6.9. Visual pathways viewed from undersurface of hemispheres.

layers of the LGN, which contain small cells, probably receive predominately W- and X-type input.

In the LGN, ganglion cell axons synapse with relay neurones which project via the *optic radiations* to the primary visual cortex—the *striate cortex*. The function of the large number of LGN interneurones (10% of the total cell number) is largely unknown. They may contribute to the powerful lateral inhibition which is found here, to the strong opponent colour properties of these cells and, finally, perhaps to the centrifugal control of this relay station which is exercised by striate cortex and the reticular formation.

Centrifugal control

There is a diffuse projection from the reticular formation which can reduce transmission through the LGN considerably, for instance during periods of inattention and during rapid eye movements. The LGN also receives a topographically organized efferent projection back from the striate cortex. The same afferent neurones which project from the LGN to a particular point in the striate cortex receive corticofugal efferents from that point. This mechanism may underly one's ability to attend selectively to a particular visual detail, by actively suppressing signals from surrounding regions.

Visual cortex

The map of the visual world which is found in the striate cortex is a rather peculiar one. First, it is upside down and left and right are transposed, a consequence of the reversing optics of the eye. Secondly, it is highly distorted because the amount of cortex devoted to each part of the visual field is proportional to the number of ganglion cell axons leaving the corresponding part of the retina. More fibres leave the fovea than the periphery; more LGN cells transmit their information to the cortex. Thus, a proportionately much greater area of cortex is devoted to foveal input. The *magnification factor* (amount of cortex per unit area of retina) is about 10:1 for the fovea in the striate cortex whereas it is only 1:10 for the retinal periphery. Thus the fovea is 100 times better represented in the cortex than the periphery (Fig. 6.10).

From the striate cortex (Brodmann's area 17) fibres pass to prestriate cortex (areas 18 and 19), also known as V2 and V3; and thence to inferotemporal cortex (areas 20 and 21). Another projection takes fibres destined to help control movement to the superior temporal sulcus and posterior part of the parietal lobe. The fibres project topographically from V1 to V2, so that the representation of the dividing line between left and right hemifields (vertical meridian) at the edge of area 17 projects to the adjacent part of

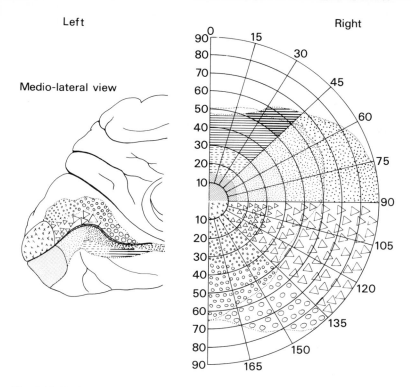

Medio-lateral view

Fig. 6.10. Projection of visual fields to calcarine fissure (Brodmann's area 17) showing cortical 'magnification' of central 10° (after Holmes G. (1945) *Proc. Roy. Soc. Lond. B.,* **132**, 349).

area 18; thus the striate representation of the centre of the visual field projects to the posterior part of area 18 while the periphery of the hemifield, even more compressed than in area 17, projects to anterior area 18. In area 19 the process is repeated, so that the periphery is represented in the posterior part of 19 adjacent to 18; and the vertical meridian is represented anteriorly. After this, strict topographical representation disappears, so that in the superior temporal sulcus, inferotemporal cortex and posterior parietal cortex, visual receptive fields are very large and not clearly mapped. This is to be expected, since visual perception and visual control of behaviour must eventually be independent of the actual position of an object on the retina. A table is a table, whether seen in the left upper quadrant of the visual field or the right lower one.

Efferent projections of visual cortex

The efferent projections from visual areas of the cortex onwards may reveal much about the way in which that information is used. The destinations of fibres leaving the occipital cortex may be both cortical and subcortical—to areas specialized for visual identification, memory or the control of movement. The striate cortex projects to other cortical visual areas, to the lateral geniculate nucleus and to the superior colliculus, in a topographically organized way. One can therefore view its efferent connections as being entirely concerned with the administration and internal organization of the visual system. But other areas, such as area 18, the superior temporal sulcus and the parietal cortex, project mainly to motor centres and probably do not preserve retinotopic topography. These pathways link visual centres with the cerebellum, basal ganglia and frontal 'premotor' areas. Inferotemporal cortical areas 20 and 21, on the other hand, probably project onwards towards the limbic system, where the visual analysis achieved by these areas is perhaps associated with emotional values, drive states, etc.

PATTERN DISCRIMINATION

In general, light levels *per se* are of little interest to an animal, and our ability to measure absolute luminosity is rather poor. What matters more are changes in light intensity across the visual field, for these discontinuities outline the shape of objects and their movements, signifying dangerous predators or attractive prey. We will first deal therefore with analysis of such spatial discontinuities—the visual discrimination of pattern.

Lateral inhibition

Bipolar cells

Although individual receptors merely register, by hyperpolarization, the presence of light of the particular wavelengths to which they are 'tuned', at the horizontal and bipolar cell stages the process of enhancing discontinuities in the visual scene by lateral inhibition has already started. The receptive fields of bipolar or horizontal cells consist of a central area in which illumination causes a change in membrane potential, surrounded by a ring in which illumination causes the opposite potential change (Fig. 6.7).

Ganglion cells

Ganglion cells have more highly developed surround inhibition; on-centre neurones receive input from depolarizing bipolars in their receptive field centres and from hyperpolarizing bipolars in their surrounds, and vice versa for off-centre cells. Their inhibitory surrounds are so effective that combined stimulation of both centre and surround can completely stop a ganglion cell from discharging. The amacrine cells connect neighbouring ganglion cells in the inner

nuclear layer. These probably also help to mediate lateral interactions, since they discharge briskly both when a light directed at
receptors situated on either side of them is switched on, and when it
is switched off.

The concentric organization of ganglion cell receptive fields is not
the result of a carefully demarcated changeover from excitatory to
inhibitory inputs at the boundary of the excitatory centre; rather,
both inhibitory and excitatory inputs are wired into the ganglion
cell. In the centre, the excitatory inputs predominate but these
gradually give way to inhibitory inputs in the surround. Since the
inhibitory area is larger than the excitatory area, illumination of the
whole receptive field can silence the cell completely. However,
during dark adaptation the excitatory centre widens and surround
inhibition diminishes, eventually disappearing. This implies that
excitatory inputs arise from the surround, even though under
photopic conditions they are swamped by inhibitory inputs, supplied, perhaps, only by cones.

As mentioned in Chapter 5, the size of individual ganglion cell
receptive fields is not of crucial significance because the spatial
resolution of the visual system is determined by the degree of
overlap of neighbouring receptive fields, rather than by their size.
Counts of ganglion cell numbers give an indication of their density
in any area of the retina, and hence of their degree of overlap. In the
foveal region of the cat eye, the average size of ganglion cell receptive fields is about 12' of arc. However, the number of ganglion cells
in the central 5° is about 20 000 along any one diameter, so a resolu-
tion of $5/20\,000° = 2.5 \times 10^{-4} \times 60 \times 60 = c.\ 1''$, rather than 12', of arc is
theoretically possible.

LGN

In the lateral geniculate nucleus, receptive fields show even more
powerful surround inhibition than in the ganglion cell layer; these
further enhance local peaks of activity corresponding to edges in the
environment, signalled by the array of neurones leading from the
eye.

Visual cortex

Simple cells

In the striate cortex, however, the shape of receptive fields under-
goes a very significant change. Instead of being concentric, like
those of the LGN afferents which arrive in cortical layer 4, they are
cigar shaped (Fig. 6.11a), so that lines and edges with the same
orientation as this long axis become the most effective stimuli. The

(a)

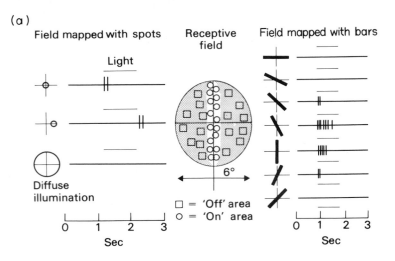

(b)

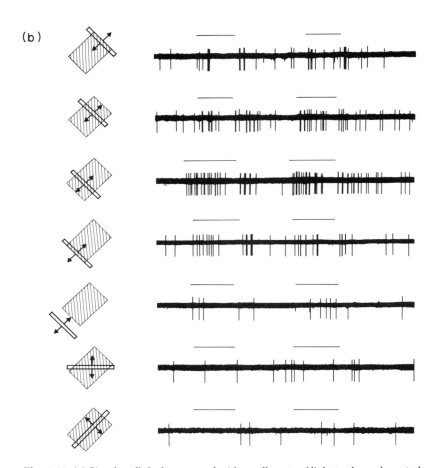

Fig. 6.11. (a) Simple cell. Left—mapped with small spots of light to show elongated 'on' centre and 'off' surround. Right—mapped with bars to show efficiency of correctly orientated bar. (b) Complex cell. Correctly orientated bar elicits response if moved over any region of large receptive field. (After Hubel D.H. & Wiesel T.N.).

shapes of the receptive fields of these *simple cells*, as they are called, can still, however, be mapped with small spots of light, though mapped in this way their receptive fields appear less elongated than when mapped using bars and edges. Hubel and Wiesel, who discovered this novel feature of cortical receptive fields, speculated that they might be constructed from inputs provided by rows of LGN neurones whose concentric fields lie alongside each other on the map of the visual world in the LGN. If they then converged upon a single cortical cell, this would explain why the cell's receptive field is oblong. However it now appears that this suggestion oversimplifies the matter considerably.

There are many different types of simple receptive fields, some with inhibitory surrounds, some with inhibitory centres, some with antagonistic fields on either side of their long axes (Fig. 6.11); but they all share the property of having an elongated, orientated receptive field.

Complex cells

Deeper and more superficially, in layers 2, 3, 5 and 6 of the striate cortex, simple cells give way to *complex cells*. In these, the optimum stimulus is also a bar or edge with the correct orientation, but their receptive fields cannot be mapped using single spots of light. They are larger and a correctly orientated stimulus positioned anywhere within the field may elicit a large response (Fig. 6.11b). Complex cells, therefore, represent a first stage in the process of abstracting the property of 'orientatedness' from its immediate spatial surroundings, discussed earlier. They also are more sensitive than simple cells to a moving stimulus; some are 'directionally selective', responding best to one direction of movement but less strongly or not at all to the other. Hubel and Wiesel suggested that these cells receive their input from several simple cells with the same preferred orientation.

Hypercomplex cells

A further stage in the abstracting process is found in some cells in area 17 and more in area 18, called *hypercomplex* cells by Hubel and Wiesel. The optimum stimulus for these cells is again a correctly orientated bar or edge. However for hypercomplex cells the bar must not exceed a certain critical length. This requirement for a particular length implies that the neurone is able to detect the right angles at the ends of the stimulus. In *higher-order hypercomplex* cells, the angle required to excite the cell maximally can, in fact, be an angle other than a right angle.

Hierarchical (series) processing

Hubel and Wiesel's conception was that the properties of simple, complex and hypercomplex cells are the result of 'hierarchical' processing—an orientated line of LGN cells exciting a single simple cell, many like-orientated simple cells converging on a single complex cell and complex cells with orientation specificities at right angles to each other converging on a single hypercomplex cell. However it is now clear that this is a great oversimplification. Sillito has shown, using the GABA antagonist bicuculline, that many of the properties of cortical cells (in particular orientation and direction selectivity) depend upon inhibitory processes occurring within the striate cortex itself, and therefore cannot be determined solely by the orderly convergence of lines of LGN inputs. This is rendered unlikely also by the wide ramification of LGN terminals; some of these extend 1 mm or more whereas the size of individual simple cells is no more than 50 μm.

Furthermore, it is now clear that simple cells do not form the only input to complex cells. They receive direct input from a class of rapidly conducting LGN axons known as Y cells, which arrive at a slightly different layer of cortex and confer on them a shorter latency to visual stimuli than simple cells together, presumably, with their greater sensitivity to movement.

Hence, unfortunately, Hubel and Wiesel's original postulate of a simple hierarchy of analytical stages progressively abstracting orientations, angles and lengths from shapes in the environment, separating them from any dependence on their immediate spatial location and eventually leading to the identification of objects in the outside world, is probably incorrect. To envisage that such hierarchical processing continues to the point where there would have to be a unique cell specialized to detect each and every possible object in the outside world is unsatisfactory. Attempts to specify orders of visual neurones higher in the hierarchy than hypercomplex have been rather unconvincing. If one thinks about this idea, the existence of such hyperspecialized trigger features seems most unlikely. A system which demanded a single cell for all possible sensations would be astronomically huge and wasteful. Would one need a special cell for such unlikely events as a pink elephant on a white background? Surely not.

Parallel processing

As discussed in Chapter 5, the cerebral cortex probably extracts general features of an object such as its shape, colour, movement, etc. by separate parallel processes taking place in different visual areas; and then attempts to match the neural patterns so generated with stored patterns, in order to identify what the object is and what to do about it. This leaves it open to intepret patterns quite broadly and to incorporate new patterns when they are encountered. The mechanism of the matching process is, of course, as yet quite unknown.

Columnar organization

The specialization of different areas of cortex for different types of analysis, such as colour, movement and shape, has its counterpart at the microscopic level in the specialized organization of cortical 'columns'. The six layers of the cerebral cortex are characterized by vertical connections with limited horizontal diffusion of signals. Input from the LGN arrives mostly in layer 4 and passes, via pyramidal cells with predominately vertical processes, to layers 1, 2, 3, 5 and 6.

Orientation columns

This anatomical organization of cortical cells in columns is the substrate for a vertical organization of function. All neurones encountered when driving a microelectrode downwards, normal to the surface of the cerebral cortex, deal with the same part of the visual world and have the same preferred orientation, whether they

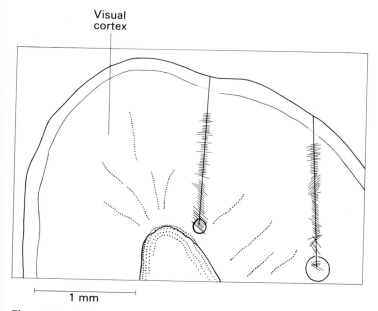

Fig. 6.12. Columnar arrangement of neurones having similar orientation preferences. The left-hand electrode track is not quite normal to the cortical surface and passes through two columns. The right-hand track passes through five. (After Hubel D.H. & Wiesel T.N. (1962) *J. Physiol.*, **160,** 106.)

are simple, complex or hypercomplex types (Fig. 6.12). One can therefore think of such a column as an orientation-abstracting unit for that local region of space. Neighbouring columns deal with progressively larger angles at about 10° intervals; so that one can discern 'hypercolumns' which deal with the full 360°. These are about 2 mm wide.

Orientation columns have recently been visualized in a striking way using the radioactive deoxyglucose technique mentioned in Chapter 2. This is taken up by neurones when they are activated, but it cannot be fully metabolized. Active cells which have absorbed deoxyglucose can then be detected by autoradiography. Thus, if the visual system is stimulated using a grating of vertical bars, neurones with vertical preferred-orientations are stimulated and take up the radioactive deoxyglucose; these cells can then be identified in appropriately prepared sections of the brain. One can actually see the columns of neurones which were selectively activated by the grating in life as a series of dark columns on the slide. This is direct evidence that visual information is segregated in the striate cortex on the basis of the orientation of contours, and not only on the basis of locus in one half of visual space. This is the start of pattern recognition.

Commissural connections

Areas 17, 18 and 19 all contain clearly discernible retinotopic maps of one half of visual space, preserving at each stage correspondence between points on their surfaces and points in the outside world. However, the two halves of the visual world are segregated in opposite hemispheres. What happens about the representation of objects which cross the mid-line, as most do when looked at directly (foveated)? Such objects are 'stitched together' across the mid-line by fibres passing in the posterior part (splenium) of the corpus callosum and anterior commissure to the opposite hemisphere. Neurones representing the midline vertical meridian project fibres to corresponding points on the other side, so that the integrity of the representation of the visual field across the mid-line is preserved.

The central 5–10° of the visual field is thus bilaterally represented. The connections between these representations may be *homotopic*, i.e. points representing 1° to the right in one hemisphere maybe connected with points representing 1° to the left in the other, 2° right with 2° left, and so on. The consequence of this is that the spatial pattern of signals representing small objects may be reversed in traversing the commissures. Presumably, the normal person learns to compensate for this mirror effect of the visual commissures; but it has been suggested that it might partially account for the mirror-image errors which are so characteristic of children learning to read and of some who fail to learn to read—dyslexics.

Inferotemporal cortex

Eventually, analysis of the shape of objects and pattern recognition must become independent of retinotopic coordinates. The 'chairness' of a chair must become an abstract rather than a spatial quality, not dependent upon where on the retina the chair is viewed. Hence, visual areas anterior to the striate cortex progressively lose their retinotopic mapping. In posterior parietal area 7 (see Chapter 20) and inferotemporal cortex, visual receptive fields are huge, and they are not mapped retinotopically at all. Gross and Mishkin found that many neurones in inferotemporal cortex receive from both visual hemifields, employing interhemispheric transfer via the splenium of the corpus callosum and the anterior commissure to acquire visual information about the ipsilateral hemifield. The trigger features of these neurones, some of which seem to be extraordinarily specific, are similar throughout this large receptive field. This observation has provided the first neurophysiological correlate for a classical psychological problem—the perceptual equivalence of stimuli despite their impingement on different parts of the retinae—despite 'retinal translation'.

Lesions of the inferior temporal cortex in monkeys result in profound deterioration in visual learning, probably because the subject can no longer effectively compare stimuli impinging on different parts of the retina in order to make reliable discriminations. If care is taken to ensure that the stimuli are always seen on the same part of the retina, the difficulties disappear.

The highest level of purely visual pattern and shape recognition therefore seems to reside in inferotemporal cortex. Cross-modal associations between visual, somaesthetic and auditory inputs, however, probably take place in the lateral parts of the parietal lobe and superior temporal cortex.

STEREOSCOPIC VISION

It has so far been argued that differences in light intensity reflected from adjacent parts of the visual world are crucially important for discerning the shape of an object. However, visual space perceived by one retina is only two-dimensional, and therefore flat. To achieve the third dimension, that of depth, we need two eyes and interaction of the information supplied by each. Although some distance cues are provided monocularly—by the shadow and apparent size of familiar objects; by movements of the head and eyes causing 'parallax'; by the degree of confergence required to fixate objects

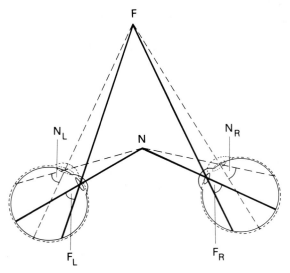

Fig. 6.13. Retinal disparity. When the eyes converge on a near object N, rays from the far object F fall at angle F_L in left eye and F_R ($= -F_L$) in right eye, i.e. there is a large disparity between the positions of the images of F in the two eyes. When the eyes are converged on F, similar arguments apply to the object N, so a particular disparity implies different distances, depending on the convergence of the eyes.

at different distances, etc.—a full stereoscopic effect requires measurement of binocular disparity. This is the difference between the positions of the images of a single object on the two retinae (Fig. 6.13).

Binocular cells

The requirements of a disparity detector are analogous to the requirements for edge detection. Neurones must respond to the difference between corresponding inputs from the two eyes to signal depth, whereas to signal the position of an edge they respond to the difference between the outputs of neighbouring retinal elements.

Ocular dominance columns

Hubel and Wiesel found that inputs to the striate cortex from the layers of the LGN serving one eye enter the cortex alongside, but never in the same place as, those arriving from the other eye. Along one strip of cortex, therefore, there are columns exclusively serving the contralateral eye (contralateral ocular dominance). Columns serving the ipsilateral eye (ipsilateral ocular dominance columns) are arranged in neighbouring strips on either side. Between them there are columns receiving inputs from both eyes, dominated by one or the other eye or with equal inputs from both.

Barlow, Blakemore and Pettigrew found that many binocular cells are sensitive to the disparity between the images of an object in the two eyes. Columns of cells respond best to particular disparities; hence they are 'tuned' to detect objects at particular distances away. One problem for this system is that the 'meaning' of the disparity to which a particular neurone is tuned, in terms of the distance away from the observer of the object stimulating the cell, is dependent on the degree of convergence of the eyes. If the eyes are converged at a near point N, an object at N elicits zero disparity; whereas an object F at some distant point elicits a large 'crossed' disparity (F_R–F_L; since F_L is negative this equals $2F_R$) (Fig. 6.13). If the eyes now converge on F, then N elicits a large crossed disparity and F elicits no disparity at all. Clearly the distance signified by any particular disparity must be recalibrated each time the eyes are reconverged. How this is done is not known, but the cerebellum is probably involved.

TEMPORAL RESOLUTION IN THE VISUAL SYSTEM

The next characteristic of the visual system we must consider is its timing. Although photoreceptor potentials begin to start and stop when a light stimulus does, they already introduce their own time distortions; these are even more intrusive at the horizontal and bipolar stages. The bipolars' hyperpolarizations or depolarizations diminish even when a stimulus is maintained; and when the stimulus is turned off they may generate a transient potential in the opposite direction. Their response to light shone on their surrounds is, of course, the inverse of this. In amacrine cells, these slow potential changes are converted into action potential signals (the first neurones in the retina to do this), which show even greater transient effects.

Sustained and transient ganglion cells

The discharge of ganglion cells serves as the final common pathway for all retinal output to the brain. They were originally classed as *on*, *off* or *on/off* cells according to whether they discharge in response to switching on or switching off a light in the centre of their receptive field, or to both; but it has now become apparent that there are two broad classes of each of on, off, and on/off cells according to how fast their discharge decreases during a maintained stimulus. The very fastest, constituting about 10% of ganglion cells, are termed *transient* or Y cells; they have large cell bodies, large receptive fields and high conduction rates. They serve to detect the occurrence of new events in the environment, since their discharge falls to zero even when a light stimulus is maintained (Fig. 6.14). The slower *sustained* or X cells are present in much greater numbers. They are probably more important in pattern recognition since their receptive fields are smaller and overlap more; and they do not adapt as quickly to a maintained stimulus (Fig. 6.14). Transient (Y) cell axons project branches both to the deep, (large-cell) layers of the LGN and to the superior colliculus, where they play a role in helping to control head and eye movements. Sustained (X) cells project mainly to the super-ficial (small-cell) layers of the LGN, and thence to striate cortex layer 4, where they probably participate in building up the simple, complex and hypercomplex fields we have discussed already. Y neurones project to different layers of the cortex and probably contribute to the movement sensitivity of complex cells, often by-passing simple cells altogether. In the cat but not in primates, Y cell output from the LGN can pass directly to complex cells in area 18, since the latency to activate complex cells there after a stimulus is shorter than for simple cells in area 17. In both cats and primates, additional Y cell signals can project to prestriate visual areas taking a totally different route—via the superior colliculus and pulvinar (the 'second' visual system).

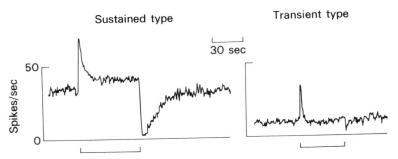

Fig. 6.14. Sustained (X) and transient (Y) ganglion-cell responses. During illumination sustained cells maintain a firing level higher than their spontaneous level, whereas the transient cell response adapts to base level completely.

Movement sensitivity

We shall now consider the movement sensitivity of cortical cells. This is first noticeable in some simple and complex cells, for which correctly orientated bars are more effective if they are moved across the receptive field. Some of these cells, particularly those in area 18, are directionally selective, i.e. they respond best if a correctly orientated bar is moved in a particular direction across their re-ceptive field, and are inhibited by movement in the opposite direction. The other important characteristic of these movement-sensitive neurones is that they often respond optimally to particular rates of movement—*velocity tuning*. Of course, the faster a stimulus moves across the receptive field, the shorter the time in which the neurone has to fire; and the larger the receptive field of the cell, the longer the time it has in which to fire. A true measure of velocity sensitivity takes this into account, for example by counting of the number of spikes per unit time the stimulus was in the receptive field.

Columns of cells sensitive in these ways to particular directions and velocities of movement are found predominantly in area 18. This specialization for movement detection is carried further in columns found in a part of the superior temporal sulcus which receives most of its input from area 18. Here, most neurones cannot be driven at all by stationary targets; they are all directionally selective and velocity-tuned and may respond to movement in depth as well, by detecting either changing disparities, or change in size, or mirror movements of the images of an advancing object in the two hemifields. It is of great significance that the main efferent projections of these movement-sensitive areas are to motor structures such as premotor cortex, basal ganglia and cerebellum. Since perhaps 70% of our movements are triggered or guided by vision this is not surprising. One might at first think that the motor cortex would be an obvious place for such projections, but it is far down the hierarchy of motor areas (for some neurones it is only one synapse away from the muscles themselves). The motor cortex has a detailed 'hard-wired' map of limb movements, whereas visual information about movements might be needed any-where, by eyes, head, trunk, hands or legs; thus it enters the system at an earlier stage, via premotor cortex, cerebellum or basal ganglia.

Flicker fusion

The Y ganglion cells enable the retina itself to follow light flashes as fast as 100 c.p.s. However, this ability is lost by the cortex, pre-sumably because of the convergence of X and Y systems at this level; so the visual cortex, and hence the visual system as a whole, cannot follow white light flashes faster than 30 c.p.s. and follows coloured flashes only much more slowly.

Cortical analysis of movement

Posterior parietal lobe (area 7)

Hyvarinen and Mountcastle have produced evidence that a further stage of this visuomotor transformation takes place in area 7. Neurones here again have very large, often bilateral, visual recep-tive fields, but the activity of cells is greatly enhanced when the animal attends to a visual stimulus in their receptive field, particularly if the animal is about to make a movement towards the stimulus. Indeed, many neurones in area 7 fail to respond to any but very powerful visual stimuli, unless the stimulus is going to be a target for an eye or limb movement. These neurones also receive input from area 5 concerning the current position of the limbs, which is provided by the motor and proprioceptive systems. Lesions in area 7 temporarily prevent an animal from making accurate eye or limb movements towards objects. Unfortunately, other pathways can very quickly assume this function, so that techniques for reversibly inactivating area 7, such as local cooling, which reduce the chance of other pathways taking over, reveal the normal actions of the posterior parietal lobe more convincingly.

These results all suggest that area 7 neurones are involved in associating visually defined information about the position and movement of objects with the position and movements of eyes and limbs, and in using this information to direct movements.

'SECOND' VISUAL SYSTEM

The importance of movement detection to animals is attested by the fact that there is a 'second' visual pathway, carrying mostly Y cell (movement) information, to the prestriate cortex via the superior colliculus and pulvinar of the thalamus.

Superior colliculus

Eye movements

Each superior colliculus contains a map of the contralateral visual hemifield, like the LGN, but receives almost exclusively from Y-type ganglion cells. Electrical stimulation of the superior colliculus causes the eyes to move in order to foveate the region of the visual world represented on the superior colliculus at the point stimulated. Of course, when the eyes have moved, the collicular point now represents retinotopically a different region of visual space; so if stimulation is continued, the eyes move again to refixate the new visual focus, and a staircase of rapid eye movements—*saccades*—ensues in an attempt to refixate the illusory object represented at the the stimulated site. Pathways to the extra-ocular muscles leave from the deeper layers of the superior colliculus, whilst visual input is delivered to the superficial layers. For the organization of normal eye movements, command signals, perhaps derived from the frontal or posterior parietal lobes, must switch the visual input through to the oculomotor system.

For objects outside the range of normal eye movements, head-turning may be necessary as well; so it is not surprising to find that the part of the superior colliculus which represents the periphery of the visual field (which eye movements alone cannot reach) gives rise to the *tectospinal tract,* which ends on and around neck moto-neurones. Thus, stimulation of the tract gives rise to head, as well as eye, movements.

Visual, auditory and body space

The deeper layers of the superior colliculus also contain maps of auditory and somaesthetic space, in register with the visual map. Of course, these representations can only correspond usefully when the eyes, head and body are all pointing straight forward, since visual space is defined by the position of the eyes, auditory space coordinates by the position of the head, and somaesthetic space by the direction of the body. Perhaps this is the reason why orientation of the head almost always follows eye movements; it may also be one reason why we always look towards the source of a sound even though we would maximize time and intensity differences, optimiz-ing correct localization, by directing one ear towards and the other away from it.

COLOUR ANALYSIS IN THE VISUAL SYSTEM

Further investigation of the Young–Helmholtz trichromatic theory of colour had to await technical advances in measuring light of different wavelengths—spectrophotometry—which enable the measurement of the *absorption spectra* of the pigments *in vitro* and *in vivo,* even in single cones (Fig. 6.15). A most important advance was the introduction of *retinal densitometry* by William Rushton. By shining known amounts of monochromatic light upon the retina and measuring the amount reflected, the quantity of light absorbed at any wavelength could be determined. Rushton first bleached the retina with different coloured lights of high intensity, and then measured the resultant absorption spectrum for the whole retina. Thus he was able to deduce, from the differences in the spectrum before and after bleaching at different wavelengths, the absorption spectrum of the three cone pigments; these are now called cyanolabe, erythrolabe and chlorolabe. These measurements cor-respond well with results obtained using single cones and extracted pigments studied *in vitro.*

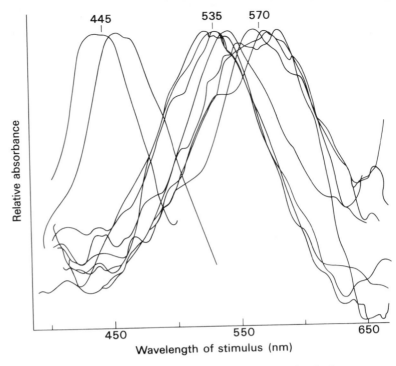

Fig. 6.15. The absorption of lights of different wavelengths by single cones.

Opponent colour coding

Though there is now abundant evidence that there are three different sorts of cones, there are many more types of bipolars, etc. Simple trichromatic coding is abandoned as soon as the signal passes from the receptors. As mentioned above, Hering championed a rival theory to that of Young and Helmholtz— opponent colour coding. Modern electrophysiological evidence has lent abundant support to Hering's ideas, for all stages of visual processing beyond the receptors themselves. The slow potential changes in colour-type horizontal cells result in depolarization in response to light at one end of the spectrum and hyperpolarization following exposure to light with a wavelength at the other end. The colour sensitivity of many bipolars is reversed in their antagonistic surrounds. These cells, therefore, combine sensitivity to the position of a stimulus within their receptive fields (by having an antagonistic surround) with sensitivity to its wavelength (opponent colour responses). Thus, they signal not only the rate of change of intensity with respect to position (dI/dx) but also change in wavelength as a function of position ($d\lambda/dx$). A proportion of ganglion cells also demonstrate combined spatial and opponent colour properties (red v. green, green v. blue and blue v. yellow). Their centres and surrounds usually have narrower spectral tuning than

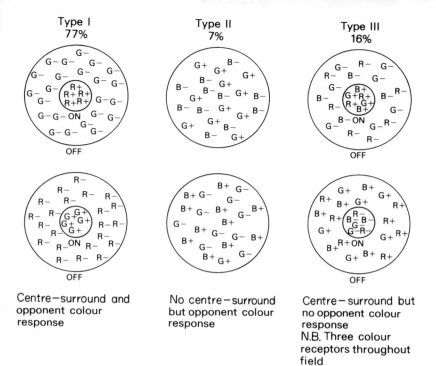

Fig. 6.16. Types of receptive field found in lateral geniculate nucleus (After Wiesel
T.N. & Hubel D.H. (1966) *J. Neurophysiol.*, **29**, 115).

cone pigments; this is presumably a consequence of the opponent
colour properties of the horizontal and bipolar cells which serve
them.

LGN

In the superficial X cell layers of the LGN, opponent colour coding
is even more prominent. Sharp colour tuning is shown by 85% of
neurones located there. De Vallois found that the degree of colour
resolution shown by these cells goes a long way towards explaining
human colour discrimination. He identified four main types of
opponent colour cells: red on/green off; green on/red off; yellow
on/blue off and blue on/yellow off. Hubel and Wiesel found, in
addition, blue on/green off and green on/blue off cells. They also
demonstrated that many cells combine opponent colour properties
with surround inhibitory spatial properties, for example, 'on'
responses to red light and 'off' responses to green light shone in
their centres, but 'off' responses to red and 'on' responses to green
in their surrounds (Fig. 6.16); this was the most common type but
most of the possible combinations of centre–surround and
opponent colour properties have been found.

Visual cortex

In the striate representation of the central 15° of the visual field, opponent colour coding is found in some 30% of the orientation-selective simple, complex and hypercomplex cells, as befits this area which is specialized for contour detection and the early stages of pattern recognition. These colour-coded cells are presumably the ones which project onwards to visual area 4 in the depths of the superior temporal sulcus. Zeki found that every cell in this area is highly colour-specific, and that cells responding to the same colour are organized in columns, as we have come to expect.

CONCLUSIONS

In the visual system none of the four basic characteristics of a stimulus (intensity, locus, colour and timing) is signalled individually. The properties of retinal neurones ensure that signalling of discontinuities in the visual environment with respect to space and time receive most attention. The rates of change of intensity and colour with respect to time and position are selectively detected and enhanced by operations such as lateral inhibition and opponent colour responses. In the visual cortex, important properties of the stimulus are simultaneously abstracted by specialized analysing units operating in parallel. The outputs of these cortical regions are consistent with their specialized processing roles. Areas 17, 18 and 19 project pattern information to inferotemporal cortex, which we know is concerned with aspects of visual memory and pattern recognition and feeds the limbic system; whilst area 18, the superior temporal sulcus and area 7 project movement information to the cerebellum, basal ganglia and motor cortex.

Chapter 7
Auditory System

Fundamental differences between hearing and vision follow from the differences between sound and light. Sound is carried by longitudinal waves (vibrating in the same direction as they propagate) which cause a series of compressions and rarefactions of the atmosphere (Fig. 7.1). Because of the long wavelength of these waves, any obstruction can serve as a secondary (reduced) source of the wave (cf. diffraction of light waves), so that they can, in effect, travel round corners. Also, dense materials reflect most of the sound reaching them (cf. the absorption of many of the wavelengths in white light by coloured objects). The kinetic energy of sound waves enables the ear to use a mechanical transducer. However, the ease with which sound waves can be bent and reflected by objects in the environment means that the direction of sound waves entering the ear is a very poor guide to the location of their source. Hence, there is no advantage in having the mechanoreceptors of the ear laid out, like the retina, in topographical correspondence to spatial relationships in the outside world in order to represent auditory space in the CNS. Instead, the disposition of cochlear *hair cells*, the ear's sound transducers, serves a different purpose, to code the frequency components of a sound, namely its tone, pitch and timbre or quality.

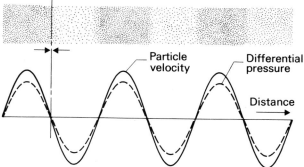

Particle velocity

Differential pressure

Distance

Fig. 7.1. Longitudinal sound waves carried by compressions and rarefactions of air molecules.

In the visual system three different types of receptor are used to signal the different wavelengths (or frequencies) of light, but in the auditory system only one type of receptor, the hair cell, is necessary; different frequencies are signalled by the location on the cochlear

115

basilar membrane of the hair cell at which the sound causes maximum vibration. This is known as the 'place' theory of frequency discrimination.

The location of a source of sound is reconstructed by integrating signals from the two ears, rather in the same way as depth is reconstructed binocularly by the visual system. The direction of an object in relation to the observer is calculated by making use of interaural differences of amplitude or timing—these vary according to the angle from which the sound is coming. Our preliminary consideration of the psychophysics of hearing must deal with the four fundamental characteristics of all sensory stimuli—intensity, quality, timing and location—bearing in mind that the auditory system differs from vision in two important ways: the frequency of sounds, rather than auditory space, is mapped in the central auditory pathways (*tonotopic* mapping); and the auditory system makes use of only one type of receptor.

AUDITORY PSYCHOPHYSICS

Intensity

As with the visual system, our ability to measure the intensity of sound is rather poor, though the range of intensities over which we can hear is enormous. Our subjective estimates of the loudness of a sound differ from measurements of its true physical intensity because sense of loudness, like brightness, varies with the logarithm of sound pressure changes, rather than linearly. The absolute threshold for hearing a tone of about 2000 Hz (where our hearing is best) is an air pressure change of only 2×10^{-4} dynes mm^{-2}. Since subjective loudness increases as the log of changes in air pressure, sound levels are measured in log units, called bels after A.G. Bell the inventor of the telephone and gramophone (and founder of I.T.T.). One decibel is $10 \times \log$ (sound power/threshold) $= 20 \times \log$ (sound amplitude/threshold). The maximum sound intensity that can be withstood for short periods without physical damage to the cochlea is 130 decibels—about 100 dynes mm^{-2}. The ear has a very wide 'dynamic range' and the smallest increment of sound intensity which can be appreciated as an increase in loudness is about 0.1 decibel.

Frequency

The quality of a sound is determined by its frequency components. Musical tones have components which are all harmonics (i.e. integral multiples) of the fundamental frequency of the note, whilst everyday noises, speech sounds, etc. have less orderly frequency spectra. It is easiest to measure the ear's frequency range and resolution using pure tones, but this can sometimes give misleading results when applied to natural sounds such as speech.

The range of frequencies which the human ear can hear is from about 40 Hz to 1500 Hz, though sounds of lower frequency can actually be felt as vibrations, particularly by Pacinian corpuscles in the abdomen. Cats are said to be able to feel the thud of the tiny feet of a passing mouse with their tummies, such is the sensitivity and number of Pacinian corpuscles in their abdomen. Children and many animals can hear frequencies much higher than adults. Dogs can hear frequencies up to 50 000 Hz, an ability of which Francis Galton made celebrated use in the soundless but effective dog whistle that he fitted into his walking stick, much to the amazement of his contemporaries. Some bats emit ultrasonic squeaks containing frequencies higher than 100 000 Hz. These bounce off obstructions in their environment and insect prey; bats detect the reflected waves and use them for navigation and hunting. Australian oil birds also live in pitch darkness at the backs of caves. The clicks which they emit for navigation are audible to humans.

A very few fortunate individuals possess 'absolute pitch'—they can determine the absolute frequency of a tone. Only completely 'tone-deaf' people fail to be able to discriminate whether one note is the same as another. Interestingly enough, even tone-deaf people are as good as those with absolute pitch at detecting the complex frequency variations which make up everyday speech. Everybody is therefore capable of detecting *changes* in frequency. At best (around 1500 Hz) a change of only 0.1% in frequency (i.e. a difference of only 1–2 cycles per second) can be detected by humans. However even this degree of frequency discrimination does not approach the acuity of spatial resolution of which the visual system is capable. Above 5 kHz frequency discrimination becomes ten to twenty times worse, probably because the auditory system then has to rely entirely upon detecting the place in the basilar membrane which is maximally activated, without any help from 'phase locking'. At these frequencies, discharge of auditory nerve fibres in phase with a sound stimulus disappears completely.

Audiometry

A standard clinical method for recording the performance of the auditory system in humans is to measure a subject's threshold for hearing pure-tone frequencies in the normal audible range—pure-tone audiometry (Fig. 7.2). The common disorders of hearing leave tell-tale imprints on the audiometry curve. Presbycusis, the cochlear degeneration of old age, affects the upper frequencies first, whilst middle-ear sclerosis (otosclerosis), which causes 'conduction' deafness, affects the lower frequencies first. However, more subtle deficiencies of hearing are often not detected by pure-tone audiometry. Comprehension of speech, for instance, depends upon recognizing different patterns in a sound: its frequency content, the relative amplitudes of different frequencies and, perhaps most important of all, changes of frequency and amplitude with time. Measurements of these are very difficult to standardize, but techniques for 'speech audiometry' are being developed and will probably contribute greatly to the diagnosis and treatment of disorders of hearing and speech.

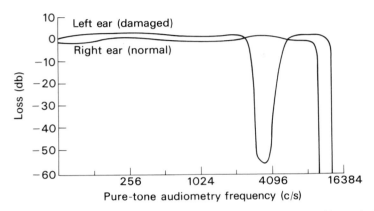

Fig. 7.2. Sensitivity of the ear to pure tones. Left cochlea damaged by explosion.

Timing

It takes a relatively long time to identify even a simple sound. About 200 ms is required to identify a pure tone. Presumably, this is the time required by the CNS to determine which cochlear hair cells are being stimulated most strongly and to detect their phase locking. Thus discrete tone bursts delivered faster than five times per second are heard not as distinct pips, but as a continuous tone with a 'vibrato' or apparent 'frequency modulation' (FM) at 5 s^{-1}. Frequency modulations are changes in frequency with respect to time; the rate at which these changes occur can itself be expressed as a frequency—the modulation frequency. Above a modulation frequency of 5 c.p.s. (i.e. an increase and then a decrease of frequency from the initial 'carrier' level occurring five times per second (Fig. 7.3)) we do not clearly perceive the rise and fall of the tone. Instead we experience a distinct auditory sensation, vibrato, which is not mimicked by simultaneously sounding all the frequencies swept through during the modulation. Thus there is something about the rate at which sound frequencies change which is itself detected, and which presumably therefore carries information of importance to us. Advantage is taken of our enhanced perception of frequency-modulated tones in police sirens (FM *c.* 2 Hz), which have a peculiarly nasty quality, and referees' whistles (FM 20 Hz), which sound shrill and authoritative.

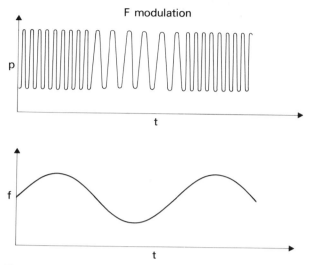

Fig. 7.3. Frequency modulation—sinusoidal increase and decrease in frequency of sound.

FM channels

What has been said so far about FM detection by the auditory system suggests that we possess neuronal mechanisms capable of detecting changes of frequency and perhaps specific 'channels' for analysing the rate of change of frequency. The existence of the former have been confirmed by neuronal recordings made from experimental animals. The latter, FM channels, have recently been demonstrated psychophysically by Kay, using the technique of selective adaptation which we encountered in the analysis of spatial frequency channels in the visual system. If a loud, 'adapting', frequency-modulated tone is delivered to a subject for a few minutes and then his sensitivity for detecting softer frequency-modulated tones is measured, it is found that the threshold for hearing frequency modulations at the rate of the adapting tone is very much raised, whilst that for detecting modulations at different rates remains unaffected. Fatigue of the channels analysing the rate of frequency change chosen for adaptation presumably desensitizes the subject's system for detecting audio-frequency changes of that rate, even if the carrier frequencies around which the modulation takes place are different. Thus these FM channels do not merely detect the change from one frequency to another, but are truly sensitive to the rate of change of frequency, independently of the frequency range employed.

The neurones responsible for this feat are analogous to the complex cells of the visual cortex, in that they respond not to the absolute position in the cochlea of the receptors stimulated, but to a higher-order consequence of the stimulation of a whole array of receptors. In the case of the complex visual cell, this is the orientation of a bar or edge over a wide area of visual space. In the case of the auditory system, the important characteristic seems to be the rate of change of frequency—the speed with which pitch changes—and not the absolute pitch. Such neurones have yet to be completely characterized in the auditory cortex of animals.

Position

Our ability to detect the source of a sound depends on both monaural and binaural cues. Monaural aids include the estimation of the amplitude of a sound at the ear and, knowing its likely amplitude at source, calculating its distance by the attenuation. Some animals are able to move their ears to maximize the loudness of a sound by pointing them towards its source. We also monitor the filtration, distortions and colourations introduced by the pinna, since these are greater for sounds coming from behind than from in front.

Binaural reconstruction of the position of a sound source is more reliable. It involves measuring either intensity difference between the two ears, as the head acts as an effective attenuator at high frequencies, or for frequencies below 1500 Hz, estimating the time difference between the arrival at the two ears of air compressions (Fig. 7.4a). As the ears, like the eyes, are horizontally separated, a sound from the left will reach the left ear (at t_L) slightly before the right, $t_R = t_L + t_H$. This information can be used in two ways. For clicks, tone bursts, etc, the onset time difference between the two ears (t_H) gives the horizontal angular direction of the sound. For continuous tones the time interval between the arrival of successive compressions at the two ears can be used to indicate their direction (Fig. 7.4b). In electronic engineering the timing of the peaks and troughs of one wave with respect to another of the same frequency is expressed as a proportion of its period (and termed the 'phase' angle). It has been shown that for low frequencies the auditory system can make use of such phase differences for locating sound. Humans are able to interpret phase differences corresponding to time intervals between the two ears of only about 25 μs, and can thus determine the source of low-frequency sounds to within 5° or so. The head does not attenuate low frequencies significantly because the wavelength is too long. Nevertheless, quite large phase differences have very little effect on what a tone actually sounds like, so phase information is used almost exclusively to determine the source of a sound and not for any other perceptual function.

(a)

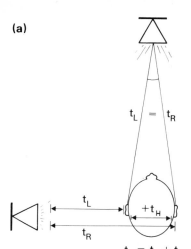

(b)

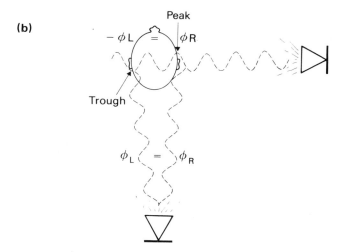

Fig. 7.4. (a) Onset tone difference. The click reaches the left ear before the right. The difference (t_H) helps to indicate the origin of the sound. (b) Phase difference. A peak reaches the right ear when a trough reaches the left ear. The phase difference between the two ears helps to locate the source.

PERIPHERAL AUDITORY APPARATUS

Impedance matching

External ear

The external ear is shaped in such a way that it funnels air towards the *tympanic membrane,* and the pinna acts as a filter and colourer of sounds coming from behind the animal. Ultimately, sound waves are used by the auditory system to vibrate hair cells floating in aqueous endolymph within the bony labyrinth. The compressions and rarefactions of the air involve the movement of large numbers of air molecules, but have little force. However water, being much heavier than air, has high inertia and needs higher forces to make it vibrate. Of the energy of sound waves arriving at a simple air/water interface, 90% is reflected. The main function of the outer and middle ears is therefore to transform the large-amplitude, low-energy movements of air molecules into smaller-amplitude, but more powerful, displacements of the faceplate of the stapes at the oval window, with a force sufficient to get the endolymph of the cochlea moving (Fig. 7.5). This is called 'impedance matching' in acoustics. The outer ear begins this process by funnelling air towards the tympanic membrane (Fig. 7.5a).

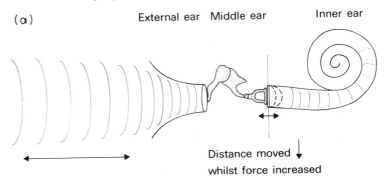

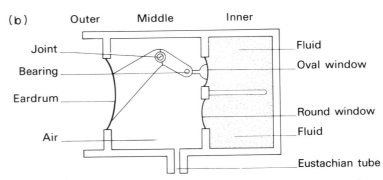

Fig. 7.5. (a) Air funnels into the external ear. The eardrum (tympanic membrane) is 16 times larger than the oval window and the mechanical advantage of the ossicles is 1.3:1. Hence acoustic movement of large quantities of air is reduced to a small movement of the stapes with much greater force. (b) Schematic structure of ear.

Middle ear

The tympanic membrane is set in motion by the movements of the air in the auditory canal. Its vibrations are transferred to the oval window by a series of small bones in the middle ear, the *ossicles,* known as the malleus, incus and stapes. These provide a small mechanical advantage between tympanic membrane and oval window (about 1.3:1). Most of the increase in force at the expense of distance moved is achieved by the difference in the area of the tympanic membrane and the oval window (about 16:1). By these means, up to 95% of sound energy incident at the external ear is utilized to vibrate the endolymph and hence the basilar membrane in the inner ear.

Middle-ear muscles

The ossicles of the middle ear are provided with two muscles, heavily endowed with length receptors (muscle spindles), the stapedius and the tensor tympani muscles. These are under auditory control and their actions can be assessed in humans by measuring the 'acoustic impedance' (mechanical resistance at different sound frequencies) of the middle ear, under various conditions. The muscles enable the middle ear to act as a mechanical filter with alterable properties, particularly for attenuating responses to a person's own voice which would otherwise sound very loud being so close, and also for enhancing speech comprehension. Much of the information contained in speech is carried by consonants which have characteristic frequencies above 2000 Hz. The tympanic membrane has two parts: the pars flaccida, which is most easily vibrated by low sound frequencies, and the pars tensa, which responds best at higher frequencies. The tensor tympani is attached to the handle of the malleus where it is bound to the centre of the tympanic membrane. When it is slack, the malleus transmits both high and low frequencies equally well, but when the tensor tympani is activated, the pars flaccida is tensed and low frequencies are attenuated, thus relatively enhancing higher frequencies. The stapedius probably acts similarly at the other end of the ossicular chain.

The tensor tympani and stapedius are usually described as having only a protective function—limiting the amount of vibration to which the cochlea is subjected during very loud sounds. However, the fact that they can only respond some time after a loud sound would already have begun to damage hair cells makes it seem more likely that their main function is to filter out low frequencies. Very little is known about how the mechanism operates or what activates it, but it may be a partial explanation for the 'cocktail party phenomenon'. When listening to someone's conversation at a convivial cocktail party one can usually make out what is being said amidst the hubbub of surrounding conversations; yet if one listens to a tape recording of the same conversation one can seldom make anything out at all. During the cocktail party, all one's capacities for selective auditory attention, including the middle ear muscles, have been tuned to the particular frequency characteristics of the voice one is listening to. Later, listening to the tape recorder, it is much more difficult to select out the qualities of a particular voice amidst the hubbub.

Cochlea

The inner ear or cochlear duct contains three fluid-filled sacs wound into three and a half turns of the petrous temporal bone. These transmit vibrations delivered at the ferestra ovale (oval window) by the foot-plate of the stapes to transducer hair cells sitting on the basilar membrane in the Organ of Corti (Fig. 7.6). Vibrations at the foramen ovale are transferred to the perilymph in the scala vestibuli and across the scala media and basilar membrane to the scala tympani and the round window, which opens back into the middle ear. The wave travelling up the cochlea is affected by reflections from the walls of the bony labyrinth and by waves travelling back down from the top. The resultant complex vibration of the basilar membrane is further modified by the fact that it is narrower and a hundred times stiffer at the base than at the apex.

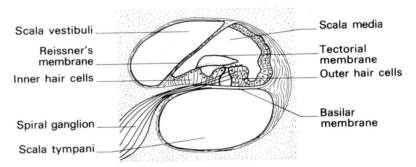

Fig. 7.6. Cross-section through cochlea.

Place theory

Von Bekesy examined the cochlea of the guinea pig (which can be more easily exposed than that of most other animals) and employed stroboscopic light of the same frequency as that of sound stimuli he used in order to observe the vibrating basilar membrane. He found that the end result of these interacting influences is that the whole basilar membrane vibrates at very low frequencies, but only the basal turn responds at high frequencies (Fig. 7.7). As the frequency of sound is reduced, the point at which the basilar membrane vibrates with greatest amplitude advances along the cochlea. If the amplitude of the tone is increased, the excursions of the basilar membrane become larger but the point of maximum movement remains in the same place. That is why this theory of frequency discrimination by the basilar membrane is known as the 'place' theory.

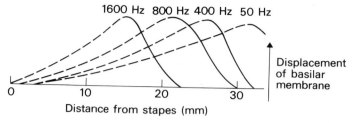

Fig. 7.7. High frequencies vibrate only the basal turn of the basilar membrane, whilst low frequencies vibrate the whole basilar membrane.

Volley theory

An alternative explanation, put forward by Rutherford, was that the frequency of a sound is signalled by the frequency of impulses in the auditory nerve and the basilar membrane itself does not respond differently to different frequencies at all. This simple theory had to be abandoned when it became clear that auditory nerve fibres could never discharge at higher than 1000 impulses per second. It was then suggested that individual fibres might respond to every fifth wave, for example, so that five fibres, each delayed by one wave with respect to the next, could signal a sound frequency of 5000 Hz. This is known as the 'volley' theory. There is evidence that sound frequencies below 5 kHz are signalled in this way, as well as by detection of the part of the basilar membrane which is caused to vibrate most strongly. Impulses in auditory nerve fibres do discharge in phase with sound pressure changes; even at low frequencies discharge is probabilistic, occurring randomly every one, two, three or four cycles (Fig. 7.8). This is, of course, essential for phase-encoded location of sound sources.

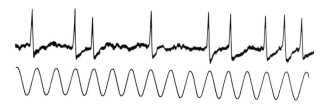

Fig. 7.8. Probabilistic phase locking of impulses in VIIIth nerve fibre on every first second, third or fourth peak of the sound wave.

Resonator theory

Another suggestion was that cochlear hair cells are actually tuned much better than is required by the place theory, each hair cell resonating only at one frequency. This 'resonator' theory was favoured by Helmholtz, who was convinced that different auditory frequencies were somehow laid out topographically along the basilar membrane by the evidence of 'boiler-maker's disease'. Boilermakers spend their lives in a very, very noisy environment—inside steel drums. Their ears are therefore subjected to loud sounds over a limited range of frequencies, defined by the material and size of the boilers. They lose their hearing selectively at these frequencies; furthermore, when examined post-mortem, only a small region of their basilar membrane is found to be damaged. This does not necessarily mean, as Helmholtz thought, that only the damaged portion vibrates at the frequency of the boiler, but rather that this region experiences the most violent vibration (to an extent sufficient to cause damage) as suggested by the place theory. However, recent intracellular recordings from hair cells of the turtle cochlea suggest that they do, after all, behave to some extent like resonators better tuned than the basilar membrane, as Helmholtz believed.

Transduction

We now know something of how vibration in the basilar membrane is converted into electrical charge movements. On the basilar membrane stand some 4000 inner hair cells close to the spiral lamina and, further out, around 20 000 outer hair cells arranged in three or four rows. The hair cells are highly charged with respect to their immediate extracellular fluid environment—80 mV with respect to the endolymph contained in the scala media. Endolymph is a further 70 mV more negative than perilymph, so that the interior of hair cells is some -150 mV with respect to the under-surface of the basilar membrane on which they are supported. Bending of the hairs occurs when the basilar membrane vibrates, as they are embedded in the tectorial membrane above; this shifts a region at the top of the hair cell known as the 'cuticular plate' in relation to the basal body, perhaps exposing a pore through which Na^+ ions can leak to generate the receptor potential.

Cochlear microphonic

Summed receptor potentials, chiefly from the outer hair cells, can be recorded very easily as the *cochlear microphonic* (CM) potential. This gives a faithful electrical representation of whatever sound is played into the ear and its magnitude at any point along the basilar membane alters with frequency, in just the same way as the basilar membrane's own vibrations change; indeed the CM is a very convenient way of recording excursions of the basilar membrane.

Hence at high frequencies the potential is maximal at the base, and at low frequencies it is largest at the apex. Like the basilar membrane, the CM is poorly tuned, i.e. at any point on the basilar membrane a wide range of frequencies centred on a best frequency will elicit it.

This potential is easier to interpret than the electroretinogram, partly because the cochlea has far fewer neural elements than the retina (it has no interneurones at all), and partly because hair cells modulate synchronously with each vibration of the basilar membrane, whereas rods and cones respond asynchronously to continuous light. However, it is not at all clear how the receptor potential is communicated to the nerve fibres of the VIIIth (auditory) nerve. A chemical transmitter, thought by some to be acetylcholine, is probably involved, as the bases of the hair cells contain abundant vesicles.

Innervation of hair cells

The hair cells are arranged in inner and outer rows (Fig. 7.9). About ten cells in the outer row, representing ascending frequencies, are connected to each fibre of the spiral ganglion nerve as it courses from apical towards basal basilar membrane, but each inner hair cell is supplied by its own private VIIIth nerve fibre. Thus, although there are five times as many outer as inner hair cells, half as many nerve fibres serve them. Outer hair cells move a greater distance than inner hair cells as they are positioned further away from the anchorage point of the basilar membrane on the spiral lamina. Hence their frequency response, and that of the fibres leaving them,

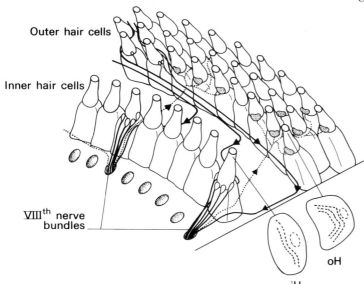

Fig. 7.9. Afferent and efferent innervation of hair cells together with pattern of hairs on inner and outer hair cells.

is probably not as well tuned as that of the inner hair cells. They probably indicate the general area of the basilar membrane which is vibrated and signal intensity of a sound; whilst the inner hair cells may differentiate more sensitively between adjacent frequencies.

Electromechanical tuning of hair cells

It is likely that hair cells are tuned better than the basilar membrane on which they rest. This is because each seems to behave as an electromechanical resonator with a high quality factor (Q). This extra tuning of individual hair cells then operates on the broad tuning of the basilar membrane to produce the sharper tuning curves found in VIIIth nerve fibres. The extra tuning cannot be attributed to synaptic interactions between neighbouring receptors (e.g. lateral inhibition) in the cochlea, as no synapses of the right sort have been seen and no electrophysiological evidence of their existence has been obtained.

Olivocochlear bundle

Although the amount of automatic peripheral processing of auditory information in the cochlea is limited in comparison to the retina, which has so many interneurones, unlike the mammalian retina the cochlea is placed under direct CNS control by a centrifugal pathway, the olivocochlear bundle. This arises in the superior olive, one of the important brain-stem nuclei involved in audition, and projects to both inner and outer hair cells. Many outer hair cells receive synapses from one centrifugal fibre as it courses from apical towards basal cochlea, in much the same way as from the corresponding afferent fibres of the VIIIth nerve; whilst a single olivocochlear fibre innervates each inner hair cell. These efferent fibres are probably inhibitory, employing GABA as their synaptic transmitter. Hence, stimulation of the whole bundle damps down discharge in the VIIIth nerve (Fig. 7.10), and stimulation of discrete regions of the superior olive may inhibit discrete regions of the Organ of Corti. Thus the olivocochlear bundle can be used by the CNS to change the overall level of transmission through the cochlea and also to adjust its response to selected frequencies. Like the middle-ear muscles, therefore, it can tune the frequency response of the peripheral auditory apparatus to enhance sound features of special interest.

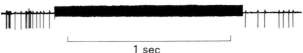

1 sec

Fig. 7.10. Inhibition of VIIIth nerve fibre discharge during stimulation (black artefact) of olivocochlear bundle.

Auditory nerve fibre tuning curves

The additional tuning of hair cells reveals itself in the *tuning curves* of individual auditory nerve fibres. A range of frequencies is tested and the amplitude of the sound at each frequency which is just sufficient to excite the fibre is recorded. A plot of this threshold against frequency (Fig. 7.11) gives the tuning curve. As would be expected from the fact that some VIIIth nerve fibres are primarily supplied by single inner hair cells and others by several outer nerve cells, some show much finer tuning than others. At high sound levels, however, the frequency spread of even the most finely tuned fibre is very much wider than the selectivity that the whole auditory system can achieve psychophysically.

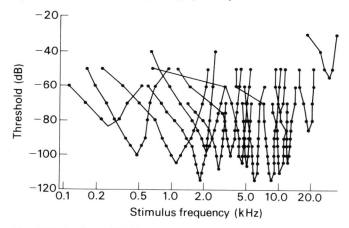

Fig. 7.11. Auditory (VIIth) nerve fibre tuning curves.

Two tone inhibition

This tonal acuity is accounted for by inhibitory processes in the central auditory pathways. Lateral inhibition is as important in the central auditory system as in any other sensation. It manifests itself psychophysically as 'two tone inhibition'. If you listen to two sounds whose frequencies are very close together, you hear waxing and waning of the amplitude of the lower tone at a frequency equal to the difference between the two, as in-phase and antiphase waves interact. These are known as 'beats'. More widely separated frequencies give rise to beats which, although they do not themselves constitute a frequency component of the original sound, nevertheless may be heard clearly as a separate tone ('the missing fundamental'). Beats contribute to the harmony of some chords and the disharmony of others. These are essentially physical phenomena. Physiologically, however, another process contributes to auditory perception. The response of a neurone to a particular tone is depressed when another tone of similar frequency is sounded at the same time—the phenomenon of two tone inhibition. In Fig. 7.12, a neurone in the cochlear nucleus is responding at its 'best' frequency of 5.3 kHz. At the point indicated by the arrow, a 4.5 kHz tone is sounded simultaneously. This powerfully inhibits the cell. Psychophysically, a similar phenomenon may be demonstrated. The detection of one tone is greatly reduced by simultaneously playing another tone close to it in frequency. These effects are the result of lateral inhibitory connections between frequency-sensitive neurones in the CNS. These are arranged as tone maps—'tonotopic' neural representations of sounds in the auditory centres of the brain-stem and cerebral cortex. Successive stages of lateral inhibition within the CNS can therefore enhance the slight differences in the firing of auditory nerve fibres between those stimulated at their optimum frequencies and their neighbours not so optimally stimulated. These processes progressively sharpen the tuning characteristics of neurones as the auditory system is ascended. As in the visual system, such mechanisms serve to identify peaks of activity in the array of fibres leaving the basilar membrane. It is presumably the detection of the pattern of these peaks together with the phase locking of individual fibres which underlies our eventual perception of the quality of a sound.

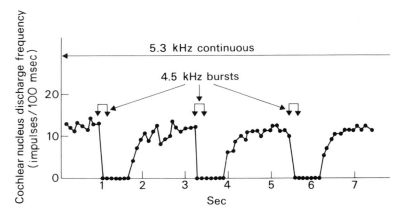

Fig. 7.12. Two tone inhibition.

Cochlear nucleus

Ventral division

The auditory nerve enters the ventral cochlear nucleus (Fig. 7.13), which is divided anatomically into anterior (VCNa) and posterior (VCNp) nuclei and a small interstitial region. Each axon bifurcates into an ascending and a descending branch, high-frequency fibres lying above low-frequency fibres. The descending branch passes on to the trilaminar dorsal cochlear nucleus (DCN). Representation of

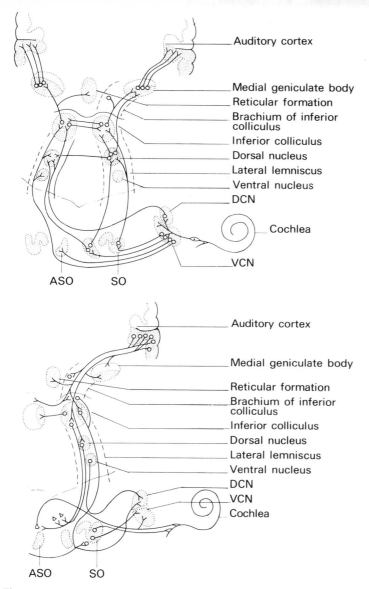

Fig. 7.13. Afferent (top) and efferent (bottom) connections of auditory systems.

pure tones within the three main divisions of the nucleus, VCNa, VCNp and DCN, is tonotopic, with high frequencies found dorsally and low frequencies ventrally (Fig. 7.14).

The anterior part of the ventral nucleus contains large and small spherical neurones which project chiefly to the superior olive, trapezoid body and central nucleus of the inferior colliculus. They respond to pure tone stimuli at an optimum frequency with an initial peak of activity followed by a gradual decline to a lower, sustained level (Fig. 7.15a). Auditory (VIIIth) nerve fibres similarly adapt slowly in this way; hence these responses are called primary-like.

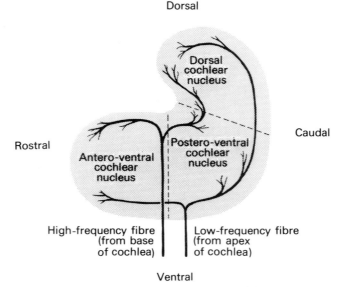

Fig. 7.14. Mapping of pure tones in cochlear nuclei.

However the tuning curves of VCNa neurones are sharper, and two tone inhibition is much more powerful than for VIIIth nerve fibres. The posterior part of VCN contains neurones known as octopus cells, from their striking appearance. They are *transient* cells, adapting rapidly to a maintained stimulus at their optimum frequency

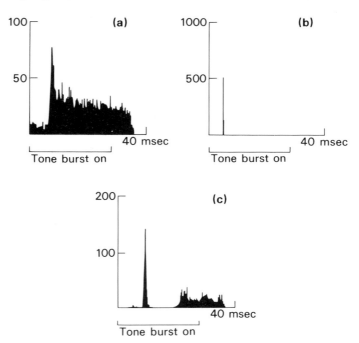

Fig. 7.15. (a) Primary-like response in ventral cochlear nucleus. (b) Transient cells. (c) 'Pauser' in dorsal cochlear nucleus.

and silencing after only a few milliseconds (Fig. 7.15b). Hence they probably signal the start of a sound rather than its frequency.

Dorsal cochlear nucleus

Patterns of discharge in the fusiform and giant cells found in the dorsal cochlear nucleus are even more complex. In some, rapidly adapting onset responses are followed by a pause and then return to a sustained level of discharge if the stimulus is continued. In others, bursts of impulses occur with a period equal to an integral multiple of the period of the frequency employed (Fig. 7.15c). Furthermore, in the DCN but not in the VCN, responses to sounds varying in frequency or amplitude with time are often complex. They cannot be predicted from the response to single tones. Frequency and amplitude modulations cause adaptation rates to be faster, inhibitory pauses to be longer, and tuning of the cell to become sharper; this is because time-dependent inhibitory processes are powerful here.

'Second' auditory system

The distinctly different properties of neurones in the dorsal as opposed to the ventral cochlear nucleus, together with their rather different projections, suggest two separate functions for these regions reminiscent of the 'first' and 'second' visual systems. The ventral cochlear nucleus projects via the superior olive, the central nucleus of the inferior colliculus and the ventral part of the medial geniculate nucleus to auditory area 1 in the superior temporal gyrus, forming a pathway primarily concerned with auditory perception; whilst the DCN projects via the nuclei of the lateral lemniscus, external nucleus of inferior colliculus and the dorsomedial divisions of medial geniculate to the secondary auditory cortex areas, and may be involved in focusing attention on auditory stimuli and in controlling movements in response to sound.

Superior olive

Fibres of the ventral cochlear nuclei project to the superior olivary complex via the trapezoid body. This again is made up of several nuclei, some of which exhibit tonotopic organization. The chief interest of this region is, however, that it is where binaural convergence onto single neurones first takes place. Neurones in the nucleus of the medial superior olive have two sets of dendrites (Fig. 7.16). The lateral of these receive inhibitory inputs from the ipsilateral cochlear nucleus, whilst the medial receive excitatory projections from the contralateral cochlear nucleus. This enables olivary cells to respond differentially to sound arriving at the two ears. The discharge rate of low-frequency neurones is influenced by interaural phase differences—the tiny difference between the time of arrival of compressions at the two ears. Each neurone has a characteristic preferred delay which means that it can respond selectively to sounds coming from a particular direction. Above about 1500 Hz such time differences become too small to be detectable, but the head begins to be more effective as a filter at higher frequencies. Hence high-frequency neurones in the superior olive are sensitive not to time differences but to intensity differences between the two ears. Thus they too give information about the direction of a sound source.

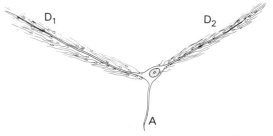

Fig. 7.16. Binaural neurones in medial superior olive.

Inferior colliculus

From the superior olive, fibres pass via the lateral lemniscus to the inferior colliculus, where some fibres synapse and others pass straight through to the medial geniculate nucleus. The inferior colliculus has three subdivisions: central (ICC), external (ICX) and pericentral (ICP) nuclei. The ICC is laminated and organized tonotopically, whereas the others are probably not. However, the responses of neurones in the ICC are more complex than at sites lower down the auditory system. Some neurones exhibit sharper tuning than encountered before, but their responses change if amplitude or frequency-modulated tones are used. In the ICX and ICP it is not possible to demonstrate tonotopic organization at all, because the cells do not possess pure-tone tuning curves of the sort we have so far discussed. They are much more sensitive to temporal features of a stimulus—frequency and amplitude modulations— and they habituate rapidly. Lesions in these areas lead to loss of selective attention in the auditory sphere. They are therefore probably part of the 'second' auditory system referred to earlier.

Medial geniculate

In the medial geniculate nucleus of the thalamus a similar division of function is discernable. The ventral MGN is laminated and contains characteristic *glomerular* synaptic complexes like those of the other two principal thalamic sensory relay nuclei [the lateral geniculate nucleus (for vision) and the ventroposterolateral nucleus (for somaesthesia)]. It is tonotopically organized; pure-tone tuning curves are sharp, with pronounced two tone and centrifugal inhibition. However, the dorsal and medial regions of the medial geniculate nucleus respond in a much more complex manner, having no clear pure-tone tuning, reacting more to the temporal characteristics of the stimulus and showing a pronounced tendency to respond less and less strongly to regularly repeated stimuli—habituation.

Auditory cortex

Tonotopicity

The primary projection area (A1) in the cortex is in the superior temporal gyrus. Layer 4 of A1 receives point-to-point projections from the laminated ventral part of medial geniculate nucleus and from contralateral A1 via the corpus callosum. Although the geniculate projection is orderly and topographic, it proved difficult to demonstrate a clear tonotopic arrangement of the best frequencies of neurones in A1. This is partly because the trigger features of the cells are more complex than can easily be summarized in a single index such as 'best frequency', partly because the anatomy of the superior temporal gyrus is so complicated but also because the responses are highly dependent on anaesthetic levels. However, it is now known that a detailed tonotopic map does exist in A1, although it is only clearly revealed under deep anaesthesia. All the cells in a cortical column show signs of having the same best frequency. In conscious animals, however, the underlying tonotopicity of A1 is almost completely submerged by its specialization for the analysis of more sophisticated aspects of sound than mere static frequency components.

Frequency modulation

As in the inferior colliculus and medial geniculate, neurones of the auditory cortex respond more to the temporal characteristics of a sound. They are specialized to respond to features such as rate of change of frequency or amplitude, the beginning or end of a tone burst, etc. They are often sensitive to particular directions and rates of frequency change, independently of the absolute frequency range chosen. Others change their response according to the previous history of the sound, discharging in response to low frequencies if the tone is ascending but more vigorously at high frequencies if the pitch is descending. In the auditory cortex of unanaesthetized animals the trigger features of most cells are so complicated that they often cannot be assessed using pure sine wave stimuli; frequency- or amplitude-modulated or natural sounds, such as vocalizations, must be employed. However, as yet no general classes of cells, such as the simple, complex and hypercomplex cells of the visual cortex, have been clearly discerned; although the columnar structure of auditory cortex is noticeable, columnar organization of trigger features is at present less apparent here than in the visual system.

Hierarchical organization

Some principles of hierarchical organization can nevertheless be borrowed from the visual cortex in order to speculate as to what types of cell we might expect to find in the auditory cortex, remembering that topographical organization in the auditory system represents sound frequency rather than external space; that the auditory transducer, the Organ of Corti, has only one type of receptor not four; and that the temporal order of sounds is relatively much more important to auditory perception than the temporal sequence of visual stimuli is for pattern recognition.

The auditory analogue of a visual simple cell is probably a neurone responding to a restricted range of frequencies (its basilar

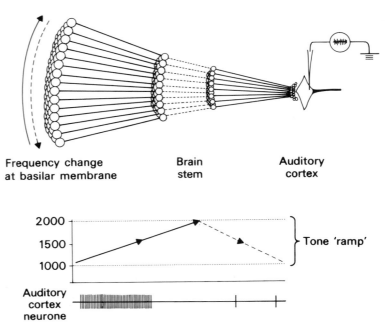

Fig. 7.17. 'Simple' A1 neurone responding to ascending frequency changes but not to descending frequencies.

membrane 'receptive field'). But because of the significance of the temporal sequence of sound frequencies, such a cell is likely to be most strongly excited by sweeping across its best frequencies in one direction (Fig. 7.17). Such neurones may then converge on 'complex' auditory cells tuned to respond best to changes in frequency at particular rates but responding equally well at their optimum modulation rate over a wide range of frequencies (this is the equivalent to the large receptive field of the visual complex cell). These would be able to detect particular frequency-modulation rates, as postulated by Kay.

Lesions

The results of making lesions in the auditory cortex support these speculations. Even if the auditory cortex is removed on both sides, an animal can continue to make pure-tone or simple amplitude discriminations reasonably well. However, animals trained to discriminate on the basis of the temporal order of tones (e.g. B-A-B versus A-B-A) lose this ability completely after auditory cortex lesions.

Similarly, the ability to respond to complex sounds depends on the integrity of auditory cortical areas. Lesions of the auditory cortex on one side cause very little deafness, owing to the multiplicity of connections between left and right auditory structures in the brain stem. However, the ability to respond to patterns of sound or to determine their direction may well be lost.

It appears probable that adjacent columns within strips having the same best frequency differ with regard to the strength of input from the two ears. It may be that a map of three-dimensional auditory space coexists in auditory cortex orthogonally with the tonotopic map. Although the initial stages of sound source localization take place at a very low level in the auditory system (superior olive), perhaps mediating very rapid orienting reflexes, accurate location depends on the integrity of auditory cortex, where amplitude and time differences between the two ears can presumably be more precisely analysed. Hence cortical lesions greatly disturb this function (which is more easily tested in animals than their responses to speech or vocalizations). Unilateral ablations of auditory cortex lead to severe mislocation of sound sources in the contralateral half of the auditory field.

Lesions of the auditory association area in the posterior part of the superior temporal gyrus on the speech dominant side (Wernicke's area) lead to a more complex deficit—sensory aphasia (see Chapter 23). Auditory perception remains sufficiently good to enable recognition of simple patterns of sound and a few words and even repeat them, but not to understand what words mean.

Auditory lateralization

Clearly, therefore, despite the large number of binaural interconnec-tions in the brain stem, a degree of lateralization in the auditory system is preserved to the level of the cortex. This is reflected in the advantage the right ear has over the left when they are in competition. This may be demonstrated in dichotic listening tests, where different verbal information is presented simultaneously to the two ears. The right ear's predominant projection is to the left (speech) hemisphere, so that its performance in such verbal tasks is superior.

Chapter 8
Cutaneous Sensations

PSYCHOPHYSICS

Modality specificity

Cutaneous sensations include touch, pressure and vibration (the mechanical senses of the skin) together with pain and temperature. These are collectively known as the *somaesthetic* senses. The use of just three words—touch, pressure and vibration—to describe the variety of mechanical stimuli we may experience through our skins is, of course, inadequate. Many other sensations, such as deep pressure, brushing of hairs and tickling, immediately come to mind. Are there necessarily different receptors for all of these? There is a plethora of histologically distinguishable receptors to choose from: eight in hairy skin and six in glabrous (non-hairy) skin. Many are named after the histologist who first described them: Merkel's discs, Krause's end bulbs, Ruffini organs, Pacinian corpuscles, hair follicle endings, Meissner's corpuscles, Golgi–Mazzoni corpuscles and Iggo's domes (a collection of Merkel's discs under thickened epidermis). Some of these are shown in Fig. 8.1. They are all thought to possess different properties; each submodality of human

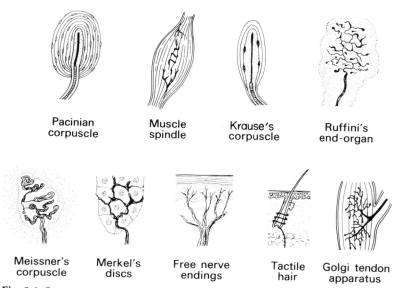

Fig. 8.1. Somaesthetic receptors.

somaesthesia was in the past enthusiastically assigned its own specific skin receptor.

In certain areas, for example the cornea, there are no specialized receptors but simply bare nerve endings, yet a wide range of sensations are perceived; and in others (e.g. the glans penis) a large range of different receptor specializations are found, yet only a few modalities register. Hairy skin has different receptors from glabrous skin, yet a similar range of skin sensations is experienced in both. The skin disease psoriasis can destroy all specialized receptor cells, yet cutaneous sensation is relatively unaffected. It is not surprising that it is in the field of cutaneous sensation that Muller's concept of modality specificity has received its hardest knocks.

Pattern theory

The alternative, 'pattern' theory proposed that differences amongst cutaneous receptors are largely histological artefacts; that in reality no receptor is modality specific. It was postulated that the CNS is able to interpret the overall spatial and temporal pattern of discharge in the array of sensory nerve fibres leaving the skin, and reconstruct all the characteristics of a stimulus from that pattern alone. Thus the difference between a cold penny pressed hard onto the skin and a warm penny pressed lightly would be signalled, not by the separate discharge of cold and deep pressure as opposed to warm and light touch receptors, but by the different ways in which non-specific, 'multimodal' receptors are stimulated in space and time by spread of heat and pressure through the skin. Leaving aside the assumption, implicit in this description, of the ability of such multimodal receptors to respond differently in some way to heat and to pressure (so that they could not strictly be called 'non-specific'), there is now abundant experimental evidence confirming that most skin receptors are more sensitive to one form of sensory energy than to others; i.e. they are modality specific. This is shown, for example, by the punctate distribution of warm and cold sensitive spots on the skin which indicate the site of specific thermoreceptors underneath. These can be mapped out easily using small hot and cold probes. Nevertheless, simple modality specificity cannot account entirely for the diversity of cutaneous sensations we experience. A less extreme version of the pattern theory is still necessary to help explain the myriad submodalities of skin sensation.

Intensity

The human sense of touch on fingers, face and lips is exquisite, particularly if exploratory movement of palpating surfaces is allowed. As usual, the system is much more sensitive to changes of skin or hair deformation than it is to steady states. A groove only one micron deep can be felt on a flat surface if the finger is allowed to move over it, and granulations even smaller than this are perceived as roughness if there is a flatter surface for comparison. However the finger cannot distinguish between smooth and much coarser sandpaper if the paper is gently placed on the skin and not moved. A single maintained prod by a fine probe will only be felt as a distinct touch at the moment of contact. However, if the prods are repeated at frequencies up to 20 c.p.s. they are felt as 'flutter', and above that frequency as vibration.

Transmission fidelity

The transmission of mechanical signals from skin receptors is remarkably faithful throughout the relays of the somaesthetic system, right up to the level of somaesthetic cortex. A proportional relationship between stimulus and response is determined by the properties of the receptors; thereafter transmission throughout the system is linear. Hence the proportional change in neural output which follows an increase in the intensity of a peripheral stimulus is the same wherever in the pathway to the cortex one chooses to examine it, though of course the absolute number of impulses varies from site to site.

What is even more remarkable is that a human subject's conscious perception of a change in stimulus magnitude (Fig. 8.2b) increases in a very similar way to that in which the discharges of monkey sensory neurones change exponentially following the same stimuli (Fig. 8.2a). Likewise, it has recently been shown that the neural threshold of rapidly adapting receptors on the fingers, recorded in conscious humans, is identical to the psychophysically determined threshold for detecting rapid prodding at that spot. This implies that none of the sensory relays or 'cognitive' processes which go into estimating the magnitude of a skin stimulus alter the basic quantitative relationship between stimulus and sensation which is determined at the level of the receptor. The scaling of a stimulus in terms of nerve impulses which takes place in the receptor is repeated faithfully all along the neuraxis.

A proportional relationship between stimulus magnitude and neural response is the rule for all sensory systems (see Chapter 5). The relationships shown in Fig. 8.2a were demonstrated in myelinated fibres innervating the glabrous skin on the fingers of primates. If the same type of experiment is performed on hairy skin, the relationship between stimulus and receptor response is again described by an exponential function with an exponent of about 0.5. On the hairy skin of the forearm also, the apparent magnitude of a

stimulus varies exponentially with its true intensity. Again,
thalamic neurones have been shown to code joint angle exponentially; they probably employ both joint receptor and muscle spindle
length signals to do this. The exponent of the equation relating
neural discharge to joint angle is approximately 0.5 and subjective
estimations of joint angle exhibit this same relationship.

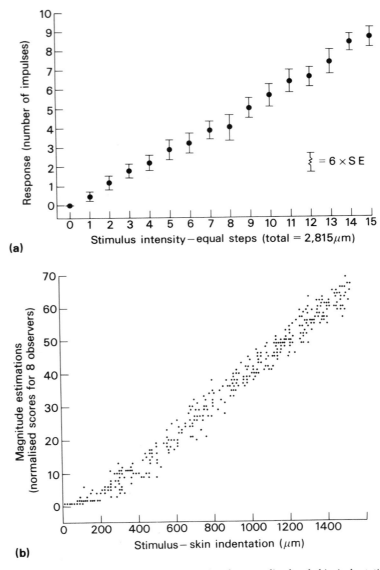

(a)

(b)

Fig. 8.2. (a) Receptor output is proportional to amplitude of skin indentation. (b)
Observer's estimation of amplitude of skin indentation shows a similar relationship.

Location

The spatial acuity of the skin varies with receptor density. It is most sensitive on the fingers and lips, and least sensitive on the back. Spatial resolution on the skin is measured clinically by the *two-point discrimination test*—determining the minimum separation of two points which can be perceived as distinct rather than as one larger one. Signalling of the location of a stimulus depends crucially upon topographic correspondence between points on the skin and a 'map' of the skin found in the postcentral region of the cerebral cortex; the resolving power of this system is enhanced markedly by lateral inhibition, as in other sensory pathways.

Temporal resolution

The study of the sensations of *flutter* and *vibration* are of special interest since they allow us to investigate the coding and signalling of temporal information by the somaesthetic system. Vibrations with frequencies ranging from one to 400 c.p.s. can be detected by humans, although their absolute frequency cannot easily be estimated. Nevertheless, very small *changes* in frequency can be perceived. Local anaesthesia of the surface of the skin raises the threshold for detecting frequencies below 30 Hz (flutter) but has no effect on that for higher frequencies (vibration), implying that a different set of receptors, deeper in the skin, is responsible for the latter. In fact the peak sensitivity of rapidly adapting mechanoreceptors in the skin lies at about 30 Hz, whereas that for Pacinian corpuscles lying in the deeper structures of the arm is closer to 400 Hz.

The fact that a frequency of 400 Hz (which is equivalent to an interval between impressions of only 2.5 ms) can be detected at all means that the somaesthetic pathway receiving from Pacinian corpuscles is capable of signalling at that rate with very high fidelity. When it is remembered that the delay at each synapse is about 0.5 ms, that this varies randomly by up to 0.25 ms, and that there are at least three synapses *en route* to the somaesthetic cortex, then this feat is seen to be even more remarkable.

SKIN RECEPTORS

Mechanoreceptors

Skin, subcutaneous and deep tissues all contain three basic types of receptor: free nerve endings, which are terminals of small $A\delta$ and C afferent fibres; endings with expanded tips which are usually slowly adapting and supplied by $A\beta$ fibres (Ruffini's endings and Merkel's discs); and encapsulated endings (Meissner's corpuscles, Krause's end bulbs and Pacinian corpuscles) which are supplied by large $A\alpha$ fibres.

Glabrous skin

In glabrous skin, free nerve endings extend through to the epidermis, while Merkel's discs (slowly adapting) and Krause's end bulbs (rapidly adapting) cluster around sweat ducts which pass through the intermediate ridges of the dermis. Lying between these, within the dermal papillae, are Meissner's corpuscles. Deep in the dermis are found Pacinian corpuscles, similar in structure to Meissner's. Both adapt very rapidly. The significance of the association of skin receptors with sweat ducts is probably that sweat released from the papillary ridges on the surface of the skin causes

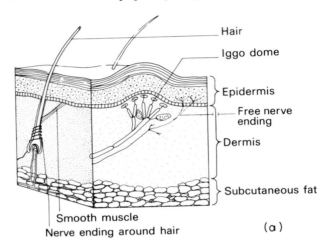

Hair
Iggo dome
Epidermis
Free nerve ending
Dermis
Subcutaneous fat
Smooth muscle
Nerve ending around hair

(a)

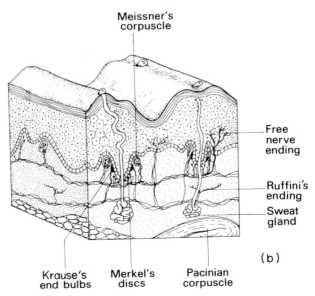

Meissner's corpuscle
Free nerve ending
Ruffini's ending
Sweat gland
Krause's end bulbs
Merkel's discs
Pacinian corpuscle

(b)

Fig. 8.3. (a) Receptors in hairy skin. (b) Receptors in glabrous skin.

the receptors to stick slightly to the palpating surface (Fig. 8.3b) and thus bends the ridge in the plane of movement. This deformation is transmitted to Merkel's and Krause's receptors beneath, and also compresses Meissner's corpuscles lying between the ridges.

Cutaneous
Sensations

Hairy skin

Hairy skin contains eight types of mechanically sensitive nerve endings, many of whose characteristics have now been established. Hairs are of two types: long guard hairs, which may act as distance receptors (particularly the very long vibrissae of rodents), and down hairs, which are the very short hairs close to the skin. The following receptors are found in hairy skin: primary (G1), secondary (G2) and intermediate guard hair receptors; down hair receptors; primary, intermediate and secondary field (F) receptors, which are situated in the skin between hairs; and bare nerve endings.

Type I and II endings

The designations 'primary' (type I) and 'secondary' (type II) were chosen by analogy with muscle spindle primary and secondary endings (Chapter 14). Primary spindle endings have high velocity sensitivity but little static sensitivity and are rapidly adapting, whilst secondary endings are mainly static and slowly adapting. In the skin, the distinction between primary and secondary endings is not quite so clear. Nevertheless, type I receptors are rapidly adapting, and hence show greater sensitivity to the rate of change (velocity) of stimulation, and type II are slowly adapting having a better response to absolute (static) level of a stimulus. Like muscle spindle endings, primary and secondary skin receptors are supplied by different-sized nerve fibres ($A\alpha$ and $A\beta$ respectively) but they receive no specialized γ-efferent control fibres.

In general, the discharge of type I fibres is more irregular than that of type II, probably a consequence of their greater sensitivity to rapid changes and their shorter refractory period. This means that their discharge must be analysed over a longish period to obtain a precise estimate of velocity. Type I receptors tend to discharge when a stimulus is removed, as well as when it is applied. They show little evidence of *directional selectivity* unlike type II fibres, which respond more strongly to one direction of movement or stretch of the skin than to others.

D receptors are supplied by $A\delta$ fibres. They respond to movement of down hairs, and to some extent to movement of guard hairs as well. They are sensitive to both rapid and slow displacements of these hairs, and also to their final position.

C fibre bare nerve ending mechanoreceptors are not sensitive to high rates of displacement at all, giving mainly static responses and fatiguing rapidly. A large proportion respond only at high levels of stimulation (high-threshold mechanoreceptive fibres) and will be considered in greater detail in the chapter on pain.

Thermoreceptors

Thermoreceptors (warm and cold receptors) respond to small changes (*c.* 0.1°C) in temperature, from a 'neutral' range around 30°C, with an increase in firing. In addition some mechano-receptors, especially those with static-position sensitivities (type II), respond with an increased discharge following cooling of their sur-roundings by 5°C or more, and with a temporary inhibition of discharge following warming by 5°C. These receptors are therefore not entirely modality specific. It may be, however, that this temperature response is actually the result of mechanical changes brought about by the variations in blood flow which thermal changes induce.

Warm receptors are predominantly supplied by unmyelinated C fibres. They show a phasic response to temperature changes up to about 35°C, only increasing their discharge during the rise in temperature and reverting to baseline firing levels if skin tempera-ture is maintained at the higher level. Thus, up to 35°C they respond to the rate of change of temperature and not to its absolute level, but above 35°C they also signal current (static) temperature up to about 45°C. Above 45°C their responses plateau at a high firing frequency of around 100 p.p.s. (Fig. 8.4). Their rate sensitivity is said to be 'unidirectional' because they respond to an increase in temperature with an increment of firing, but following a decrease in temperature they are temporarily silenced, so they give no information about the rate of temperature fall.

Cold receptors are supplied by small myelinated Aδ fibres. Their

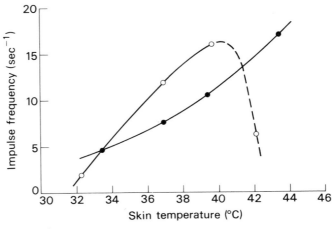

Fig. 8.4. Two types of steady-state response of warm receptors.

tonic discharge is a function of static ambient temperature over the range 15–35°C and they exhibit a bell-shaped response curve, peaking with a fairly low discharge frequency at about 25°C. Cold receptors too show unidirectional rate sensitivity in the cold direction (Fig. 8.5). A drop in temperature from 35°C to 25°C causes an increase in their rate of discharge, the initial increment depending on the rate of temperature decrease, whilst an increase in temperature temporarily silences them. Below their peak firing frequency at 25°C, their discharge only increases when the temperature is lowered, and then reverts to a lower, tonic level proportional to the new temperature. Thus they may signal temperatures above and below 25°C with the same tonic discharge frequency; this ambiguity can only be resolved by noting the differences in their pattern of discharge above and below this temperature. Above 45°C, some cold receptors give a 'paradoxical cold' response, increasing their discharge inappropriately. This may account for the sudden chill one unaccountably experiences on stepping into a very hot bath, and for the difference between warm and hot, the former comfortable, the latter threatening pain.

SOMAESTHETIC PATHWAYS (Fig. 8.6)

In the visual and auditory systems a second pathway to the cortex has only been described in recent years, but in the somaesthetic

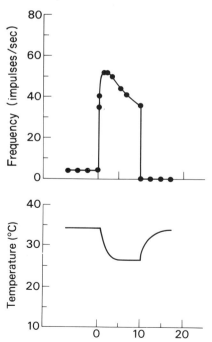

Fig. 8.5. Transient response of a cold receptor showing unidirectional sensitivity to decrease in temperature.

system separate *spinothalamic* and *lemniscal* projections have been clearly recognized for many years. The phylogenetically oldest pathway is the spinothalamic tract, which is itself commonly divided into *arch-, paleo-* and *neospinothalamic* divisions. These carry sensations of pain and temperature, together with some

Fig. 8.6. Somaesthetic pathways.

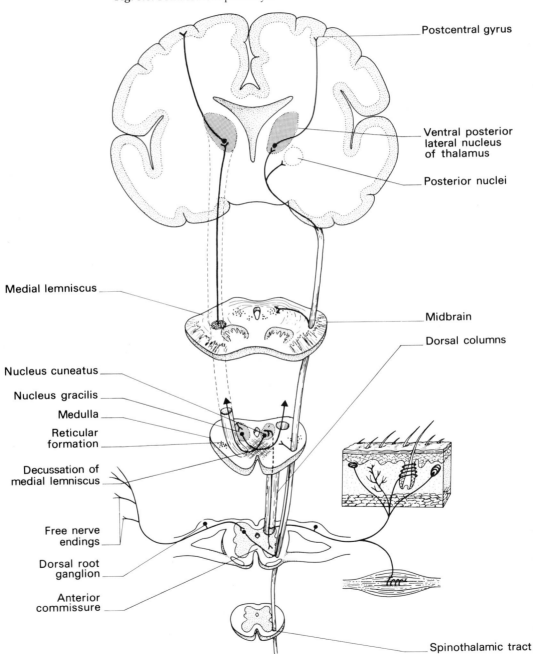

mechanoreceptor information. The extent to which this information is detailed and localizable has been the source of great controversy. Superimposed upon the spinothalamic system are the more recently evolved *spinocervical* and *dorsal column* systems, the former entirely cutaneous, the latter carrying localized touch, deep pressure, vibration and position senses.

Dorsal column system

The dorsal column system takes its name from the thick bundles of myelinated nerve fibres which travel in the dorsal part of the spinal cord. These are, in fact, the central branches of the axons of neurones whose cell bodies lie in the dorsal root ganglia. Their peripheral branches constitute the large myelinated (Aα and Aβ) axons which supply many of the receptors in the skin discussed above. In a tall man these axons may be as long as two metres, in continuity from the toes to the dorsal column nuclei, and are the longest nerve fibres in the body. They enter the spinal cord in the medial division of the dorsal root; the main axon passes into the dorsal column on the ipsilateral side after giving off collaterals which pass into the dorsal horn of the spinal grey matter (serving spinal reflexes among other functions). Fibres from the legs enter the cord first and therefore travel in the most medial part of the dorsal column, the gracile funiculus. Those from the arm arrive later, and hence travel in the lateral part of the dorsal columns, the fasciculus cuneatus (this must not be confused with the lateral column of the spinal cord, which lies lateral to the dorsal horn and contains mostly descending fibres). Throughout their course, dorsal column fibres preserve their topographical order, so that when they arrive in the dorsal column nuclei (N. gracilis and cuneatus) which lie at the junction of the lower part of the medulla and cervical spinal cord, they form a map of the body there, with the arm lateral and the leg medial. Here the axons synapse with second-order neurones which project onwards to the thalamus in the *medial lemniscus*. In the middle part of the medulla they turn medially and ventrally and change places with those coming from the other side (the 'decussation' of the medial lemnisci), ending up in the pons, just above the main motor tract leaving the cortex (the pyramidal tract).

Lemniscal fibres then pass into the ventroposterolateral (VPL) nucleus of the thalamus, where they make the next synapse. Here the arm is represented posterolaterally while the leg is dorsomedial. Thus when the third-order axons curve into the *somatosensory cortex* (SI) situated in the *postcentral gyrus* (Brodmann's areas 1, 2 and 3) the arm is represented laterally while the leg is medial, close to the mid-line. The face is represented in the extreme lateral part of the posterior gyrus close to taste and the tongue.

Dorsal column nuclei (DCN)

The distinctive property of the dorsal column/lemniscal system is that the intensity, modality, locus and temporal sequence of a stimulus are transmitted through every station with extreme fidelity. In the dorsal column nuclei the topology of the fibre projections reflects the dermatomal arrangement of cutaneous nerves; thus each dermatome is represented by a thin, longitudinally arranged sheet of cells within the DCN. Within each of these lamellae the modalities are topographically separated, so that cutaneous mechanoreceptors are represented dorsally, and joint and deep tissue receptor input is found ventrally.

The caudal cells in the dorsal column nuclei are arranged in densely packed cell nests with tight, concentrically arranged dendritic fields receiving from only one or two dorsal column afferents. They also receive pre- and postsynaptic contacts from a corticofugal efferent system of fibres descending from the primary sensory cortex. DCN receptive fields are small and well-localized; they exhibit strong surround inhibition and are modality specific.

Rostral and ventral neurones are rather different to caudal neurones. They are arranged in a looser, reticular formation. They have widely spreading dendritic trees and correspondingly large receptive fields. Many of the fibres projecting there probably come from the dorsolateral columns, and not from the dorsal columns proper. Rostral dorsal column neurones also receive corticofugal projections; in general, however, these cells do not project into the lemniscal system, but pass either to other neurones within the DCN or into the reticular formation.

In fact, in the cat only about 25% of the large ($>4 \mu$m) myelinated fibres entering the dorsal columns from the medial division of the dorsal root project to the dorsal column nuclei. The remaining 75% either synapse with neurones in the dorsal horn of the spinal grey matter or they project beyond the spinal cord and dorsal column nuclei as external cuneate fibres. These are destined for the cerebellum and reticular formation.

Surround inhibition (Fig. 8.7)

In the caudal part of the dorsal column nuclei powerful surround inhibition occurs. If the centre of the receptive field of one of these neurones is stimulated, there is a brisk response which falls off with time even if the stimulus is maintained. If the surrounding area is stimulated at the same time as the centre, the discharge elicited from the latter is inhibited. Because these neurones have a rather low spontaneous firing rate, this surround inhibition cannot easily be seen unless it is elicited during simultaneous stimulation of the excitatory centre. As explained in Chapter 5, surround inhibition is crucially important in achieving the great spatial resolution of which the somaesthetic system is capable.

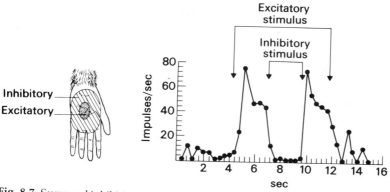

Fig. 8.7. Surround inhibition in the skin.

Corticofugal control

The other important feature of the dorsal column nuclei is that 'centrifugal' control is exerted over them by the sensory cortex. A topographically arranged projection from primary sensory cortex passes to corresponding points on the somatotopic map in the DCN. This projection supplies both excitatory and inhibitory components, enabling the sensory cortex to enhance or reduce transmission in different parts of the dorsal column system depending on the focus of attention at that moment.

Trigeminal system

The cutaneous supply from the face does not join the dorsal column or anterolateral cord systems but is provided with its own dual system, analogous to these. This private mechanism for the face presumably reflects the biological importance of the facial skin as a sense organ; this is witnessed by the fact that the two-point discrimination of the tip of the tongue is three times better than even that of the finger tips.

The cell bodies of the primary afferents from receptors in the facial skin arrive from the three divisions of the trigeminal nerve (opthalmic, maxillary and mandibular nerves) at the 'semilunar' ganglion behind the joint of the jaw. Here the skin of the face is topographically represented. On entering the brainstem, trigeminal axons divide into long descending and short ascending branches. The latter terminate within the 'main' sensory nucleus whilst the descending branches form the 'descending spinal tract'. The *spinal nucleus* of the trigeminal to which these fibres descend is divided into three parts (oralis, interpolaris and caudalis). The main sensory nucleus and spinal nucleus oralis are modality specific and somatotopically organized, and appear to be equivalent to the dorsal column nuclei of the lemniscal system. N. interpolaris and caudalis are the trigeminal equivalents of the spinothalamic anterolateral system. In the main sensory nucleus and spinal nucleus oralis, perioral and intraoral skin are represented medially, and eye and ear laterally.

The trigeminal nuclei then project towards the contralateral ventrobasal thalamus via the trigeminal lemniscus, which lies dorsomedially to the medial lemniscus. Some cells of the main sensory nucleus actually project to the ipsilateral thalamus, making up the so-called dorsal trigeminothalamic tract. These account for the ipsilateral (uncrossed) representation of the face (chiefly of the upper part) which occurs at thalamic and cortical levels. N. caudalis resembles the dorsal horn of the spinal cord cytoarchitectonically, projecting to the thalamic targets of the anterolateral system—the intralaminar and posterior nuclear groups. Section of the trigeminal spinal tract rostral to the obex (caudal to N. oralis and the main sensory nucleus of nerve V, but above N. interpolis and N. caudalis) leads to loss of facial pain and temperature sensations, but to insignificant changes in mechanoreception. This further supports our analogy of the caudal spinal nuclei of nerve V and its projections to the spinothalamic system. It clearly deals with pain and temperature for the face, as the spinothalamic system does for the rest of the body surface.

Spinothalamic system (Fig. 8.6)

Smaller Aδ and C fibres pass into the spinal cord via the lateral division of the dorsal roots. Together with collaterals of the larger Aα and Aβ cutaneous afferent fibres, some enter the dorsal horn immediately while others course up or down the cord for a few segments before plunging into it. Within the grey matter of the spinal cord, *laminae* may be observed, each containing neurones of a uniform size. These are known as *Rexed's laminae* (Fig. 8.8). Lamina I is the most superficial layer of cells, while lamina VI is the deepest layer of the dorsal horn. The collaterals of large sensory fibres passing to the dorsal columns, and Aδ and C fibres coming from the lateral division of the posterior roots, synapse with neurones in all five layers, but predominantly those of laminae I and V. Many of the axons of neurones in laminae IV and V cross over the mid-line and travel up the spinal cord in the contralateral anterior column, as the lateral and ventral spinothalamic tracts. Some fail to cross over and travel in the ipsilateral lateral column as the spinocervical tract or with ipsilateral spinothalamic tracts. It used to be taught that the lateral spinothalamic tract transmits pain and temperature signals exclusively whilst the anterior spinothalamic tract signals touch, however this is now known to be an over-simplification.

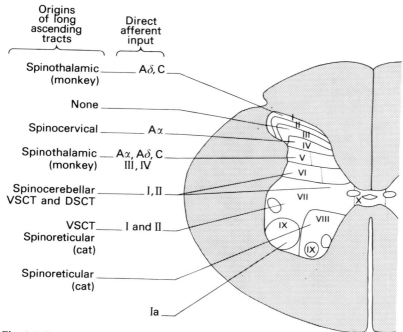

Fig. 8.8. Rexed's laminae in spinal grey matter.

Fibres from the spinothalamic tracts pass into the brainstem as the spinal lemniscus, which runs alongside the medial lemniscus; they terminate either in the reticular formation of the brainstem or in the intralaminar, posterior or ventroposterolateral nuclei of the thalamus. Those ending in the reticular formation constitute the *archispinoreticular* fibres—the most primitive somaesthetic system. Since they project only to the reticular formation, strictly speaking they should not be included with the spinothalamic system at all. Those ending in the intralaminar and posterior groups of thalamic nuclei are known as *paleospinothalamic* fibres; while those ending in the ventroposterolateral nucleus make up the *neospinothalamic* tract which, as we shall see, can duplicate to a large extent the functions of the dorsal column/lemniscal system. However, neospinothalamic fibres constitute only about 10% of fibres travelling in the spinothalamic tracts; the other 90% end in the reticular formation, in the reticular or intralaminar nuclei of the thalamus, or in the diffusely organized posterior group of thalamic nuclei. From the reticular formation of the brainstem further fibres pass to the intralaminar nuclei (hence mainly to the basal ganglia), and also to the hypothalamus.

From the thalamus two types of somaesthetic projection to the cortex emerge. The first is a coarsely somatotopically organized projection from the posterior group of thalamic nuclei to the second somatic sensory area situated behind, and lateral to, primary somaesthetic cortex. The second is the finely topographically organized pathway from the VPL nucleus to SI.

Thalamus (Fig. 8.9)

Almost all nerve fibres which bring sensory signals from lower centres to the cerebral cortex synapse in the dorsal thalamus. This received its name from fancied resemblance to a couch. Embryologically, neurones developing in this region fall into four groups: *epithalamus* which gives rise to the pretectal (visual) and habenular nuclei; *hypothalamus* which helps to conduct the hormone orchestra and directs drives and motivation; *ventral thalamus* which gives rise to the subthalamic nucleus and part of the reticular formation; and *dorsal thalamus* which acts as the gateway to the cortex.

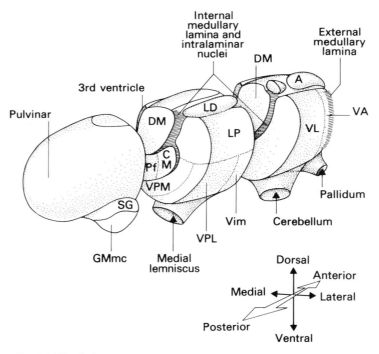

Fig. 8.9. The thalamus.

The dorsal thalamus is what most people refer to when they talk of 'the thalamus'. It contains more than a dozen subdivisions which are most easily understood if the disposition of the *internal medullary lamina* is borne in mind. This separates the dorsal thalamus into medial and lateral divisions; because it divides into two anteriorly, it encloses an anterior division as well. Within the internal medullary lamina lie the intralaminar nuclei.

The anterior nucleus receives from the mamillary bodies of the hypothalamus via the mamillothalamic tract, and projects to the cingulate gyrus which lies on the medial surface of the hemispheres.

The nuclei lateral to the internal medullary lamina consist of ventral, lateral and pulvinar groups. The ventral group is sub-divided as ventralis anterioris (VA), lateralis (VL), and posterioris (VP) (of which there are medial (VPm) and lateral (VPl) divisions, where the majority of somaesthetic lemniscal fibres terminate). The lateral nuclei are further divided into dorsal and posterior divisions.

The nuclei medial to the internal medullary lamina are divided into dorsomedial and mid-line nuclei, whilst the intralaminar nuclei (N. centralis, paracentralis, parafascicular and centromedianum) are found within it. The dorsomedial and mid-line nuclei project to the frontal lobe and the intralaminar nuclei project to the basal ganglia and hypothalamus, and diffusely to the frontal lobe. All these divisions and subdivisions may seem impossibly complicated but may make more sense if the simplified diagram shown in Fig. 8.9 is consulted.

Postcentral gyrus (Brodmann's areas 1, 2 and 3)

Lesions of the postcentral gyrus in man or other animals produce defects in somatic sensation, while stimulation there causes cutaneous sensations in conscious humans, localized to a point on the contralateral body surface corresponding to the part of the body represented at the cortical position stimulated. Stimulation here does not, however, cause movement unless the stimulus strength is so great as to cause current spread to neighbouring precentral motor cortex. There thus exists in areas 1, 2 and 3 of the postcentral gyrus a well-ordered map of skin and deep receptors according to their cutaneous site. The amount of cortex devoted to any particular part of the body is determined by the density of receptors in that area. Thus the lips, fingers and glans penis attain a large cortical representation whereas the back of the trunk or of a limb receive very little.

As in other sensory systems, different cortical areas are special-ized to deal with different types of sensory information; a modality map is superimposed on the somatotopic one. Area 2 is the most posterior of the primary receiving areas; neurones here are almost exclusively activated by joint, deep fascial and periosteal receptors. Area 1 just in front of it receives input from superficial skin mechanoreceptors with pronounced surround inhibition, while area 3 is purely cutaneous. However, area 3a, which lies in the depths of the central sulcus adjacent to motocortical area 4, receives from muscle spindles as well as cutaneous receptors, as befits its station close to the cortical motor outflow to muscles.

Sensory columns

Within the somatosensory cortex (SI), neurones are arranged in columns, as in the visual and auditory cortices. In fact it was in SI that 'columnar organization' was first clearly recognized by Powell and Mountcastle. As in other sensory systems, the evidence for columnar organization is both anatomical and physiological. Golgi staining of entire individual nerve cells shows that the majority of neurones in the cortex link adjacent layers vertically; their dendritic trees are aligned radially so that they link the cortical layers above and below them. Recording with microelectrodes shows that this vertical anatomical organization is mirrored functionally. Cells lying beneath each other on a track normal to the cortical surface all have receptive fields in the same part of the periphery; they receive in layer 4 from a single thalamic afferent fibre; they all have the same modality sensitivity, the same rate of adaptation and similar latencies following stimulation of the skin. Bands of columns receiving from slowly adapting receptors seem to interdigitate with bands receiving from rapidly adapting ones, in a manner rather reminiscent of the alternating bands found in the visual cortex receiving from ipsilateral and contralateral eyes. It is likely that subtler modes of feature extraction exist in the somaesthetic system, analogous to the orientation-selective, binocular or colour columns found in visual cortex. Probably these too will turn out to have a columnar organization, but it has not yet been elucidated.

'Barrels' (Fig. 8.10)

An interesting exaggeration of columnar structure is found in rodents, which use their vibrissae as very sensitive probes of their immediate surroundings. Local expansion of the cortical representation of each vibrissa has occurred, and the tight packing of columns of cells in barrel-shaped cortical areas can easily be seen histologically. Each whisker has its own barrel, and if a whisker is removed early in life its private barrel degenerates.

Intercolumnar inhibition

We understand only the barest outlines of how this columnar organization contributes to sensory analysis. One important mechanism is probably intercolumnar inhibition. This ensures that the column most effectively stimulated by a particular stimulus

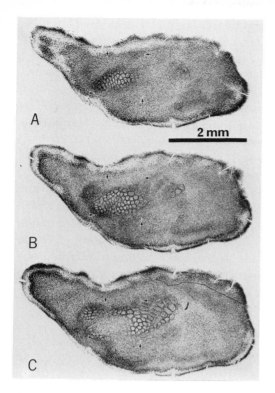

Fig. 8.10. Orderly arrangement of 'barrels' (local aggregations of columns) analysing mechanical input from each of a mouse's vibrissae. (From Woolsey T.H. & van der Loos H. (1970) *Brain Research,* **17**, 205. Elsevier Biomedical Press, Amsterdam. With kind permission.)

tends to extinguish activity in its less excited neighbours, and thus localizes consequent activity. This not only helps to identify the site of a peripheral stimulus, but because each of the many columns dealing with a particular area has its own optimum trigger features, the particular set of columns excited by a skin sensation precisely establishes the identity of that stimulus.

Second somaesthetic area (SII)

On the lateral side and posterior to SI in the superior bank of the Sylvian fissure, lies a second sensory representation (SII) discovered by Adrian. Like SI, SII is topographically organized, but it is smaller and depicts both halves of the body superimposed, so that the receptive fields are continuous across the mid-line, but for those at matched left and right skin areas. For proximal skin areas the two receptive fields are continuous across the mid-line, but for those at the distal extremities of the limbs the two receptive fields are entirely separate. In other respects SII neurones appear similar to those in SI, but only the skin surface is represented; deep receptors and proprioceptors do not project here. Neuronal responses are more labile and habituate very easily. An important feature is that high threshold (pain) receptors probably project to SII only, not to SI.

The response characteristic which is pre-eminent in SII is sensitivity to movement. This often takes the form of *directional selectivity*, i.e. the neurones in a column respond to a stimulus moving across the receptive field in one direction, but far less strongly, if at all, if it moves the other way (Fig. 8.11). In such instances the neurones sometimes respond to one direction of movement in the receptive field on one side of the body, but to movement in the opposite direction in the receptive field on the other side. Such neurones thus combine information about which parts of the body are being touched or moved over with information about the direction of movement. A branch brushing over the animal's back from one side to the other excites such a neurone maximally, but water pouring down both sides of the body simultaneously excites it minimally.

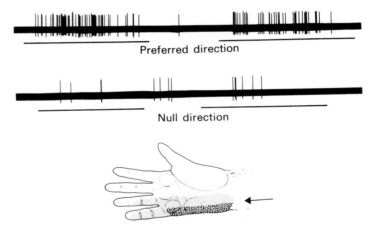

Preferred direction

Null direction

Fig. 8.11. Directional selectivity of a neurone in SII.

PARALLEL PATHWAYS

In the somaesthetic system then, there are many parallel pathways carrying information from the skin towards the cerebral cortex. We have come to expect that such parallel arrangements will be found in all sensory (and motor) systems. The classical description of these separate pathways for somaesthesia suggests that there is a complete separation of function in the spinothalamic and dorsal column systems, the former carrying pain and temperature signals, whilst the latter carry precise mechanoreceptor information—touch, vibration, superficial and deep pressure, and kinaesthesia. However, all but the most subtle touch discriminations achieved by active palpation may still be made after both dorsal columns have been sectioned; a famous lady in whom one dorsal column was severed in an accident was reputed still to be able to play Beethoven sonatas, though the quality of her playing is not recorded. Neospinothalamic pathways must therefore be able to carry relatively precise mechanoreceptor information; strict modality separation between dorsal columns and spinothalamic pathways is not found.

'Active' touch

The dorsal columns have evolved alongside the pyramidal tract and motor cortex, which are primarily concerned with fine control of the digits. It appears that the chief function of the dorsal column/ lemniscal system may be to inform the motor cortex, via postcentral sensory cortex just behind it, about sensory conditions in the limbs, in order to facilitate precise somaesthetic control of palpation. Only such fine tactile guidance of the digits is completely eliminated by dorsal column section.

Chapter 9
Pain

Pain is fundamentally different from other sensations of the skin. It is not only a feeling, but always demands a reaction—both motor and emotional. If you step on a drawing pin you jerk your foot away and swear. Alterations in the emotional component of the reaction can change subjective attitudes to a painful stimulus out of all recognition. Wounded soldiers suffering injuries which would render a civilian half mad with pain often feel practically nothing in their relief at getting off the battlefield alive.

It is the subjective component of a painful sensation which makes its psychophysical study so difficult. A person's estimate of the magnitude of a painful stimulus depends very much on his personality and emotional state at the time; therefore it is not easily reproducible. The amount of an analgesic drug required to negate a painful stimulus varies uncontrollably for the same reasons, so that this ostensibly 'objective' technique for measuring pain is also unreliable.

A further complication is that pain can be evoked by any of the forms of energy to which human sensory systems are receptive—mechanical, chemical, thermal, electrical and sometimes even light. The nature of the primary stimulus and its location are often appreciated separately from the degree of pain; as if other somaesthetic sensory systems signal the nature and location of the stimulus whilst a separate pain system signals its dangerous nature. In fact there is a great deal of evidence that there is indeed a specialized pain system with its own receptors, nerve fibres and central pathways. However, this has led people in the past into the error of supposing that sensations of pain are entirely separate from others and do not interact with them at all. This is by no means the case.

Fast and slow pain

Two phases in the evolution of a painful sensation are commonly described. In the first a sharp, pricking, easily localizable sensation occurs, which does not itself cause much emotional anguish. It was called by Head 'first' or 'fast' pain. 'Second' or 'slow' pain is the burning pain which evolves sometimes long after the initial localized sensation is over. This is the really unpleasant feeling which gives rise to the autonomic and emotional reactions which are so characteristic of pain. These can often be more easily measured than the painful sensation itself by means of changes in cardio-vascular and respiratory indices which they induce.

Nociceptors

Such subjective observations indicate that there may be two systems responsible for signalling to the CNS the site and intensity of a painful stimulus. Nevertheless, whether different receptors are responsible for first and second pain is not at all clear. It has been suggested that the receptors employed for detecting both types are 'nociceptors'—receptors situated on Aδ- (myelinated) and C-(unmyelinated) fibre terminals, which respond at high threshold to any situation in which damage to the body tissues is imminent or actually occurring (derived from the Latin *nocere*—to hurt). They are unusual in being slowly adapting. The adequate stimulus for the perception of pain may, therefore, always be the destruction of tissue.

Chemical theory

Mechanical, chemical, thermal and electrical stimuli, if applied with sufficient intensity at a sufficient rate, can all cause tissue destruction; hence it is natural to suspect a common mechanism whereby they excite nerve endings. Tissue damage leads to the release of a variety of chemical agents such as histamine, 5HT and bradykinin. These may serve as intermediates for stimulating C-fibre, but not Aδ, pain endings. These chemical agents are all also potent vaso-dilator agents, so painful stimuli also cause dilatation of blood vessels; this leads to redness followed by swelling (oedema) due to exudation of fluid into tissue space—all reactions calculated to defend the skin from its injury. Within an injured area and in the surrounding area of redness, a pin prick causes more intense pain than elsewhere; local pain threshold is thus lowered by previous injury. This suggests that tissue damage causes release of chemical agents which locally facilitate C-fibre pain receptors. The latter are sometimes called mechano-heat receptors since their usual stimulus is mechanical or thermal. However it is clear that there is no single chemical which is *the* pain transmitter for the skin; it is not possible to eradicate painful sensations by inhibiting any one of the transmitters mentioned earlier. For instance, histamine- or 5HT-blockers have little effect on cutaneous pain. It is possible that a series of polypeptides synthesized in extracellular fluid as a result of the release from damaged tissue of proteolytic enzymes are often responsible for painful sensations. Bradykinin is just one of these.

Furthermore, Aδ (myelinated) pain endings do not respond at all to chemical irritants such as bradykinin. They respond minimally to firm pressure but vigorously to a damaging mechanical stimulus, and are therefore known as 'mechanonociceptors'.

PAIN PATHWAYS

Spinal cord

More is known about signalling and analysis of pain signals within the central nervous system. The small myelinated (Aδ) and unmyelinated (C) fibres carrying pain information pass into the anterolateral somaesthetic system. Severing the anterolateral white matter in the spinal cord abolishes pain on the contralateral side of the body below the lesion; whilst damage to the dorsal columns does not diminish pain, although it may alter its localization and quality. All of this suggests that the anterolateral system is primarily responsible for signalling pain. However, Aδ- and C-fibre projections travelling in the anterolateral system are also capable of responding to temperature and light mechanical stimuli, as we have seen. Hence dorsal column lesions do not entirely eliminate touch sensation, whilst the anterolateral system is not exclusively devoted to pain but can signal touch as well.

Like Aδ and C mechanoreceptor and thermoreceptor fibres, the two types of pain fibre enter the dorsal spinal cord via the lateral division of the dorsal roots and travel for short distances up and down the cord in Lissauer's tract (situated at the tip of the dorsal horn), before terminating in Rexed's laminae I, II, III, IV and V (see Fig. 8.8). It is likely that one of the excitatory substances released by small pain fibre afferents is substance P, a peptide transmitter.

The axons of a few second-order neurones in lamina I which receive directly from pain afferents cross over to the other side of the cord and project modality-specific pain fibres straight onwards, in the contralateral anterolateral tract to the brain. Both lamina II and lamina IV cells receive in addition short collaterals from large myelinated sensory fibres (Aα and Aβ cutaneous mechanoreceptor afferents); these synapse with dorsal horn neurones both pre- and postsynaptically.

Substantia gelatinosa

Laminae II and III constitute the 'substantia gelatinosa' (S.G.); this contains only small interneurones whose axons pass back into Lissauer's tract, in which they travel for a few segments before re-entering the cord. Here they synapse with other S.G. neurones, both postsynaptically and presynaptically, by axo-axonic synapses made on the small- (Aδ and C) fibre primary afferent terminals there. The chief output of the substantia gelatinosa is directed ventrally towards the neurones of laminae IV and V, where the main projection neurones of the *spinothalamic* and *spinocervical* tracts are situated. The spinothalamic axons cross over in the anterior commissure of the cord to take up their position in the anterolateral columns of white matter ascending to the brainstem; but spinocervical axons remain on the same side and pass upwards alongside the dorsal columns, in the dorsolateral columns.

Gate control

It is probable that the main function of the interneurones of the substantia gelatinosa is to control the balance of activity relayed from small and large fibres onwards to the spinothalamic system— the spinal 'gate control'. S.G. neurones have a high spontaneous level of activity, and subgroups of these cells may be either inhibited or facilitated by inputs from large-fibre mechanoreceptor collaterals, small-fibre mechanoreceptors, or small-fibre nociceptors. Their axons end presynaptically on the terminals of nociceptive primary afferents, on S.G. interneurones and on spinothalamic relay cells. They also make postsynaptic contacts with each other and with relay cells. In general, their activity is predominantly inhibitory. Cells in the lateral part of the lamina which receive from distal extremities depress spinothalamic relay cells more than medially placed ones.

When large fibres are stimulated electrically, they set up prolonged primary afferent depolarization in both neighbouring and contralateral dorsal roots (indicated by long-lasting negative dorsal root potentials). This is primarily directed at the terminals of other large fibres, i.e. it is 'modality-specific' inhibition. Similarly, if Aδ and C fibres are stimulated, the presynaptic inhibition they cause mainly affects neighbouring small fibres. However, there is now evidence for the existence of inhibitory interaction between large and small fibres—'cross-modality' inhibition—as well. This is an essential prerequisite for the so-called 'gate control' theory of pain.

The starting point for the 'gate' theory, first advanced by Melzack and Wall in 1962, is that mechanical stimulation of the skin overlying or surrounding a painful area often alleviates the pain, whilst destruction of larger myelinated afferents from an area (e.g. following trauma or amputation) often causes spontaneous (e.g. 'phantom limb') pain, as though a normal restraining influence of large fibres over small fibres had been withdrawn. Melzack and Wall therefore proposed that large fibres entering the spinal cord normally inhibit small fibres presynaptically, and that this constitutes a 'gate' which allows pain through to higher centres via the anterolateral system only if there is a disproportionate amount of small-fibre activity compared with large-fibre activity.

In its simplest original form the theory is no longer tenable, as volleys in large cutaneous fibres can by no means completely suppress the activity of neighbouring small-fibre terminals. However, inhibition of small pain fibres by large mechanoreceptor afferents is now well documented, although the presynaptic mechanism originally suggested is only part of the story. There are neurones in the deeper layers of the cord (laminae IV and V) which have cross-modality 'opponent' (touch versus pain) properties. Noxious stimuli applied to the receptive field centre excite such cells, whilst they are inhibited by low-threshold mechanoreceptor stimulation in their surrounds and occasionally also in their centres (Fig. 9.1). Axons of these cells give rise to many of the fibres of the spinothalamic and spinocervical tracts.

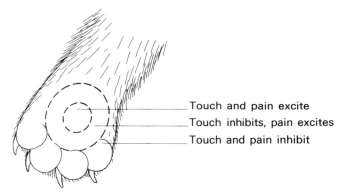

Touch and pain excite
Touch inhibits, pain excites
Touch and pain inhibit

Fig. 9.1. Cross-modality inhibition in a dorsal horn neurone.

Brainstem projections (Fig. 9.2)

As we have seen, the neospinothalamic components of the anterolateral system project to the ventrobasal part of the thalamus and from there to somatic sensory area 1, in a relatively strict somatotopic way. They are probably responsible for the localized sensations of touch, etc. which survive dorsal column section and perhaps contribute to the localizability of fast pain. The archispinoreticular component of the anterolateral system travels to the reticular formation in the medulla, pons and mesencephalon. The paleospinal pathway passes to the lateral posterior nucleus of the thalamus, which projects separately to the second somatosensory area (SII); both archi- and paleospinothalamic components project to the intralaminar nuclei and directly to the hypothalamus.

Presumably, the neospinothalamic system is responsible not only for spinothalamic touch, but also for first (or fast) pain, which may be accurately located, and is relatively precisely quantifiable but not unduly unpleasant. Second (or slow), intolerable pain is probably carried by the phylogenetically most primitive parts of the spino-thalamic system. Their projections to the reticular formation, and from there to basal ganglia, frontal cortex and hypothalamus might account for the special property of pain arousing intense activity and emotion.

Fig. 9.2. Principle pain pathways.

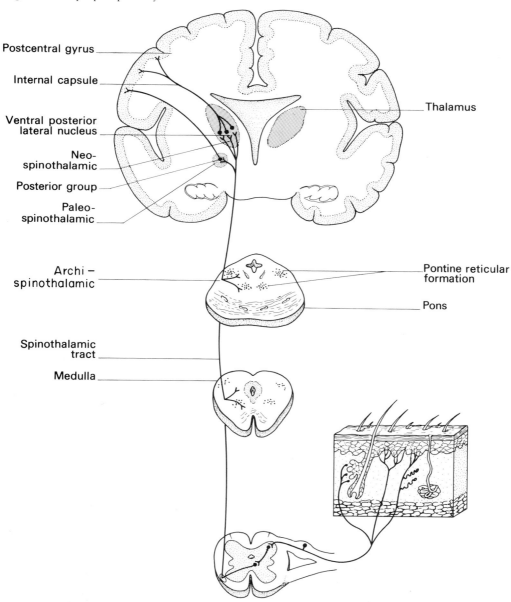

Centrifugal control

Pain pathways, like all other sensory systems, are provided with extensive centrifugal control over ascending signals. Unlike other sensory pathways, however, the dominant descending pain control system does not originate from the sensory cortex, but from the brainstem. Serotonergic fibres originating in N. raphe magnus travel down the spinal cord in the dorsolateral funiculus, and in the dorsal horn make contact with a further system of inhibitory neurones. These employ a novel class of peptide transmitter known as endorphin.

Endorphins

Endorphins were discovered as a result of attempts to identify the natural pain control mechanisms which the analgesic drug morphine so effectively usurps. The natural transmitters which morphine manages to mimic are now thought to be methionine- and leucine-encephalin. These are seven-amino-acid polypeptides (heptapeptides) split off from much larger precursor polypeptides such as β-lipotrophin (named before its relationship to the encephalins was recognized) and 'melanocyte-stimulating hormone'. These substances are collectively known as endorphins and are produced in large quantities in the pituitary gland, and probably at other encephalinergic sites as well. Encephalinergic neurones are ubiquitous and have now been identified in structures with as little to do with pain as the basal ganglia, retina, pituitary and gut. In the reticular formation of the brainstem, and more especially in dorsal horn interneurones of the spinal cord, their probable role is to inhibit pain transmission. This begins to explain how morphine controls pain.

Interestingly, it is likely that encephalins are involved in many natural situations in which pain is alleviated. For example, psychogenic analgesia produced by the expectation of alleviation when no analgesic is actually administered (known as the *placebo* effect) can be prevented by naloxone; this is a drug which specifically blocks encephalin/morphine receptors. This implies that encephalins normally mediate the analgesic effect of a placebo. Naloxone also partially blocks the analgesic effect of acupuncture. Since the efficacy of this treatment is thought to involve the activation of large fibres and the 'gate control' mechanism, it seems that encephalinergic interneurones are responsible not only for descending control over pain pathways, but also for part of the inhibitory control which is exercised by large cutaneous afferent fibres over small ones.

Lesion results

Ultimately however, a subject's reaction to pain is dependent on his whole cerebral cortex—summed up as his 'personality'. No single operation has a lasting effect on such chronic intractable pain as occurs in some types of cancer. Destruction of the posterior thalamic nuclei or of the second somaesthetic area (SII) offers only temporary alleviation, whilst lesions of the neothalamic, somatotopically organized, ventrobasal thalamic complex often lead in fact to the opposite effect—long-term enhancement of pain, 'hyperpathia'.

Leucotomy

Another technique which has been used in the past in an attempt to alleviate severe pain is performance of a 'frontal leucotomy', which consists of severing the fibres linking the dorsomedial nucleus of the thalamus to prefrontal cortex. There is no suggestion that this nucleus has anything specifically to do with the projection of pain sensations, but it is now clear that the frontal lobe and its connections with the limbic system play an important role in the control of emotions and their behavioural expression. Frontal leucotomy probably does not alleviate pain at all. What it does is to change a subject's emotional attitude to it, so that it provokes much less anxiety and distress and the patient can cope with it much better. Stimulation at the dorsomedial nucleus is alleged to result in subjects actually enjoying pain!

Unfortunately, the operation of leucotomy diminishes a person's capacity for anxiety and distress altogether—and does so irreversibly. Since these emotions of conscience are at the root of most civilized behaviour, the operation often causes drastic and unacceptable personality changes and is now seldom performed. Indeed its inventor, Monez, was murdered by a recipient of the operation, who had thereby been deprived of normal restraint to natural expression of his disappointment with the treatment.

VISCERAL PAIN

Pain caused by inflammation, distension or poor blood supply (ischaemia) of visceral organs is very useful to the clinician diagnosing these conditions. It is different from the fast, sharp, easily localized pain that informs of danger on the skin surface, and is more like the slow pain that follows actual damage. In the viscera there is no initial fast phase unless external, 'parietal' surfaces of the organs or overlying muscle and skin (all of which are supplied by somatic sensory nerves) are involved.

Appendicitis

In the later stages of acute appendicitis, inflammation passes right through the wall of the appendix and affects the peritoneum and overlying muscle. A characteristic parietal pain can then be localized on the skin at the midinguinal point. (This is often called 'McBurney's point' after the American surgeon who first clearly described the progression of symptoms in acute appendicitis and demonstrated conclusively that appendectomy was the safest treatment.) Earlier however, the pain of appendicitis has a dull, aching, throbbing quality and is poorly localized, roughly in the centre of the abdomen, nowhere near the site of the appendix (Fig. 9.3).

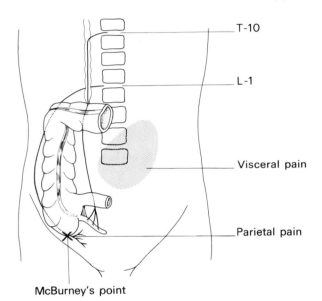

Fig. 9.3. Early, poorly localized, and later, sharp pain of appendicitis.

Localized damage to a viscus (e.g. by the surgeon's scalpel) causes very little pain because the viscera possess a low density of pain endings. However, overdistension, spasm (which simultaneously reduces blood supply and increases the requirements of the hyperactive muscle), ischaemia from other causes, and release of chemical stimuli all cause intense visceral pain like that of early appendicitis—extremely unpleasant but not localized. These diffuse and powerful stimuli recruit enough pain endings to reach perception, whereas the surgeon's scalpel affects only a few.

Referred pain

Visceral pain fibres are all of the unmyelinated C type; there are no myelinated Aδ axons. They enter the spinal cord via the white 'rami communicantes' of the sympathetic system (see Chapter 24) but pass into the substantia gelatinosa and onwards into the spinothalamic, spinocervical and spinoreticular tracts, much like the C fibres carrying cutaneous slow-pain signals. It is probable that the resulting sensations of pain are qualitatively so different and so badly localized because of the lack of Aδ-fibre projections from the viscera to the neospinothalamic system. Aδ fibres confer spatio-temporal precision on the cutaneous nociceptor system. A curious, though sometimes helpful, consequence of their absence from the viscera is the phenomenon of 'referred pain'. The pain of a visceral organ is mislocated to the surface of the body, sometimes far away from the true site of the organ, as in the early stages of appendicitis.

The site in the spinal cord to which visceral afferent fibres pass from internal organs depends on the segment of the body from which each originated during embryonic development. For instance, the heart is derived from endoderm in the neck and upper thorax, with the result that the heart's pain afferents enter the cord through dorsal roots C3–T5, and not further down, as might be expected from its eventual site lower in the thorax. Similarly, afferents from the gall bladder enter at T9 rather than at L1, its site in later life. The pain signals carried along these fibres can then often be mislocated and 'referred' to the areas of skin which supply Aδ fibres to the same segment of the cord. Thus a heart attack (causing ischaemia of cardiac muscle) can often present with pain in the left shoulder passing into the left arm—the cutaneous segments supplied by C3–T5. In the same way, an inflamed gall bladder can frequently cause pain at the tip of the right scapula, supplied by T9 (Fig. 9.3b).

Headache

Headache is sometimes, quite wrongly, said to be a prime example of referred pain. Neural tissue itself is not supplied with pain endings of any sort. However, blood vessels supporting meningeal membranes and sinuses are richly supplied by the Vth cranial nerve above the tentorium and the 2nd cervical nerve below the tentorium. The middle meningeal artery is well known to neurosurgeons as one of the most pain-sensitive structures in the body. Both Aδ and C fibres are found in these nerves; so both fast, localized and slow, aching types of pain are transmitted. However, most of the pathological processes giving rise to stimulation of the meninges and vessels, such as raised intracranial pressure following tumours, oedema provoked by trauma or surgery, dilatation of meningeal vessels (migraine) and reduction of intracranial pressure (e.g. following lumbar puncture) are all diffuse processes, so that there is no real localization of the insult anyway. Thus cerebral pain is not ill localized because it is referred, but because the processes causing it are usually not localized in the first place. Sharp, well-localized headaches are almost always extracranial, often caused by tension in scalp muscles. These often have a psychological, not an organic, origin.

Chapter 10
Position Sense and Kinaesthesia

A person's awareness of the position and movements of the parts of his own body depends on two entirely different sorts of information (Fig. 10.1). The first of these is internal feedback or *'corollary discharge'* to sensory centres about what motor structures engaged in moving the limbs have been doing. The second source is *feedback* about position from receptors in the joints, deep tissues, muscles and skin, and information from the balance organs of the vestibular system (Chapter 11). Put simply, you know where your arm is because your sensory systems are informed where you intend to put it, and you know that it got there because proprioceptors and other receptors inform you of the fact.

Fig. 10.1. Sources of information about limb position and movement.

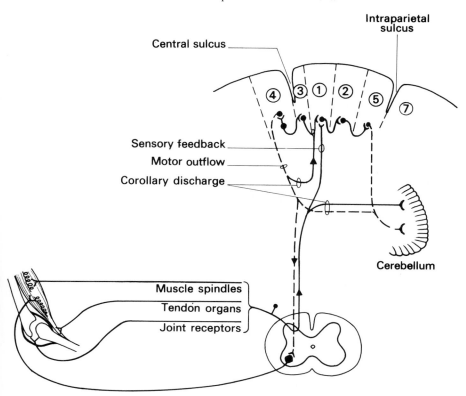

Passive position sense

The contribution of feedback from peripheral receptors to positional sense can be assessed by studying the ability to detect externally imposed movements of the limbs.

Muscle spindles

There has been much argument about which receptors contribute to passive position sense. For many years it was thought that signals from muscle length receptors (muscle spindles) do not project as far as sensory cortex, implying that they are not involved in any muscle sense, but rather are used only by the spinal cord and cerebellum for involuntary adjustment of muscle contraction. It is now known however that muscle spindle signals project to area 3a of the cerebral cortex which lies deep in the central sulcus—that was why they were so difficult to find. Moreover, it is now clear that they do contribute to limb position sense. If all the joint receptors and other local receptors in a finger are anaesthetized, leaving unaffected only the spindles in the forearm muscles which flex and extend the fingers, then a subject can indicate with fair, though not normal, precision when and by how much his finger is passively moved. Hence a sense of the position of the fingers may be derived solely from spindle discharge signalling the length of forearm muscles. If these are then silenced by anaesthetizing the forearm as well, the subject can no longer tell where his fingers are at all.

Joint receptors

However, this is an extremely artificial situation. Under normal circumstances one might expect joint receptors to be able to supply more reliable information about limb position than muscle spindles. In fact they cannot. Patients who have no joint receptors in the hip following total replacement of the hip joint are able to report the position of their artificial joint as accurately as subjects with normal joints. Most joint receptors only signal at extremes of flexion or extension, so that they cannot accurately record angles in between. Muscle spindle signals are probably more important than joint receptors for registering intermediate joint angles. During operations under local anaesthesia, if the surgeon pulls on the tendons of the long flexors of the fingers, the patient can tell which finger would have moved, in which direction and approximately by how much. Thus the muscle receptors stimulated by this procedure—muscle spindles and tendon organs—can supply all this information.

Vibration illusion

The sensorium can be tricked into thinking that a muscle is longer than it actually is by applying vibration—an exceptionally effective stimulus for dynamic (Group 1a) muscle spindle receptors. When this is done in a blindfolded subject his impression is that his limb moves to a new position, that which it would have taken up if the muscle were actually at the greater length erroneously suggested by the vibrated muscle spindles (Fig. 10.2). Information supplied by joint receptors about the true position of the arm is overridden under these circumstances. Muscle spindle discharge may therefore be used in preference to joint receptor signals to indicate the whereabouts of the arm.

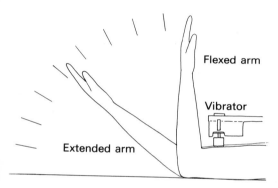

Flexed arm

Vibrator

Extended arm

Fig. 10.2. Vibration of left arm flexors excites muscle spindle Ia afferents, eliciting the stetch reflex and causing the arm to flex. Blindfolded subject reporting apparent position by matching with right arm underestimates the degree of flexion because vibrated muscle spindles signal incorrectly that the flexors are longer than they actually are.

Corollary discharge

We know very little about corollary discharge. This is the internal feedback from motor to sensory structures which indicates to the sensory systems that a limb is about to be moved, in order to permit correct interpretation of the sensory consequences of the movement. It is clear that such a system must exist, as otherwise we could never be sure whether we had moved or the world had moved us.

Eye movement

The classic example of the necessity of such feedback was first outlined clearly by Helmholtz; it is the case of active and passive eye movements. When we move our eyes 'saccadically' (the normal way of changing eye position), despite the fact that this causes images to stream across the retina in the opposite direction, the world nevertheless appears to remain satisfactorily stationary. Yet if we push our eyes around with our fingers the world seems to lurch all over the place. In the first case Helmholtz suggested that a 'corollary' discharge, or 'outflow' signal, of motor activity informs the visual centres that it was the eyes and not the world which had moved. In the second, without confirmatory evidence from motor centres, feedback from the moving eyes is insufficient to overcome the overwhelming impression from the retina that the world has moved. The world appears to move even though proprioceptors with which eye muscles are liberally endowed presumably protest that it was the eyes that were passively displaced. In this situation, corollary discharge is of greater importance than peripheral feedback.

In the limbs, matters are less complicated, since they do not feed back both retinal and proprioceptive signals which can tell different stories. Proprioceptors by themselves are usually sufficient to signal passive movement of a part, as we have seen. Nevertheless, in most situations proprioceptive feedback from the limbs interacts with corollary discharge about motor commands in order to inform us of their position.

Weight estimation

A good example of this interaction is demonstrated when we estimate the heaviness of an object. In order to assess the weight of something we must judge the amount of effort required to lift it, which involves matching the strength of the motor signals going to the lifting muscles against the information coming back from proprioceptors about the tension in the muscles and movement of the limb.

One strategy we might employ to estimate weights would be to consider only motor outflow signals, monitoring the 'sense of effort'. Proprioceptive feedback would then be used merely to signal that the limb had moved, and therefore that the motor power employed had been sufficient to overcome the weight. The amount of motor activity would then indicate the size of the weight. An alternative strategy would be to ignore motor signals and derive the weight of the object from the discharge of Golgi tendon organ tension receptors in the muscles. If we ask subjects to estimate the weight of an object, most will monitor the motor discharge necessary to lift it, concentrating on their 'sense of effort'; but if they are asked to judge the tension in their own muscles, or in springs they are required to compress, then they pay more attention to tension feedback.

When outflow sense of effort is relied upon for perception, the sensorium can quite easily be tricked into making mistakes if we interfere with the motor apparatus. Suitcases feel heavier as muscles tire, because motor systems have to generate a 'stronger' signal to achieve the same contraction from fatigued muscles. Partial curarization of a muscle has the same effect. Similarly, vibration of an antagonistic muscle causes weights to appear heavier than they are, since the vibrated muscle spindles then inhibit the lifting muscle's motoneurones by reciprocal inhibition.

On the other hand, any procedure which supplies additional excitation to the appropriate motoneurones causes a subject to underestimate weights. Thus vibration of agonist or synergist muscles, electrical stimulation of the skin of the moving part or 'Jandressek's manoeuvre' (clenching the other fist very tightly), all of which facilitate motoneurones of the active muscle, make objects feel lighter.

Posterior parietal lobe

Lesions of the posterior parietal lobe in humans cause disturbances in sensorimotor integration such as: astereognosis—inability to recognize objects by feel; amorphosynthesis—disturbance of a patient's appreciation of the parts of his own body and how they relate to each other and to the outside world; and apraxia—disorganization of the initiation and control of voluntary movements, even though similar movements may be made automatically. These disabilities have in common the loss of proper association of passive positional sense with control over the movements of parts of the body. Thus the 'parietal lobe syndrome' suggests failure to integrate corollary discharge from motor centres with sensory feedback from cutaneous receptors and proprioceptors in the limbs.

Parietal area 5

Such associations may well occur in Brodmann's cortical area 5, the superior parietal lobule, which lies immediately behind the primary sensory areas. Stimulation here causes coordinated complex movements of a whole limb, and lesions lead to deterioration of the ability to judge the shape of objects by palpation (astereognosis) and to disordered control of limb movements. They also result in an inability to judge the weight of objects. Recordings from neurones in area 5 show that they receive convergent inputs from neighbouring joints of a limb and from the skin moved by those joints; furthermore, area 5 neurones are facilitated when motor centres move the relevant limb (Fig. 10.3). Cutaneous and proprioceptive inputs to these cells probably come from the sensory cortex in front, whilst information about motor activity is derived from motor cortex and cerebellum. Thus area 5 may well be the site where corollary discharge and sensory feedback from the limbs are integrated.

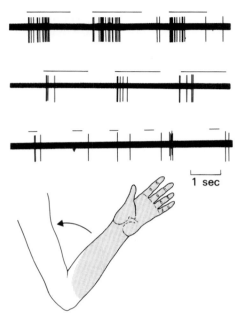

Fig. 10.3. Touching the skin of the forearm or hand (lower trace) or moving the elbow joint (middle trace) excites this neurone in area 5. Touching skin and moving elbow simultaneously excites it maximally (upper trace).

In humans the parietal lobe syndrome is complicated by *hemispheric dominance*. The very highest of mental functions—speech, language, reading, writing and calculation—are (in most people) lateralized in the left hemisphere (see Chapter 24). Lesions of the left parietal cortex therefore cause particular problems with reading and writing. The other hemisphere becomes expert in non-verbal skills such as pictorial representation and spatial thinking. Hence lesions in the parietal lobe of the 'minor' hemisphere cause complex disturbances such as 'constructional apraxia' (inability to make even simple drawings) and failure to remember or follow well-known routes successfully.

Chapter 11
The Vestibular System

The vestibular system, like the cochlea, is derived from the 'lateral line' vibration detection and balance organ of fish. It is situated within the bony labyrinth in the petrous portion of the temporal bone, at the base of the skull. The contents of the bony labyrinth (Fig. 11.1), known as the membranous labyrinth, are two large sacs (the utricle and saccule), three semicircular canals and the cochlear duct (which we have already considered in Chapter 7).

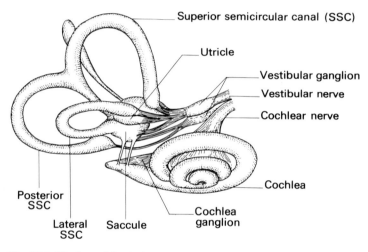

Fig. 11.1. The bony labyrinth.

UTRICLE AND SACCULE

In the walls of the utricle and saccule are two specialized regions, about 2 mm in diameter, called *maculae*. At the base of these lie two types of hair cell, disposed in a systematic array (Fig. 11.2). They are bottle shaped (type I) or cylindrical (type II), and are supplied with both afferent and inhibitory efferent nerve endings at their base. The significance of the different structures of type I and II hair cells or of their inhibitory efferent control is not yet evident. Both have a tuft of hairs emerging from their top surface, which embed in a gelatinous substance lying above them. The hairs on one side of the cell are always thinner and shorter than on the other side. The thickest and longest hair emerging from one edge is known as the *kinocilium*. It is likely that this arrangement confers on the cell its directional selectivity. The cell is excited by bending the hairs in one direction, but inhibited when they are bent in the other. Resting in the gelatinous substance lie many crystals of calcium carbonate, known as *otoliths*; so when the head is bent in any particular direction the weight of the otoliths on the gelatinous substance bends the hairs in a characteristic pattern, specific directions of head movement being catered for by the systematically organized distribution of polarization of the hair cells. The utricle appears to register mediolateral movement and the saccule registers superior–inferior movement, whilst both contribute to the signalling of anteroposterior head movements (Fig. 11.2).

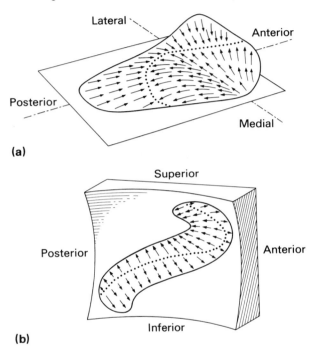

Fig. 11.2. Directional selectivity of hair cells in (a) utricle (b) saccule.

The utricle and saccule mainly provide information about the current (static) position of the head but they relay some information about linear acceleration (movements in a straight line) as well. The fibres from the saccule and utricule, which travel to the pons in the vestibular nerve, transmit a continuous stream of impulses when the head is stationary, signalling its position. When the head is moved, discharge along some fibres increases (because these are connected to hair cells whose thinner hairs fall away from the stiffer kinocilium during that particular movement of the head) whilst the discharge in others decreases. Impulse traffic in most fibres is maximal during movement and adapts to a lower level when the head rests in its new position. The increment in discharge during motion therefore signals the movement itself. Other fibres fire maximally only when the head is upright and their activity falls off when the head rests in any other position; thus they signal the static position of the head in relation to the vertical.

SEMICIRCULAR CANALS

The three semicircular canals are orientated in three planes set mutually at right angles to each other. When the head is bent 30° forwards the 'horizontal' canal (also known as the 'lateral' or 'external' canal) comes to lie truly horizontal; the anterior canal lies vertically but points 45° outwards and forwards; whilst the posterior canal also lies vertical, but points 45° outwards and backwards. Thus the anterior canal on one side is parallel to the posterior canal on the other, and the two horizontal canals are parallel to each other. The output from each side can thus act in 'push–pull' mode—rotation in one direction exciting one side and inhibiting the other (Fig. 11.3). The ampullae situated at the base of each semicircular canal contain hair cells similar to those found in the utricle, saccule and cochlea, with cilia embedded in a gelatinous body, the cupula. The canals are filled with endolymph fluid. When the head is rotated, the inertia of this fluid causes it to lag behind. Hence the ampulla moves whilst the endolymph remains stationary. This deflects the cupula whose distortion bends cilia embedded in it and thus excites vestibular nerve fibres (Fig. 11.3). All possible directions of head motion elicit

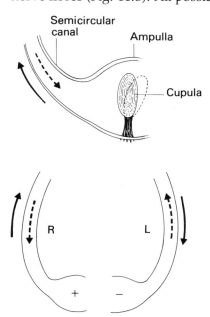

Fig. 11.3. Clockwise turning of head leaves canal endolymph behind, causing bending of cupulae to the right. This excites right vestibular nerve fibres but inhibits left. (From Lamb *et al.* (1980).)

characteristic movements of the cupulae in the six canals, resolved into two directions in each of the three planes at right angles to each other. Hence the pattern of discharge in vestibular nerves varies for each direction of head movement.

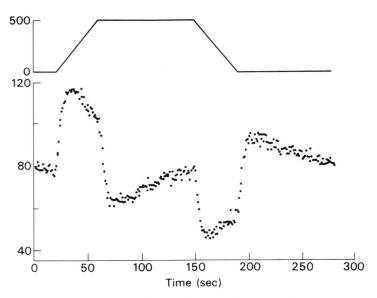

Fig. 11.4. Upper trace—angular acceleration of head in degrees s^{-2}. Lower trace—discharge of single vestibular afferent.

This inertial mechanism means that the cupulae are affected by angular acceleration of the head rather than by velocity or position. Thus when the head is stationary or has been moving at a uniform velocity for some 20 s they emit no signal. On stopping after movement, it takes about 20 s for the fully-deflected cupula to return to its resting position.

Nevertheless, the discharge in the nerve fibres leaving the semi-circular canals is usually more closely proportional to velocity than to acceleration of the head. This is because the cupula behaves like a damped 'torsion pendulum' with a moment of inertia of approximately 250 μg. cm^2. This frictional component is so great that the system is highly overdamped. Thus for the normal range of head movements, cupula displacement is actually closely proportional to head velocity. The linking of endolymphatic movements to the receptors thus acts as a mechanical 'integrator' converting head acceleration to velocity—it behaves like an integrating or 'low pass' filter with a 'short' time constant of about 2 ms (equivalent to a high-frequency cut-off of around 500 Hz) and a low-frequency cut-off at about 0.05 Hz (3 cycles per minute). Frequencies lower than 0.05 Hz therefore produce a signal which is unrelated to either velocity or acceleration of the head.

An interesting consequence of this insensitivity to very low frequencies is that very slow movements of the whole body, as occur on ships at sea or in a well-sprung car, are impossible for the vestibular system to interpret; a fact which, taken together with the close proximity of the 'vomiting centre' to the vestibular nuclei, may well offer some explanation for car and sea sickness.

Vestibular psychophysics

If the semicircular canals are stimulated artificially, subjects experience an illusion of rotating in the plane of the canal stimulated, as one might expect. When the body is rotated at a constant velocity, the semicircular canals cease being stimulated because there is no movement of the endolymph once it has caught up. If the rotation is then halted suddenly, the subject now senses rotation in the opposite direction, as the endolymph continues to move deflecting the now stationary cupula in the opposite direction. This feeling continues for about 20 seconds—equivalent to *c.* 0.05 Hz (this was one of the ways in which the low-frequency cut-off of the ampullary response was calculated).

Vestibular adaptation

Subjective sensations of rotation, however, are not simply functions of the deflection of the cupula, because the vestibular system shows the phenomenon of *long-term adaptation* to sustained vestibular stimulation. (This should not be confused with short-term, receptor adaptation—taking place over milliseconds.) If vestibular stimulation is continued for many minutes, vestibular responses are attenuated, as though a normal reference level of vestibular output against which current signals are compared is slowly shifted in the direction of any continuous displacement of the cupulae. Thus cumulative stimulation seems to be able to bias the system in one direction.

Long-term adaptation may explain phenomena as diverse as the apparent heaving of dry land after a day spent at sea; the remarkable capacity of the vestibular system to compensate completely for the imbalance caused by the loss of the input from one side (as happens for instance in Meniere's disease); and the ability of test pilots and ballet dancers to avoid passing out or throwing up! Many visual/vestibular responses may be entirely reversed after wearing inverting spectacles for a few days, but this is probably as much a property of connections with visual and oculomotor systems as of the vestibular apparatus alone.

The vestibulo-ocular reflex and vestibular nystagmus

One of the easiest ways to demonstrate the activity of the vestibular system in intact animals and human subjects is to observe the movements of the eyes which occur following vestibular stimulation. Rotation of the body leads to conjugate movements of the eyes in the opposite direction, enabling the eyes to remain fixed on a point in space (Fig. 11.4). As a result, one is able to see one's stationary finger without it blurring when making rapid to and fro movements of the head; whereas if one waggles one's finger at the same rate, the visual system is unable to process the signals fast enough and one cannot see it clearly. Continuous vestibular stimulation therefore causes 'nystagmus'. The eyes move in the opposite direction to the head (in response to a vestibular signal mimicking head movement) in order to compensate for it. This 'slow phase' is interrupted when the eyes are fully deviated by a fast phase in the same direction as the head movement, returning them to the other side of the orbit.

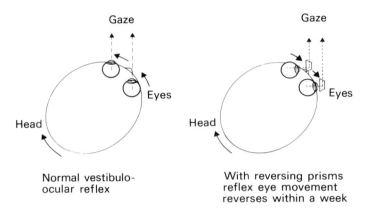

Fig. 11.5. When the head moves the vestibulo-ocular reflex helps the eyes to maintain gaze fixed in space, and can reverse its normal direction of action if necessary.

If a subject is rotated in a 'Barany' chair, the slow phase of the ensuing nystagmus is therefore directed in the opposite sense to the rotation, enabling the eyes to remain fixed on a stable point in space; the fast phase is in the same direction as the subject is spun. On halting the chair suddenly (which makes the eye movements easier to see!) these phases reverse, the slow phase now being in the same direction as the chair had been rotating and the fast phase in the opposite direction. 'Post-rotational nystagmus' continues for about 20 s, while the endolymph slows down and the elastic recoil of the cupula is completed. Damage to the labyrinth is often indicated by changes in these slow and fast phases, and in the period of post-rotational nystagmus.

Another way of investigating the function of the semicircular canals, which is altogether more convenient, is the *caloric test*. Since the horizontal canal lies close to the tympanic membrane, warm or cold water placed in the external ear induces thermal currents in its endolymph, particularly if it is made to lie vertically by bending the head back by 60°. Because only one canal is affected, the resulting nystagmus is easy to interpret; however, the test is very unpleasant for a subject with normally functioning canals, as the imbalance of signals from the two sides promotes vertigo and nausea.

Chapter 12
Smell and Taste

The sense of smell is the most primitive we possess, evolutionarily speaking, yet it receives very little attention. The importance of the chemical senses in lower animals is well recognized. A tiger moth can scent his mate as far as seven miles away, and fly to her. The way in which rats have deluded the credulous into over-estimating their visual abilities—mistaking phenomenal discriminative abilities as visual when they are in reality olfactory—is a parable of the dangers of inadequately controlled behavioural research.

We like to think that smell and taste are less important to humans, but this can hardly be so. The main impetus for many early voyages around the world was not one of pure adventure, but to obtain the powerful exotic spices from the east which could mask the evil effects of winter storage of meat in a Europe without refrigerators! Likewise, the ingredients of exotic perfumes, whose identity is a jealously guarded secret, probably have a much more basic 'animal' attraction than either their purveyors or purchasers would care to admit. Certainly one of them, musk, obtained from the anal gland of the musk deer and the civet cat, is one of the most powerful scents known to man, and is clearly judged by the perfumery trade to be able to attract mates from great distances!

SMELL

Despite the importance of olfaction little is known about its physiology. A major reason for this is the difficulty of accurately defining characteristics of the stimulus with respect to its timing, magnitude, location and quality. Only about two per cent of a puff of scent reaches the 2.5 cm^2 of *olfactory epithelium* in the upper part of the nasal cavity, and it takes an unknown time to diffuse from there into the receptor cells themselves. These cells are covered with finger-like cilia which actually increase the effective surface area of the olfactory epithelium to perhaps 600 cm^2. This no doubt helps to account for the incredible sensitivity of the olfactory system. At threshold, just 20 million molecules of the highly odoriferous substance mercaptan may reach our 40 million receptor cells. Thus each olfactory receptor needs one molecule to excite it; and stimulating half the receptor cells can produce a sensation.

The quality of an odour is another baffling problem. Humans

have been alleged to be able to distinguish as many as 4000 odours qualitatively, but no experimenter has managed to make subjects agree on the classification of more than 100. The relationship between odorant quality and chemical structure is also a mystery. Only seven single chemical elements smell (four halogens— fluorine, chlorine, bromine and iodine—plus ozone, phosphorous and arsenic). To have an odour, a substance must have a molecular weight between 17 and 300; it must be volatile; and it must be soluble in either water or lipid (because it is necessary for the olfactory epithelium to absorb it). There is no clue yet as to what chemical structures give rise to what odours.

Despite the difficulty of classifying odours, one would have thought that some broad principles would have emerged, but they have not. One is driven to conclude that in the olfactory system the idea of receptor specificity which has served so well in other sensory systems has finally let us down. Results from electrophysiology suggest that in the olfactory system at least, a 'pattern' theory has more to offer.

Olfactory bulb

Each receptor tapers down to a small (0.2 μm) unmyelinated fibre which passes through the cribriform plate in the floor of the cranial cavity.

Immediately above the cribriform plate lies the olfactory bulb. The 40 million axons of olfactory neurones converge on *mitral* and *tufted* cells in the olfactory bulb, forming globular synaptic complexes

Fig. 12.1. Olfactory pathways.

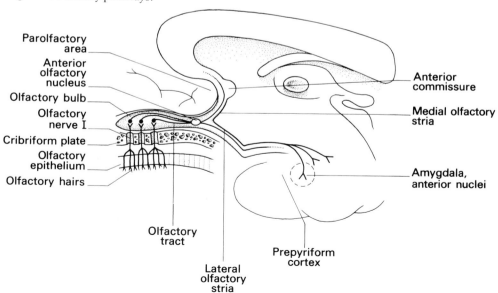

called glomeruli, in a ratio of about 250 olfactory fibres to one mitral cell; this convergence is another feature accounting for the great sensitivity of the system. The axons of mitral cells pass along the olfactory tract to the inferior region of the frontal lobe, where they divide to form the medial and lateral olfactory stria (Fig. 12.1). The medial stria projects to the medial part of the 'anterior perforated substance' in the ventral part of the forebrain, and to the septum; whilst the lateral olfactory stria terminates in the prepiriform cortex, amygdala and lateral portion of the anterior perforated substance. In addition to fibres from the receptors, olfactory bulb glomeruli receive fibres from the bulb on the other side and centrifugal efferent control fibres originating in prepiriform cortex, anterior perforated substance and amygdala, i.e. from all its projection areas.

Electro-olfactogram

A one second puff of an odorous substance wafted into the nasal cavity gives rise to a 5 mV negative potential in the olfactory epithelium, which rises and decays exponentially, taking about four seconds in all (Fig. 12.2). This is thought to represent the summed receptor potentials of all the olfactory neurones stimulated, and is known as the electro-olfactogram (EOG). The form of the EOG

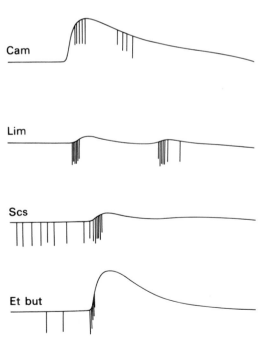

Fig. 12.2. Discharge of a single olfactory fibre superimposed on the electro-olfactogram (EOG) for different smells (camphor, limonene, carbon disulphide and ethylbutyrate). (After Gesteland H.C. (1963) In: *Olfaction and Taste* (ed. Zotterman Y.). Macmillan, New York.)

varies in its size and temporal and spatial properties according to what is being sniffed. It is presumably these changes in the pattern of electrical activity in the fibres leaving the olfactory epithelium which underly our ability to distinguish so many odours, though the precise receptor mechanisms still elude us, as does the central processing whereby these different patterns are identified.

The variation of pattern of EOG with odour is reflected in the discharge of single fibres (Fig. 12.2). Each responds only to a selection of odours though, unfortunately, the ones to which they do respond are not distinguished by any common chemical characteristic. Single olfactory neurones discharge with a different pattern following each odour of the subset to which they respond. Although no two fibres respond exactly similarly to the same odour, some eight different general patterns of activity have been identified. Again, however, no common chemical characteristic can be related to these discharge types, nor do they correspond to any subjective classification of the resultant sensations.

Synaptic organization of olfactory bulb

The olfactory bulb has been a gold mine for electrophysiologists, however; not because of their interest in smell, but on account of its convenient geometrically organized anatomical arrangements. Felicitously, the mitral, granule and tufted cells, together with their dendrites, inputs and outputs, are all arranged in highly ordered, separate layers. Therefore intimate details of their interactions can be examined more easily than in most other areas of the central nervous system.

Dendrodendritic excitation and inhibition

Powerful inhibition of mitral cells, lasting up to 100 ms, follows antidromic stimulation of their axons from the olfactory stria. This inhibition is the result of the action of granule cells excited not by mitral cell axon collaterals, as might have been expected, but by secondary dendrites of mitral cells. This was a most heretical concept at the time it was put forward, since it postulated that dendrites as well as axons are able to release transmitter and excite granule cells. Furthermore, olfactory-bulb granule cells have no obvious axon, so it appeared that granule cell dendrites are not only excited by mitral cell dendrites, but could themselves reciprocally inhibit mitral cells (Fig. 12.3). Fortunately, shortly afterwards, dendrodendritic synapses in the granule cell layer of the olfactory bulb were confirmed with the electron microscope, and dendritic release of transmitters has been observed elsewhere (e.g. from the dopaminergic cells of the substantia nigra—see Chapter 18).

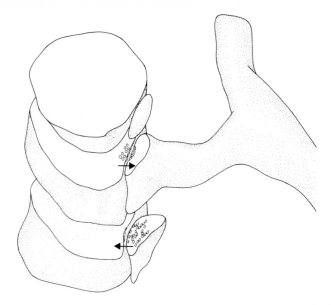

Fig. 12.3. Reciprocal dendrodendritic synapses between mitral and granule cell dendrites in the olfactory bulb.

'Odour mapping'

As in the retina, cochlear nuclei and dorsal horn of the spinal cord, the main business of this first relay in the olfactory system, the olfactory bulb, is probably to effect lateral inhibitory 'sculpturing' of incoming sensory information in order to enhance the peaks of activity in the array of olfactory fibres. Little is known about how these mechanisms, which have been so successfully dissected electrophysiologically, actually effect odour analysis. A clue is given by the observation that responses to different classes of odours (again unfortunately not linked by any chemical similarity) are segregated in different regions of the bulb, rather in the same way as different frequencies are laid out in different regions of the cochlea, or different modalities in the sensory cortex. As we have seen, it is a general principle within sensory systems that the processing of the different qualities of a stimulus takes place in parallel in separate regions of the nervous system.

Limbic system (Fig. 12.4)

One reason for paying particular attention to olfaction is that it is the sense which is most closely linked to the emotional and drive systems of the brain, presumably because correct identification of the smell of food, enemies and mates is so important to survival. In fish and amphibians the forebrain is dominated by the olfactory system, which projects to the primitive *hippocampus* medially and to *piriform* cortex laterally. Throughout the phylogeny of the mammals, an initially small dorsal area between these two areas expanded enormously to form the *neocortex*; so that both hippocampus and piriform cortex (represented by hippocampal and cingulate gyri) end up on the medial surface of the resulting cerebral hemisphere. These olfactory areas are often collectively known as the *rhinencephalon* (Greek for 'smelling brain'), even though only a small part (the anterior perforated substance, amygdaloid nuclei and prepiriform part of the anterior end of the hippocampal gyrus) actually receives directly from the olfactory striae. Another name that has often been used for these areas is the *limbic system* (from the Latin *limbus*—an edge), conceived as the ring of grey matter surrounding the interventricular foramen. The list of structures that have been included under this heading is long: cingulate gyrus, induseum griseum, hippocampus and dentate gyrus, piriform cortex, septum, amygdaloid nucleus, orbitofrontal cortex and hypothalamus. The list is so extensive that one is inclined to doubt whether there is any rational basis for considering them all part of the same system. Of all these structures only the prepiriform cortex is essential for the discrimination of odours. The others are specialized for other functions. However, they are all linked

Fig. 12.4. The limbic system.

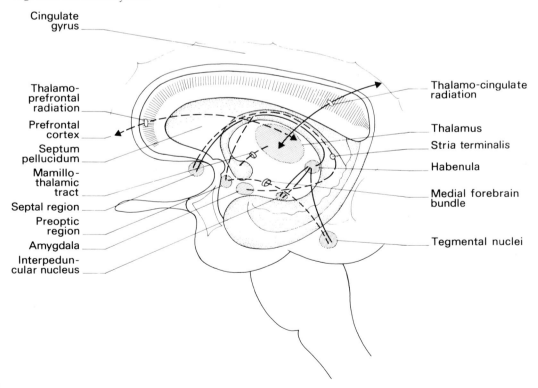

Cingulate gyrus

Thalamo-prefrontal radiation

Prefrontal cortex

Septum pellucidum

Mamillo-thalamic tract

Septal region

Preoptic region

Amygdala

Interpedun-cular nucleus

Thalamo-cingulate radiation

Thalamus

Stria terminalis

Habenula

Medial forebrain bundle

Tegmental nuclei

anatomically in what is known as the 'Papez' circuit, and electro-physiological techniques have confirmed their relationships to each other. The role of this system in drive-related behaviour and memory is considered in Chapter 25.

TASTE

Like the sense of smell, that of taste has not really received the attention it deserves from physiologists, despite the importance most people attach to the taste of their daily food. The myriad magical flavours and gastronomic miracles with which gourmets titivate their palates depend not only on the taste buds of the tongue and pharynx, as these can discriminate no more than four basic tastes (sweet, sour, salt and bitter), but also upon the sense of smell—upon the odours which simultaneously assail the olfactory organs. For the nose can make much more subtle distinctions than the tongue and the taste and smell of food are inextricably entangled.

Taste buds

The taste system is some 25000 times less sensitive than that of smell. This is probably because the *taste buds,* each of which contain up to twenty *gustatory cells* (Fig. 12.5), are situated inside small elevations (papilla) on the tongue and pharynx and only communicate with the surface through small pores which make up a tiny percentage of the tongue's surface.

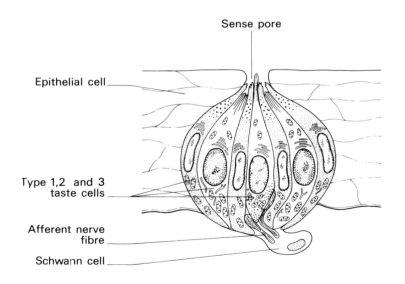

Sense pore

Epithelial cell

Type 1,2 and 3 taste cells

Afferent nerve fibre

Schwann cell

Fig. 12.5. Taste bud.

For some reason, taste buds have a very short lifespan—less than one week. New gustatory cells are continually formed at the periphery of the bud and migrate towards its centre. The fifty or so gustatory nerve fibres entering each taste bud are not renewed in the same way so they have to cope with their receptor cells being replaced at a high rate. Nevertheless, the pattern of each fibre's response to sweet, sour, salt and bitter substances (which differs from fibre to fibre) remains constant. If it did not, the central processing mechanisms would find it well nigh impossible to interpret the changing pattern of impulses received. Each nerve fibre probably imposes upon the receptor cell with which it happens to be temporarily in contact the particular pattern of responses it will exhibit.

Evidence that sensory nerve terminals control the response characteristics of gustatory cells in this way is provided by sectioning these nerves. Immediately afterwards, taste buds disappear completely; they reappear only when the nerve regenerates. Hence the nerve fibres probably exert 'trophic' control over the whole taste bud. It is likely therefore that individual fibres exert similar control over the chemical specificity of the receptor cells with which they are in contact.

Gustatory pathways (Fig. 12.6)

Gustatory axons pass from the front of the tongue, via the chorda tympani, to the VIIth (facial) cranial nerve; from the back of the tongue to the IXth (glossopharyngeal) nerve; and from the pharynx to the Xth (vagus) nerve. The taste fibres in these nerves all eventually find their way to the nucleus of the solitary tract, in the medulla oblongata, to which project also the vascular chemoreceptors found in the aortic and carotid bodies and the gut chemoreceptors supplied by the vagus nerve. Second-order fibres pass from there not only to the thalamus, and hence to the tongue area of the sensory cortex, but also to the locus coeruleus, reticular formation and limbic system, where integration of taste and the chemical state of the body fluids with the sense of smell presumably occurs.

Tastes

More is known about the underlying chemical characteristics of the basic taste sensations (sour, salty, sweet and bitter) than is the case for olfaction, but still there are many mysteries. All acids taste sour to humans and their degree of sourness depends on pH. All inorganic anions taste salty. However, not only do sugars such as sucrose, glucose, etc. taste sweet but so, mysteriously, do beryllium salts, chloroform, amides of vitamin C, lead salts and some proteins such as saccharin (which is 100000 times as sweet as sucrose). Another protein, miraculin, alters the taste of acids so that they too begin to taste sweet. The bitter taste of quinine, strychnine and other alkaloids is well known, but urea, magnesium, calcium and ammonium salts also taste bitter. Furthermore, it seems that

Fig. 12.6. Gustatory pathways.

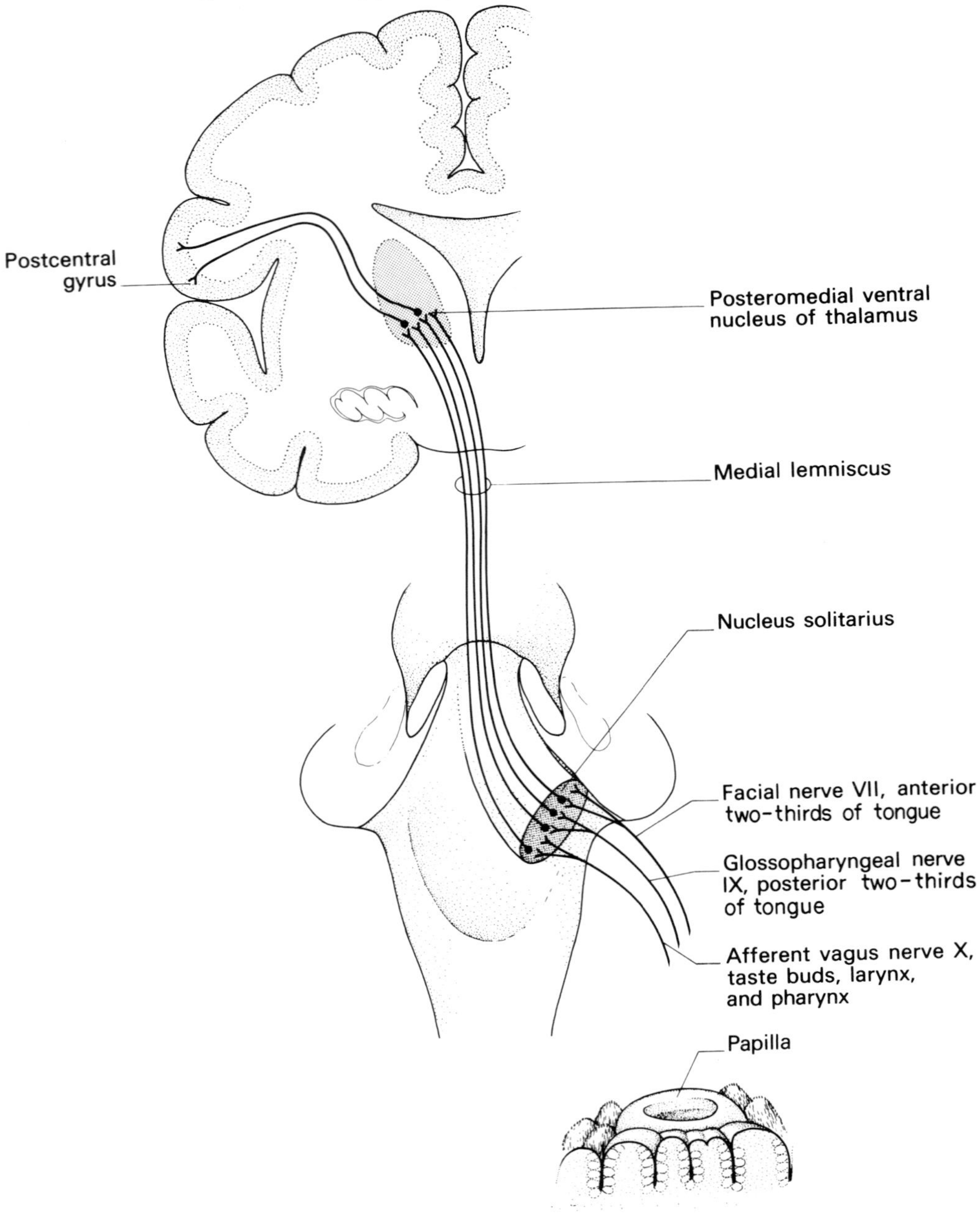

many animals—not including man—have a fifth, very sensitive taste for pure water, which may explain their ability to detect it at very great distances.

Taste mapping

As with olfaction, the central processes underlying taste discrimination are unclear. The fibres leaving individual taste buds often discharge following application of all four classes of sapid substances, though with a different pattern of discharge for each. Sweet substances give larger responses in fibres leaving the tip of the tongue; the sides of the tongue are more sensitive to salty and sour; whilst bitter substances elicit most activity from the back of the tongue. Thus the pattern of discharge from the whole of the gustatory receptor surface must be assessed by central mechanisms when identifying a taste. It is likely that inhibitory mechanisms analogous to lateral inhibition in the other sensory systems classify the patterns into peaks and troughs, and thus help in transferring the spectrum of tastes encountered by the tongue into a *spatial map* of tastes in N. tractus solatarius.

Olfactory and gustatory stimuli seem to enjoy a very direct pathway to the roots of our personalities and the springs of our actions, presumably as a result of their intimate connections with reward systems and the limbic pathways of emotion. A rather attractive theory to account for our otherwise inexplicable ritual of kissing is that it evolved as a means of tasting and smelling prospective partners!

Chapter 13
Introduction to Motor Control

TECHNIQUES

Investigation of the way in which the CNS controls movement has proved very much more difficult than the study of sensation, so that our present knowledge is very incomplete and much of the theory that follows cannot easily be tested experimentally. First, movements are very much harder than sensory stimuli to describe precisely and quantitatively. Secondly, unlike sensory processing, voluntary movements cannot be studied in anaesthetized animals. Thirdly, whereas the many parallel sensory pathways carry different types of information which are relatively easily identified, the different motor pathways also operating in parallel do not have such clearly separable roles, and so understanding them is thus much more difficult.

Quantification of movement

We may consider the problem of the movements of the thumb as an example of the difficulties in describing movements fully and precisely. It is the exceptional properties of this digit which give the human hand much of its dexterity. The thumb itself can move in three planes: flexion and extension (curling and uncurling); adduction and abduction (sideways movement to and from the side of the index finger); and opposition (rotation of the base of the thumb to touch the finger tips). The hand on which the thumb is mounted can move in nine additional planes: three at the wrist (flexion, abduction and rotation), one at the elbow, and three at the shoulder (again flexion, abduction and rotation). So the tip of the thumb has some 27 different planes of movement. Just to describe these mathematically in terms of the movement of the individual joints would require an expression with at least ten variables, but the problem is worse even than this. Movements in each plane are effected by at least two (*agonist* and *antagonist*) muscles and influenced by many other *synergists*. For any given action of the thumb, therefore, we have to consider the timing and magnitude of length and tension changes not only in prime movers, but also in all the other antagonistic and synergistic muscles operating on the upper limb. In fact some 126 muscles act on the shoulder and arm, so a full description of the movements of the thumb would clearly be a truly formidable undertaking.

Compared with this, sensory stimuli can be defined with great ease. For example, in the visual system only four variables (colour, location, intensity and timing) need to be specified; these can, in principle, be completely controlled by the experimenter, and the behaviour of neurones at successive stages in the visual system correlated with each of them. A 'sensory trace' (a change in electrical activity of neurones which is locked in time to the peripheral stimulus) can be followed through many synapses into the CNS. Such simplicity is denied the motor system physiologist. There appears to be no such thing as a 'movement trace' which can be identified within the CNS and followed out to the spinal cord motor neurones.

What has served sensory physiology so well has been the vigorous simplification of the stimuli used, which enables the neuronal responses to them to be more easily interpreted. It would be difficult if not impossible, for example, to identify a sensory trace corresponding to a complete visual panorama, but it is relatively to observe the response to a simple orientated bar. Expecting to be able to isolate a motor trace for a complete movement may be like attempting to identify a simple neural counterpart in the visual cortex for the experience of viewing the Mona Lisa! Our current knowledge of the visual system should convince us that that is impossible at present.

Spinal reflexes

Successful investigation of motor physiology requires a strategy similar to that which has been so useful in studying sensation—simplification of the movement under study. Research on spinal cord reflexes may be seen as a step in this direction. 'Higher' motor centres are removed in the operation of *decerebration.* In addition to removing the animal's ability to feel pain, making the use of anaesthetics unnecessary, decerebration limits the repertoire of movements which the animal can make to spinal cord and brainstem reflexes alone. The pain centres in the thalamus and cerebral cortex are completely removed in the standard 'mid-collicular' decerebration; the remaining reflex behaviours may then be subjected to detailed analytical study.

A reflex is an involuntary, stereotyped and therefore highly predictable motor response to a particular sensory stimulus (Fig. 13.1). The invariance of reflex responses implies underlying invariance of the connections in the spinal cord among the neurones which execute it. Of course motor activity of intact animals is not stereotyped like this. Teleceptors, cortical receiving and association areas and higher motor centres, particularly the cerebellum, basal ganglia and motor cortex, enable the parameters of basic reflex organization to be altered, substituted and even reversed in the light of prevailing circumstances and the needs of the animal at the time; they liberate an animal from its reflexes.

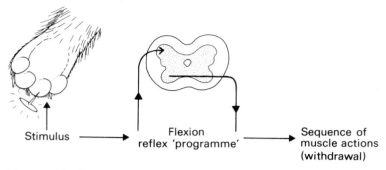

Fig. 13.1. The flexion reflex.

The influence of higher centres, however, makes underlying spinal mechanisms less easy to study. Decerebration allows examination of the complete pathway for many reflexes, from receptors through the spinal cord and then back to the muscles. The lessons learnt from these artificially simplified systems can then be applied to the much more complex situation found in conscious, moving, intact animals. It must never be forgotten however that the description of any reflex is a convenient abstraction. It is a means of 'dissecting' the intact control system, but the process of dissection alters normal operation. Hence the study of reflexes can only give a partial insight into the normal control of movement.

Electroanatomy

The initial stages of sensory processing remain unaffected by anaesthetics; so in anaesthetized animals features of a stimulus may be correlated with the neuronal responses recorded along the appropriate sensory pathway. But since anaesthetized animals cannot move voluntarily, voluntary movement cannot be studied in this way. Using anaesthetized animals the electrophysiologist interested in movement is really limited to confirming the existence of pathways described by neuroanatomists—the study sometimes known rather disparagingly as 'electroanatomy'. Nevertheless, this technique is essential for obtaining details about such things as the quantitative importance and conduction velocity of pathways and, most important of all, for finding out which connections are predominantly excitatory and which inhibitory.

A most useful technique for investigating movement control is to make lesions, to destroy putative motor centres in the brain, either physically or pharmacologically, and observe what changes in movement control ensue. It is often necessary to train animals beforehand to make particular types of movement, chosen to reveal expected deficits clearly. However, lesions, even if accurately positioned, almost always disrupt fibres travelling through the region from structures quite removed from the intended target. The results may thus have little to do with the structure supposedly ablated.

Deficiency and release symptoms

The results of lesions are relatively easy to interpret if the affected area has a predominantly excitatory effect on motor pathways. The lesion then removes some motor ability, giving rise to 'deficiency' or 'negative' symptoms. However, if the ablated structure normally holds another motor centre in check, the result of its destruction may often be extra, 'involuntary' movements or distortions of posture. These are known as 'release' or 'positive' symptoms. They are usually much more difficult to interpret because pathological activity may emanate from any of the large number of areas with which the ablated structure communicates. This is a particular problem in the case of elucidating the functions of the basal ganglia but because the motor systems are organized as a hierarchy, with higher levels both restraining and potentiating lower levels, the interpretation of release symptoms is a common problem in motor physiology.

Plasticity

An even more formidable problem is presented by the way in which the central nervous system can compensate very rapidly for lost tissue, alternative 'parallel' motor pathways taking over missing functions. This plasticity of the CNS is a fortunate corollary of one of its main characteristics—long-term adaptation to changes in the outside world—but it means that the final results of a lesion do not always tell us a great deal about the normal functions of a structure, but more about the functions which are exclusive to it and cannot be taken over by other parts of the CNS. Recently developed techniques for temporarily inactivating certain areas (pharmacologically or by local cooling) may however enable us to learn more about the normal functions of an area.

Recording in conscious trained animals

Study of movement control in the intact unanaesthetized animal is much more difficult. What is required is to induce an animal to make a simple movement repeatedly, keeping all other muscles and joints in a constant state, whilst recording from appropriate parts of the nervous system. This can now be partly achieved using painless recording techniques in conscious animals trained to perform movements as stereotyped as the decerebrate's spinal reflexes. For instance a monkey can be trained to move a lever, using a simple wrist movement, within 250 ms of a light signal (Fig. 13.2). The activity of neurones in motor cortex, basal ganglia, cerebellum, etc., can then be timed and correlated with this simple action and with the visual stimulus triggering it. These techniques are still in their infancy and the problems of correlating neuronal activity with even the simplest of movements are formidable; but eventually a combination of recording from conscious animals and training them by operant conditioning to perform the types of movement thought to be regulated by structures under investigation promises to be as fruitful to the study of motor physiology as Hubel and Wiesel's use of line and edge stimuli has been to the understanding of visual processing.

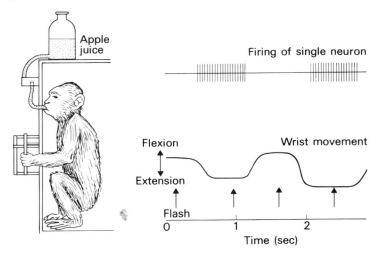

Fig. 13.2. Recording from motor cortex in a conscious monkey rewarded for moving the wrist following a light flash (from Evarts E.V. (1968) *J. Neurophysiol.*, **31**, 14).

MOVEMENT 'MODALITIES'

That there are some five or six different sensations and several modalities within each sensation goes a long way to explaining why there are so many parallel sensory pathways; though the existence of 'second' sensory pathways with slightly different functional roles somewhat complicates this simple picture. On the motor side, however, we have not yet been able to sketch even a simplified picture to explain the several parallel motor pathways. Unfortunately, they probably all contribute to the control of every movement, rather as separate sensations all contribute to a complete sensory experience; this naturally makes understanding their different functions very difficult.

Distal v. axial muscles

It is probable, nevertheless, that each motor pathway performs a different function; the problem is to identify it. What are motor equivalents to the different senses such as hearing and vision? One approach to this question has been anatomical; movements are classified according to whether the prime movers are axial (trunk), proximal or distal limb muscles (Fig. 13.3). The separate sites of these muscles may be analogous to the anatomical separation of sensory surfaces (e.g. photoreceptors situated in the retina and

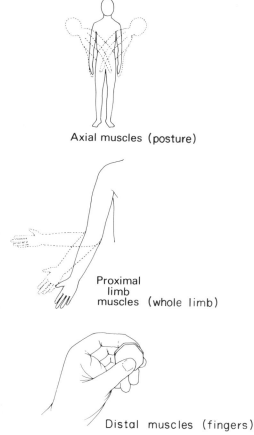

Axial muscles (posture)

Proximal limb muscles (whole limb)

Distal muscles (fingers)

Fig. 13.3. The 'anatomical' classification of types of movement.

auditory mechanoreceptors in the cochlea). As we shall see, there is now ample evidence that axial, proximal and distal muscles are controlled by largely separate descending systems.

Automatic v. voluntary movements

Another classification of movements divides them into voluntary and postural (automatic). Although it is quite clear that we make postural adjustments unconsciously and automatically all the time, without necessarily making any voluntary movements, the converse is never the case; we can never make voluntary movements without corresponding postural adjustments. Indeed, appropriate postural changes usually anticipate voluntary movement. When one leans over to grasp an object the first muscles to increase their force of contraction are those in the thigh, anticipating changes in the centre of gravity.

A hierarchy of motor levels

It is important to realize that there is a whole spectrum of possible movements ranging from the most automatic (postural) to the least automatic (voluntary). Not only are postural movements mostly carried out by axial and proximal muscles served by 'medial' descending systems, whilst voluntary movements all involve distal muscles in the limbs served by 'lateral' descending pathways, but also the most automatic adjustments may often be carried out by the lowest centres in the spinal cord, such as those mediating the stretch reflex. Voluntary movements, however, require participation of higher levels of the nervous system—cerebral cortex and upper brainstem.

Anatomical overview

The motor cortex and lateral corticospinal (pyramidal) tract are thought to be primarily concerned with voluntary control over the most distal muscles, controlling, for example, independent finger movements and curling of a prehensile tail. The red nucleus and lateral reticular formation of the brainstem, together with their laterally descending projections, are chiefly concerned with proximal (voluntary and postural) movements of the limbs, e.g. shoulder, elbow and wrist movements. The vestibular system, medial brainstem reticular formation and medially descending pathways are thought to be responsible for controlling axial musculature, and hence automatic control of body posture. The cerebellum is said to contribute to all three systems: lateral cerebellar cortex and dentate nucleus cooperate with motor cortex in evolving the strategy for voluntary movements of the extremities; intermediate cerebellar cortex and interpositus nucleus work with the red nucleus to organize detailed execution of whole limb movements; whilst vermis and fastigial nucleus relay to the vestibular system and medial reticular formation to help control body posture. The basal ganglia are sometimes said to be concerned only with posture and to play no part in voluntary movement. However, this takes no account of the major projection from the basal ganglia to motor cortex, whose importance explains why one of the cardinal symptoms of Parkinson's disease (of the basal ganglia) is inability to make voluntary movements.

Corticospinal system

Clearly the above scheme is highly oversimplified. For example, the role of the corticospinal system is more complex. Although the main function of the corticospinal system (pyramidal tract) appears to be to control contralateral distal musculature (particularly that of the forelimb in primates), in order to achieve this the motor cortex has also gained considerable control over more proximal muscles of the forelimb. Accurate positioning of the fingers clearly requires prior positioning of the shoulder, elbow and wrist. Thus when movements of these joints are required for precise finger action the motor cortex can institute them. It can execute this control by making use of its 'extrapyramidal' connections with the basal ganglia, cerebellum, red nucleus and reticular formation, and also by using pyramidal tract connections in the spinal cord which influence motoneurones supplying proximal muscles, as well as those supplying distal muscles. The attention of the motor cortex then is by no means confined to distal motoneurones. Similarly, vestibulospinal projections are not entirely confined to proximal motoneurones.

Ballistic and feedback control (Fig. 13.4)

Another promising way of approaching this problem of defining separate functional roles for different parallel motor pathways is to consider the methods employed to control movement. An important distinction is between 'open-loop', 'feedforward' or 'ballistic', and 'closed-loop', 'feedback' or 'pursuit' modes of control.

Ballistic control (open loop)

Ballistic movements are those which are completely 'preprogrammed' before they start; so that they are completed independently of whatever may happen during their execution. The

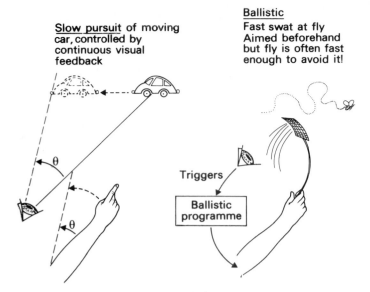

Fig. 13.4. Pursuit and ballistic control of movement.

word is derived from the Latin *ballista*—a catapult. The science of ballistics is devoted to predicting the course of a projectile after it leaves its projector from prior knowledge of its velocity, weight, elevation, etc. The flight of a stone from a catapult is predetermined by these factors; it is preprogrammed. Similarly, the course of a ballistic movement is set, following a central 'programme'. A control signal is fed to the muscles effecting the movement without the benefit of feedback information during its execution (Fig. 13.3). This arrangement has the advantage that it can act very quickly and powerfully. However, being stereotyped, such a system cannot compensate for any disturbances whether they are external (e.g. changes of load) or internal (e.g. muscle fatigue).

Pursuit control (closed loop)

Guided missiles, unlike catapult projectiles, may be controlled by signals derived from their target or even from the ground. Likewise the *pursuit movements* made by animals are continuously controlled by feedback from their intended target and from the moving limb. A 'closed' control loop is formed linking target to control mechanism, control mechanism to limb, and limb to target (Fig. 13.4). Sensory signals about the actual position of the target and the limb are compared and used to match the movement of the limb to that of the target. The advantage of this mode of control is that negative feedback can readily compensate for unexpected disturbances. However, it is slow.

Since the nervous system conducts relatively slowly in relation to the speed at which many movements have to take place (e.g. the rapid eye movements known as saccades), none of the most rapid movements of which an animal is capable can be controlled by continuous sensory feedback; such actions have to be preprogrammed ballistically. Often however, ballistic performance of a fast movement may be improved by incorporating information about how it went off last time. Fast movements of large amplitude are usually performed in two stages, consisting of a relatively crude ballistic jerk in the general direction of the target, followed by a much more precise corrective movement homing in on it. Incorporation of 'historical' feedback concerning the results of past movements and current feedback necessary for corrections at the end of a movement is probably an important function of the cerebellum. Only slow movements (e.g. those made when tracking a moving target) can be controlled by continuous feedback throughout their course. Even such slow movements require some sort of central programme to initiate them.

Predictive control

Not even slow movements, then, are entirely feedback controlled nor, in fact, are all fast movements entirely ballistic. For instance, some slow movements are not made in pursuit of an object and therefore cannot derive target movement signals to guide them. An 'internal programme' must exist somewhere in the nervous system to generate the sequence of signals which causes the muscles to execute the movement. An example of this is the case of 'predictive' movements—e.g. matching the position of a limb to the expected position of a target which is temporarily blanked out. Here, information about the previous trajectory of the object is used to form a prediction of where it is likely to move to in the future. The only movements which are entirely preprogrammed are those made to express some idea or emotion; most others are at least *triggered* by some external event, such as a visual or auditory stimulus, and then may proceed ballistically, often ending with a final, slower, feedback-controlled corrective movement onto the target.

Cerebellum and feedback control (Fig. 13.5)

There is, as yet, no agreement among physiologists about which parts of the nervous system are responsible for these different movement strategies. However, the evidence suggests that the cerebellum, along with its associated structures (pontine nuclei, inferior olive, etc.), is the highest centre concerned chiefly with using feedback, projected from brainstem, cerebral cortex and spinal cord, to control current movements and perhaps also with acquiring 'skill', using feedback about the past results of a particular movement to improve its execution in the future.

Basal ganglia and ballistic control (Fig. 13.5)

The highest centres concerned with ballistic control are probably the basal ganglia. On instructions from the cerebral cortex these are probably able to generate preprogrammed trains of signals for the execution of crude ballistic movements, which are released to motor centres following appropriate cues. The cerebellum probably contributes skill and precision to these basic patterns, on the basis of feedback information gained from previous movements and stored.

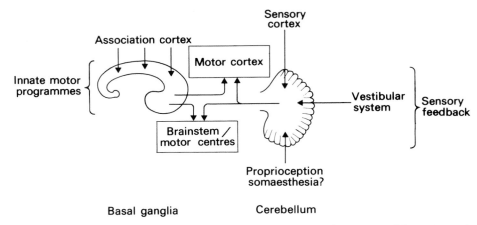

Fig. 13.5. The basal ganglia probably provide innate 'programmes' for movement, whilst the cerebellum is involved in feedback control.

Motor cortex (Fig. 13.5)

Both cerebellum and basal ganglia employ motor cortex and brainstem motor structures to execute their actions. Thus the motor cortex is now judged to be rather low down in the anatomical hierarchy of motor structures; some of the pyramidal tract neurones within it are only two synapses removed from the muscles themselves. However, under certain circumstances direct connections from skin and muscle receptors to motor cortex and its monosynaptic projections to spinal cord motoneurones enable it to override all other elements in the hierarchy. This underlies the 'long loop' or 'cortical' stretch reflex discussed in Chapter 14.

Movement initiation

It is now clear that the motor cortex is not the site of 'free will' as was somewhat naively believed by some of the people who first stimulated the region and saw movement of the extremities. Expressions such as 'the Will to move', 'the conception or idea of movement', 'initiation' and 'command' abound in the literature on movement control. Clearly, it was thought by early workers in the field that electrical stimulation might indicate where these things happen. However, movements are initiated in response to all sorts of external and internal triggers. It is highly unlikely that one could ever find a single anatomical site where all motor activity could be said to commence. Rather, the initiation of movements depends on their stimulus—visual association areas relay signals for visually triggered movements; auditory areas for responses to sound; limbic system for drive-reducing behaviour, etc. Hence the purely verbal convenience of referring to 'initiation' of movement, as though it were a process common to all movements, probably does not correspond to any single, definable neurophysiological process or specific neural structure. The responsibility for initiating and commanding movements is probably distributed over a large number of structures whose precise identity varies with the current stimulus for movement and the type of movement to be made.

Initiation as decision

The phrase 'initiation of movement' is often used in a rather different way, however, to refer to the decision-making process which must precede movement. The anatomical pathways which link visual, auditory and somaesthetic processing areas to motor structures, although permanent, are only employed when an animal 'decides' to move—when it allows a sensory stimulus to trigger or regulate activity. This opening of appropriate pathways is probably a function of the limbic system, which directs behaviour according to internal drive states.

VISUAL CONTROL OF MOVEMENT (Fig. 13.6)

We can exemplify these considerations by examining visually controlled movements (which constitute perhaps 70% of all human actions). Vision may be involved in the control of movement in three ways. A movement may be triggered by a visual stimulus, such as when one smiles on recognizing a friend; visual information may be used to calculate the required trajectory of a ballistic movement; or it may be used in the control of a pursuit movement, allowing continuous correction in response to visual feedback.

Visual phase

First, an object of interest is identified by the visual system. As described in Chapter 6, the visual cortical areas have two main executive outflows, dorsally towards movement-sensitive areas in superior temporal sulcus and the parietal lobes, ventrally towards the temporal lobe and limbic system. The former carries information about the position and movement of objects, and of the position and movement of the eyes. These pathways are of obvious significance for controlling an animal's movements in relation to an object, but are only activated if 'switched on' in some way. The route into the limbic system carries information about the nature of an object independently of its position or movements, probably classifying its 'significance' to the animal in terms of danger, nutrition, etc.

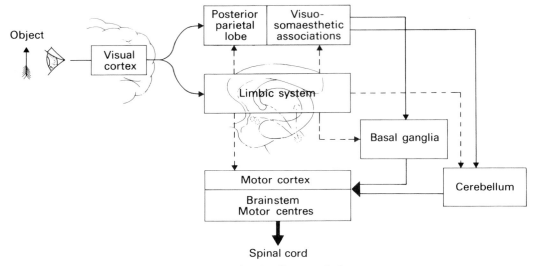

Fig. 13.6. Main routes for visually controlled movement.

'Limbic gating'

The next stage in the organization of a visually controlled movement is the 'gating' or switching-on of motor systems. This probably depends on whether the object is of interest or not, and is presumably decided by the limbic system according to the object's drive-reducing potential, as noted earlier. Very little is known about the process, except that it happens. Many sensori-motor connections in the cortex and brainstem are facilitated only if an animal is going to move. Thus the limbic system 'initiates' movements in this rather non-specific sense of facilitating prewired sensory motor pathways. It would be difficult to identify an 'initiating signal' by conventional electrophysiological techniques because this facilitation probably does not take the form of a discrete electrical signal locked in time to eventual movement; rather it enables motor systems to operate if called upon, perhaps employing long-term 'neuromodulators' such as catecholamines.

Sensory associations

Before the motor system can formulate a signal to move the hand to grasp an object, it must first calculate where the limb is currently positioned in relation to it—position of limb and object must be *associated*. This probably first takes place in posterior parietal areas 5 and 7. Cutaneous and proprioceptive records of limb position reach area 5 and signals about the position of objects, derived either from the retina or from the position of the eye inspecting them, are delivered to area 7. Ablation of these areas prevents accurate reaching for objects. Area 7 has been called the initiator or 'command centre' for visually controlled movements. It is now clear, however, that association of visual and proprioceptive inputs proceeds here all the time; but parietal neurone activity is enhanced and gated through to lower motor centres only if the animal is going to move. So the decision to move is probably made elsewhere— probably in the limbic system.

Subcortical phase

The next stage of movement control probably involves descent to *subcortical* motor structures, particularly the cerebellum which receives a large projection from movement-sensitive areas of the visual cortex and from parietal regions 5 and 7; perhaps the basal ganglia are also involved, they receive visual and parietal projections. The direct cortico-cortical projection from visual cortex to frontal lobe is less important. It passes to prefrontal rather than motor cortex and is probably chiefly concerned with the control of eye movements by the frontal eye fields (area 8).

Motor cortex and brainstem

The lateral part of the cerebellum and part of the basal ganglia project back to the motor cortex via the ventro-lateral nucleus of the thalamus. However, both basal ganglia and cerebellum also project directly to brainstem motor structures, bypassing motor cortex. Movements of a whole limb thus involve activation not only of the motor cortex but also of the red nucleus, reticular formation, vestibular system, etc., all of which cooperate in engineering them. The sole function that it seems only the motor cortex can perform is fine control of the contractions of the most distal muscles which effect precise movements of individual digits. Since such control is only necessary during the final phases of a whole-limb movement, it is probable that the motor cortex, far from planning and initiating voluntary movements, actually participates only at a relatively late stage in their execution. This conclusion is supported by recent results of recording electrical activity and local blood flow (another index of the activity of a region) in the motor cortex. These only increase just prior to a movement, whereas prefrontal cortex, sensory association areas and supplementary motor cortex all show changes much earlier.

Spinal cord

The final common path upon which all this cerebral activity ultimately is concentrated consists of the motoneurones lying in the ventral horn of the spinal cord. These receive from the corticospinal (pyramidal) tract both directly and indirectly, via local interneurones, and from medial or lateral 'extrapyramidal' descending pathways. Extensors lie dorsal to flexor motoneurones, and those supplying axial (postural) musculature lie medially to those supplying distal muscles. The smallest motoneurones which supply the most slowly contracting muscle fibres are recruited most easily, and therefore discharge first when a muscle is activated; the largest supply the fastest, phasic, muscle fibres and discharge later. During moderate contractions therefore the largest motoneurones may never be activated at all. The dependence of the order of discharge of motoneurones on their physical size is known, logically enough, as the 'size principle'. The size principle may well be an automatic device for ensuring that the contraction of both fast and slow muscle fibres is finally synchronized; the slower contraction of some fibres being compensated by the earlier recruitment of the small motoneurones supplying them.

CONCLUSIONS

As a result of the enormous difficulties involved in controlling and quantifying movements, motor systems are far less well understood than their sensory counterparts. However, it will be useful to the reader in the following chapters to attempt to make comparisons between motor and sensory systems. It will also be useful to bear in mind whether axial (postural) muscles or distal (voluntary) muscles are predominantly involved in a movement under consideration, since medial descending systems control axial muscles, while lateral systems control distal muscles. Furthermore, it is important to distinguish between feedback and ballistic 'feedforward' systems, as the neural systems involved may again be different. Finally, it is unrealistic to try to make too hard and fast distinctions between sensory and motor processes. Sensory inputs are used in many different ways in the control of movement: as cues or triggers; to calculate the parameters of a ballistic movement; or during negative feedback control to make continuous comparisons as a movement proceeds. However, movement itself can often become an important input for sensory systems; for example, movement of the eyes to a new position indicates to the visual system where objects identified on the fovea are actually situated in space; movement of the hand over a three-dimensional object indicates where one edge lies in relation to another. Furthermore, conversion of input from sensory receptors into motor output is not a series of discrete steps but a continuum. There is no point where sensation stops and movement begins. It is thus counter-productive to spend a lot of time attempting to define what is truly sensory and what is motor.

Chapter 14
Spinal Cord, Muscle Receptors and Spinal Reflexes

The technique of decerebration enabled Sherrington and his successors to discover an enormous amount about the basic principles of operation of the brainstem and spinal cord. Many of the concepts derived from these studies may be transferred piecemeal to the intact nervous system. The advantage of the decerebrate preparation results from eliminating cortical and brainstem descending influences, which allows uncomplicated reflex activity of the spinal cord to be studied.

REFLEXES

The sensory inputs to the spinal cord which arrive along the dorsal roots (from cutaneous, muscle, joint and deep fascial receptors) not only provide information for ascending sensory pathways, such as the dorsal column and spinothalamic systems, but may also elicit reflex responses, employing collateral connections which they make with interneurones and motoneurones in the grey matter of the spinal cord.

A reflex may be defined as an *involuntary, stereotyped* but *co-ordinated* motor response to a sensory stimulus. It was thought by the ancients that the sensory energy contained in the stimulus flowed towards the centre and was physically 'reflected' from there back out to the muscles. The important point about reflexes is that their *predictability* indicates an underlying stability within the CNS of the anatomical connections which are responsible for them. Co-ordinated programmes for appropriate muscle actions and their regulation by feedback from the periphery are 'hard-wired' into the spinal cord. In the case of some of the best-studied, such as the stretch, 'claspknife' and flexion reflexes, this spinal cord wiring has been elucidated in great detail.

Open-loop and closed-loop reflexes

In the same way as we can distinguish between 'open-loop' and 'closed-loop' modes of overall motor control, so we can make a distinction between open- and closed-loop reflexes. An open-loop reflex is one in which the stimulus triggers a sequence of actions whose course is not controlled by the stimulus and which do not themselves affect it. For example, a painful stimulus elicits the 'flexion' reflex, which is a coordinated sequence of contractions of most of the muscles of the limb, withdrawing it from the danger. The flexion reflex is not regulated by the stimulus during its execution, nor does it have any feedback effect on the painful stimulus itself; thus it forms an open loop. In contrast, the stretch reflex is a closed loop; the stimulus (muscle stretch) both regulates the degree of muscle contraction and is itself affected by the response, which feeds back on the stimulus thus reducing it.

Stretch (myotatic) reflex

The simplest reflex is achieved by just two neurones, a sensory afferent projecting directly to a motoneurone, which it excites (Fig. 14.1). The properties of the stretch reflex were first described in 1924 by Liddell and Sherrington. Sherrington was studying the phenomenon of 'decerebrate rigidity'. Division of the brainstem at the standard midcollicular level leaves an animal in which the physiological extensors (antigravity muscles) are powerfully contracted. This condition has been called 'a caricature of normal standing' (Fig. 14.2). Any attempt to stretch these muscles causes them to resist the stretch by contracting even more. Section of the brainstem lower down in the medulla yields a flaccid 'spinal' animal, suggesting that the excitation of extensors which underlies decerebrate rigidity originates higher up, in the midbrain and pons.

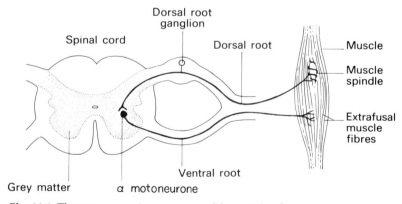

Fig. 14.1. The monosynaptic component of the stretch reflex.

Local sign

Careful study of decerebrate rigidity showed that it has pronounced 'local sign'. Even after severance of all cutaneous and muscle nerves to a limb except the afferent and efferent fibres to the muscle under study, stretch of that muscle excites its own 'autonomous' motoneurones, inducing reflex contraction (Fig. 14.2). The stretch

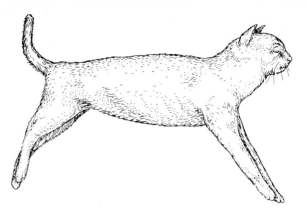

Fig. 14.2. Decerebrate rigidity—a caricature of normal stance.

receptors mediating the reflex are, therefore, to be found in the contracting muscle itself. They were subsequently identified as *muscle spindles*. As would be expected, cutting the dorsal roots which carry the spindles' stretch signals to the spinal cord leads to collapse of decerebrate rigidity by abolishing the stretch reflex.

Stretch of any of the muscles which normally contract together (synergists) causes a large response in the stretched muscle together with a smaller reflex response in its neighbours and inhibition of antagonists operating the other side of the joint. This is known as *reciprocal inhibition*. Thus a muscle's stretch reflex is excited most strongly by spindles within it (local sign) and to a lesser extent those in synergists, and it is inhibited by spindles in antagonistic muscles. This arrangement tends to fix muscles at a constant length and to resist any attempt to change that length; clearly, therefore, it could contribute to the maintenance of stable posture.

Passive elastic tension

Cutting the ventral roots carrying motor nerves to a muscle leads to collapse of its activity. Although this observation is not in itself very illuminating, since a muscle deprived of motor nerve supply obviously cannot exhibit reflex activity, cutting the motor nerve supply to a muscle does enable one to assess afterward the contribution made by passive elastic properties of the muscle to the total tension which it achieved when fully innervated.

Monosynaptic component

It was shown by Lloyd that the very first component of the stretch reflex probably only has time to traverse one synapse, so that the initial component of the reflex is mediated by a monosynaptic two-neurone arc. Cajal had already suggested this arrangement on the basis of Golgi studies which had shown the possibility of direct connections between collaterals of the large, myelinated dorsal root afferents and ventral horn motoneurones. In fact it has now been found that each myelinated spindle afferent makes at least one synaptic contact with every motoneurone supplying the muscle in which it is situated.

Tendon jerk—dynamic stretch reflex

The rapid, monosynaptic, *phasic* component of the stretch reflex is utilized daily by physicians testing their patients' tendon jerks in order to establish the integrity of afferent and efferent connections to muscles and of the excitability of the spinal cord synapses between them. A sharp tap applied to the patella tendon suddenly stretches the quadriceps muscle together with the muscle spindle endings sensitive to rapid stretch within it; these communicate the stretch to the spinal cord which therefore excites thigh muscle motoneurones, in part monosynaptically, to jerk the leg. However, later components in the e.m.g. show that longer-lasting poly-synaptic pathways, some travelling as far as the sensorimotor cortex and back, are also involved in the tendon jerk.

Tonic stretch reflex

The *dynamic*, or phasic, component of the stretch reflex is only part of the story, however. Even when the length of a muscle is kept constant, muscle spindles return a signal of this static length to the spinal cord; this underlies the *tonic*, or static, stretch reflex which acts continually, particularly in extensor muscles. Although there is recent evidence to suggest that spindle endings, which are sensitive to the current length of a muscle, also make monosynaptic connec-tions directly on to motoneurones, the major role in the tonic stretch reflex is probably undertaken by polysynaptic pathways engaging many spinal cord interneurones. These pathways enable the excita-tion to greatly outlast muscle spindle input. Confusingly, however, in some decerebrate preparations the predominant action of muscle spindle secondary endings is inhibitory and contributes to the clasp-knife reflex.

Ia inhibitory interneurones

Reciprocal inhibition of muscles antagonistic to a stretched muscle is mediated by a disynaptic pathway. Muscle spindle endings excite Ia inhibitory interneurones by releasing glutamate or aspartate. These interneurones are located in Rexed's lamina IX, dorsal to the α- and γ-motoneurones supplying antagonistic muscles. They probably inhibit the motoneurones by releasing GABA. All the neuronal pathways which excite α- and γ-motoneurones, such as Ia, cutaneous, rubrospinal and corticospinal inputs, also excite the Ia inhibitory interneurones, and thus ensure reciprocal inhibition of antagonists.

Renshaw cells, which are activated by cholinergic motoneurone collaterals and exert recurrent inhibition on these motoneurones to limit their firing rate, also inhibit Ia interneurones, thus removing inhibition of antagonistic muscles and helping to limit the excursion of a limb.

MUSCLE SPINDLES

All sorts of questions were thrown up by the discovery of the stretch reflex, many of which still remain unanswered. Which receptors are responsible and how do they work? How does the phasic component of the reflex relate to the maintained tonic contraction responsible for decerebrate rigidity? Most importantly, since most muscles (with the notable exception of eye muscles) are endowed with a stretch reflex, what is its role in posture and how is it modified to allow movement? It is easy to see how myotatic maintenance of a constant muscle length could assist in regulating posture, but less easy to understand how it could contribute to the changes in muscle length which are required if a limb is to be moved.

All striated muscles contain stretch receptors situated alongside the main muscle fibres, in parallel with them, so that when the muscle is lengthened they discharge, but when it shortens they are 'unloaded'. Thus, in principle, they signal the length of a muscle rather than its tension. These stretch receptors are situated within their own fibrous sheath or capsule, shaped like a spindle of thread—hence their name.

Intrafusal muscles

Muscle spindles contain their own specialized *intrafusal* muscle fibres, which place them under central control. These intrafusal muscles are of three types: 'nuclear bag' 1 and 2 and 'nuclear chain' (Fig. 14.3). Each spindle contains at least two nuclear bag fibres (bag 1 and bag 2) and up to ten nuclear chain fibres. These fibres are so named on account of the arrangement of their nuclei: either in a central 'bag' or in line along the middle of the fibre. Only the ends (known as 'poles') of intrafusal muscle fibres contract. Their sensory nerve terminals are situated on the central, non-contractile, 'equatorial' region, and are therefore stretched when intrafusal muscle fibres contract. The two types of fibre contract at different rates—nuclear bag fibres contract slowly and nuclear chain fibres contract fast. Their contractile poles are supplied by specialized *fusimotor, γ efferent* nerves which terminate on nuclear bag fibres as 'plate', and on nuclear chain fibres as 'trail', motor end plates. Aγ axons (3–8 μm in diameter) constitute some 30% of all the motor nerves supplying a muscle; the other 70% are the Aα axons (9–17 μm) which innervate the main muscle fibres (known, in this context, as *extrafusal* fibres since they lie outside the spindle). A few Aβ fibres divide to innervate both intrafusal and extrafusal fibres.

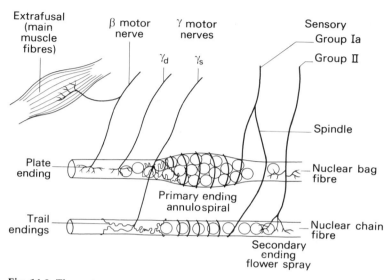

Fig. 14.3. The main components of the muscle spindle.

Receptors (Fig. 14.3)

Encircling the middle of both chain- and bag-type fibres lie the *annulospiral* endings, branches of a single, large, group-Ia *primary* afferent nerve; whilst on nuclear chain fibres, two *flowerspray* endings of the small, group-II *secondary* afferent nerves lie on either side of the annulospiral terminal. These arrangements confer on spindle primary endings both a high sensitivity to the rate at which muscle length changes (*dynamic response*), particularly for small movements (<0.1 mm), derived from their attachment to nuclear bag fibres, and a weak sensitivity to instantaneous length (*static response*) provided by nuclear chain fibres (Fig. 14.4b). However, the discharge of secondary endings is proportional to the actual (static) length of a muscle alone, and not to changes in length.

Control of dynamic and static sensitivity

The separate arrangement of plate and trail fusimotor nerves and bag and chain intrafusal muscle fibres allows the dynamic and static

sensitivities of a spindle to be varied independently by CNS centrifugal control. Dynamic fusimotor efferents (γd) cause contraction of
the polar regions of the slow nuclear bag 1 fibres, in effect increasing
their viscosity but not causing them to shorten, so that changes in
muscle length are more sensitively conveyed to the annulospiral
endings (Fig. 14.4d); whilst the steady-state length signal provided
by secondary endings situated on nuclear chain fibres is not altered
much. Static fusimotor efferents (γs), on the other hand, cause rapid
contraction of the poles of fast nuclear chain fibres and also of bag 2
fibres, so that the sensitivity to static length of a muscle, signalled by
both primary and secondary receptors, is enhanced but dynamic
sensitivity is unchanged (Fig. 14.4c).

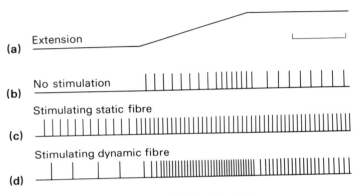

Fig. 14.4. Responses of muscle spindle Ia afferent fibre.

The picturesque terminology employed by muscle spindle
histologists gives emphasis to the highly elaborate neuromuscular
machinery contained in spindles. It seems to be incredibly
complicated—just to measure muscle length! Why do we need
separate static and dynamic signals concerning length, and why do
we need separate central nervous controls over their sensitivities?
As explained in Chapter 4, dynamic sensitivity of receptors is
desirable in order to help to compensate for time lags in negative
feedback systems—preventing instability and 'hunting'. One can
see that knowing the rate at which a muscle changes its length might
enable a control system to predict where the muscle will be at some
future instant, and thus avoid overshoot. The dynamic response of
muscle spindle primaries could well provide 'damping' of this sort
(indeed this function for the stretch reflex was suggested early in its
history (see Fig. 5.8)), but this is a far cry from understanding
precisely how the dynamic information is used by the spinal cord
and supraspinal machinery to achieve this end. The most we can say
at present about the mechanism by which damping is achieved is
that both velocity and position feedback affect the spinal cord. The
dynamic receptors (primaries) subserve the rapid phasic stretch

reflex, whilst the static secondaries probably underlie its slower tonic
component.

Role of fusimotor control

During active contraction of a muscle its spindles become unloaded,
so they cease firing and as a result become useless as length
transducers. Hence the simplest explanation for the existence of
fusimotor control of muscle spindles is that γ efferents effect
intrafusal muscle contraction in order to enable them to 'keep up'
with extrafusal muscle contraction, and not to become silent just
when they are needed most. However, this explanation actually
raises many more questions than it answers. Efferent fusimotor
control causes the output of a spindle to become a function not only
of muscle length but also of fusimotor activity. Each time intrafusal
contraction occurs, therefore, the 'meaning' of a spindle's discharge
changes in terms of the real length of a muscle. Presumably spindle
signals must be continually 'recalibrated' centrally, but we have no
inkling of how this is done.

Servo-action

The Second World War forced great advances in theoretical understanding of feedback control systems designed to shift the aim of
heavy guns, searchlights, etc. Since so much of physiology is taken
up with attempting to understand the body's control systems, it is
not surprising that physiologists soon took over many of the same
ideas. One of the problems to which they were first applied was the
stretch reflex.

Regulators and servo-mechanisms (Fig. 14.5)

Feedback control systems can be divided into two broad categories:
regulators in which a variable, such as muscle length, the temperature of the body or blood pressure, is to be held at a constant

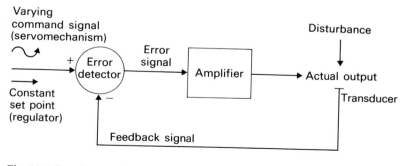

Fig. 14.5. Regulators and servo-mechanisms—negative feedback control systems.

set-point; and *servo-mechanisms*, where the variable to be controlled, such as the desired position of a limb, must be allowed to change, so the control mechanism is designed to follow variations in a *command signal* in a servile fashion.

For the regulation of posture one can view the stretch reflex as working in the regulator mode, since the maintenance of an upright position clearly requires a control system which will keep muscle lengths constant. However, for voluntary movement or for any change of posture, the tendency of the stretch reflex to hold a muscle at a constant length is obviously unhelpful. Either the stretch reflex must be suppressed during movements or it must be used in a different way—as a servo-mechanism.

The 'follow-up length' servo hypothesis

Eldred, Granit and Merton suggested in 1953 that supraspinal control over fusimotor outflow might enable the stretch reflex to be employed as a servo. They suggested that the command for a muscle to shorten passes not to α-, but to γ-motoneurones. These would cause spindle intrafusal muscle fibres to contract, exciting primary and secondary afferents which in turn would excite α-motoneurones by the mono- and polysynaptic connections of the stretch reflex. α-discharge would therefore 'follow up' the γ-signal and cause the main muscle to contract until spindle discharge ceased (Fig. 14.6). The advantage of this apparently cumbersome *gamma loop* mechanism would be *load compensation*, although it would act slowly.

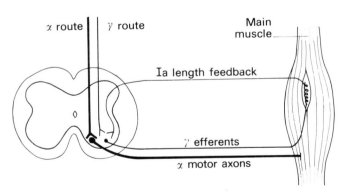

Fig. 14.6. The 'follow-up length' hypothesis. A command signal passes to γ-motoneurones which set the length of spindle intrafusal fibres. Length feedback then excites α-motoneurones until the main muscle length equals the value set by the muscle spindles.

Load compensation

Muscle spindle intrafusal fibres experience essentially constant load, for they lie in parallel with the main muscle fibres and have no connection with an external load. They contract only at their poles and are free to slide within the spindle sheath. Thus they produce no external tension and no overall shortening of the muscle, only stretch of spindle afferent endings. Thus a given γ-efferent signal produces a reliable amount of intrafusal muscle contraction of a predictable magnitude whatever happens to the extrafusal fibres. The main muscle, on the other hand, has to develop varying amounts of force, depending on the load to be shifted and the speed with which it must move. Furthermore, the amount of force which a muscle can produce in response to identical neural signals depends on its length at the time and the velocity with which it is moving, as a result of the non-linear length/tension and force/velocity characteristics of skeletal muscle. The CNS must elaborate motoneural signals which can compensate for these factors, even though many are unpredictable. The intrinsic characteristics of a muscle vary from one to another and are altered by fatigue, etc., whilst unexpected weights, changes in load and impediments to movement may occur externally.

A γ-loop mechanism would offer many advantages. Intrafusal muscle fibres would shorten to an accurately calibrated length; this would then cause the extrafusal main muscle fibres to shorten by a controlled amount just sufficient to eliminate the mismatch between the new length of the intrafusal fibres and their own. This would make muscle contraction independent of changes in load, fatigue, etc., because not until the muscle had achieved its new length would the discharge of muscle spindles exciting α-motoneurones and hence the extrafusal muscle fibres return to normal. In short, the system would then be an effective 'follow-up length, load-compensating servo-mechanism'.

Evidence for servo hypothesis

Three crucial sorts of evidence must be provided in order to verify this servo hypothesis. First, the γ-signal must be shown to *lead* the discharge of α-motoneurones, since the two are alleged to be causally related. Secondly, spindle afferent signals must be shown to be quantitatively proportional to the length of a muscle during movement. In the simplest possible scheme, spindle output should fall to zero when the desired length of the muscle had been attained, but should indicate muscle length until then. Finally, if the reflex is to be worth anything as a load-compensating device it must have a high 'gain', i.e. every impulse emitted by the spindle should cause a large extrafusal muscular contraction, in order to eliminate mismatch. Unfortunately, existing evidence in all these areas is equivocal.

γ-lead

First let us consider the problem of γ-lead. Indirect evidence suggested that under some circumstances muscle spindle discharge might precede movement. Immediately after electrical stimulation of the nerve supplying a muscle the electromyogram (e.m.g.) of that muscle falls silent for a short time, suggesting that its normal level of electrical activity is supported by continuous muscle spindle afferent discharge. When this discharge is removed (because the artificially induced contraction unloads the spindles), e.m.g. silence ensues. However, electrically induced muscle contraction is hardly normal movement. It is now clear that muscle spindle signals seldom, if ever, precede extrafusal muscle contraction, rather they lag behind it. In man and experimental animals it is possible to record from muscle spindle afferents during various voluntary movements. In all the situations where it has been exhaustively studied, the first muscle spindle discharge occurs concurrently with or after the onset of the main muscle contraction and never before it (Fig. 14.7).

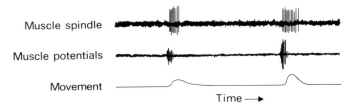

Muscle spindle

Muscle potentials

Movement

Time ⟶

Fig. 14.7. Muscle spindle discharge never precedes but follows onset of a voluntary movement. (After Vallbo Å.B. (1971) *J. Physiol.*, **218**, 405.

α/γ coactivation

The fact that muscle spindles discharge at all during muscle shortening indicates that γ-motoneurones must have been activated in order to counteract unloading of the spindles. In fact α- and γ-motoneurones are often coactivated by the same descending signals; since γ-motoneurones are smaller, the size principle ensures that they are recruited first, to some extent compensating for their slower conduction velocity to the periphery. Thus spindle signals often parallel the force output of a muscle rather than its length, since γ-motoneurones, causing the spindle to discharge, experience the same descending control as α-motoneurones causing the muscle to contract. One might begin to wonder whether muscle spindles do in fact measure length during active shortening at all.

During passive extension of a muscle, however, there is no doubt that they do record muscle length; this may give a clue to the true function of muscle spindles during active contractions. Ia afferents are at their most sensitive during very small stretches and longer extensions elicit disproportionately less discharge. It is possible, therefore, that spindles (and hence the stretch reflex) may provide 'servo-assistance'—effecting load compensation at spinal cord level following small disturbances of muscle length—very quickly. Slower systems involving monitoring of the situation by higher centres may look after the longer-term consequences of larger perturbations, load changes, etc. One should perhaps think of the stretch reflex as the first line of defence against perturbations, 'setting up' the spinal cord quickly in order that higher centres, particularly the motor cortex and cerebellum, can take over compensation later.

Gain of stretch reflex

It seems, therefore, that fusimotor activity seldom precedes that of the main muscle, so that the stretch reflex cannot normally act in the follow-up length servo mode. Furthermore, as a result of α/γ co-activation, the output of a muscle spindle is not always proportional to the length of the muscle in which it is situated. These features would not necessarily prevent the reflex providing servo-assistance in response to unexpected stretches of a muscle during movement. However, for such servo-assistance to be useful, the gain of the stretch reflex under these circumstances must be very high; yet it is extremely difficult to show that this is so. The strength of the spinal stretch reflex is probably rather low during most voluntary movements and even in the advantageous circumstances found in decerebrate animals, reflex tension is often only moderate. Bizzi found that load compensation in monkeys during head movements was almost as good following dorsal root section, which eliminates the stretch reflex, as before it; this implies that the stretch reflex is quantitatively rather unimportant under these circumstances. This has also been shown for many voluntary limb movements in humans. In fact the 'shortening reaction' is made more common in relaxed humans. In this reaction the muscle increases its activity when passively shortened rather than when stretched.

In fact, it appears that we have been carried away by the ease with which the isolated stretch reflex can be studied under the artificial conditions of decerebration into attributing too great an importance to it. As we shall see, the stretch reflex is probably only a part of a more complex spinal cord control system, involving Golgi tendon organs as well, which regulates the stiffness, or its inverse the compliance, of a muscle. This is so that supraspinal mechanisms can rely on a given descending motor command signal to produce a predictable change in the tension or length of a muscle, whatever the initial state of that muscle may be, despite the non-linear relation between muscle length and the tension it can achieve at each length.

GOLGI TENDON ORGANS (GTO)

Golgi tendon organs are situated within the tendons connecting muscle to bone, in series with the muscle fibres, so they are excited both when the muscle contracts actively and when it is passively stretched (cf. muscle spindles, which are situated alongside the main muscle fibres in parallel with them, so that they are only stretched when the muscle is stretched but are 'unloaded' when the muscle shortens actively).

About 10–15 muscle fibres are attached to each GTO and it is able to monitor the tension produced by each such small bundle of fibres; thus there are hundreds of GTOs in each muscle. They signal both rate of change of tension and the static, tonic level at which a muscle's tension is maintained (Fig. 14.8). Their signals pass continuously to the spinal cord via '1b' myelinated afferents. These are only slightly thinner than the 1a afferent fibres from muscle spindle primary endings. 1b fibres terminate on inhibitory interneurones in the ventral horn of the spinal cord. Like Ia inhibitory interneurones, the latter probably provide a common inhibitory service for many pathways descending from brainstem and cortical motor areas and also for the inhibitory components of spinal reflexes. Ib inhibitory interneurones receive excitatory input from corticospinal and rubrospinal tracts and also from cutaneous and joint afferents. Each makes contact with many hundreds of other interneurones and motoneurones, so that the effect of stimulating one Golgi tendon organ is distributed much more widely than that of spindle afferents.

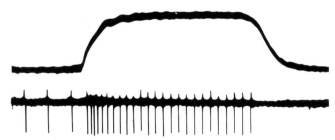

Fig. 14.8. Golgi tendon organ. Upper trace shows tension in a slip of muscle to which the GTO is attached. The GTO responds to both change in tension and new steady-state tension.

GTO ('clasp-knife') reflex

Until recently it was thought that the only function of the GTO was protective, mediating the lengthening or 'clasp-knife' reflex. The

GTO was believed to contribute nothing significant during normal stretching or contraction of a muscle unless the combination of active and passive tension on a tendon reached a dangerous level. Then when the muscle might be in imminent danger of tearing or ripping its tendon out of bone, GTOs finally discharged and inhibited the muscle's motoneurones. This then caused the collapse of active tension and the muscle relaxed and lengthened, avoiding damage (rather as the tension required to close a spring-loaded clasp-knife suddenly collapses when the knife springs shut). This is also known as the 'lengthening' reaction

Tension feedback

However, the idea that Golgi tendon organs contribute nothing useful during most of the life of an animal was always rather unsatisfactory and this view is now untenable, as it has been shown that they discharge even when the muscle fibres connected to them are contracting only slightly, for example in response to stimulation of a single ventral root efferent. Ib inputs therefore exert a continuous inhibitory effect on autogenous motoneurones and probably provide the afferent information for a 'tension servo'.

Precise control over the magnitude and timing of contraction of a muscle requires not only information about length, but also information about tension—which can clearly be supplied by GTOs. Tension feedback is also necessary to help the stretch reflex to compensate for the non-linear length/tension relationships of muscle fibres. A muscle can produce very different tensions in response to the same neural signal, depending upon its length at the time. This is an unavoidable consequence of the sliding arrangement of the contractile filaments but it makes precise limb control very difficult because a given amount of motoneurone discharge may have totally different peripheral effects depending on whether the muscle happens to be long or short at the time.

CONTROL OF STIFFNESS

It is probable that tension feedback from Golgi tendon organs and length feedback from spindles combine to help control muscle stiffness (the ratio of tension to length). In the original servo hypothesis of Eldred, Granit and Merton, load compensation was considered to be the result of forceful control of muscle length; any change in length apart from that dictated by the γ-signal would be powerfully resisted by the stretch reflex. Another way of describing such a mechanism would be to say that 'reflex stiffness' of the muscle is maintained at a high level, opposing any change of length. However, as we have seen, this is not the case—stretch reflex gain is rather low.

Another possible strategy would be to regulate muscle tension alone. The tension in a muscle is registered by GTOs, and any increase causes the GTOs to inhibit motoneurones supplying the muscle in which they are situated; similarly, any decrease disinhibits these motoneurones. Thus muscle tension tends to remain constant as a result of the Golgi tendon organ reflex.

However, it is physically impossible to keep both muscle length *and* tension constant when external forces vary. For example, when an increased load is applied it stretches a muscle and stimulates the stretch reflex to increase muscle tension in order to resist the stretch. The Golgi tendon organ reflex would tend to counteract this by inhibiting the muscle in response to the increased tension; hence simultaneous regulation of both length and tension is impossible. The solution to this conundrum appears to be that neither length nor tension is in fact fixed individually, but rather the ratio between the two (i.e. the stiffness) which the muscle and its reflexes present to mechanical loads is controlled. This offers some degree of regulation of both length and tension but, more importantly, has the effect of making linear the length/tension relationship of a muscle, so that descending control systems can operate on the musculature more reliably. As shown in Fig. 14.9, if a muscle is activated at a constant level at a length below its optimum (around Ⓐ in Fig. 9.14), any lengthening generates a disproportionately large increase in tension. However, this excites GTOs which therefore reduce motoneurone discharge (arrows at Ⓐ). Similarly, above the muscle's optimum length, when stretch would cause a smaller increase or even a decrease in muscle tension, GTO excitation diminishes,

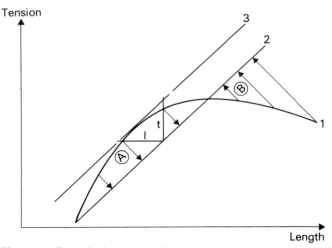

Fig. 14.9. Control of muscle stiffness. Non-linear length/tension characteristic of muscle (1) may be converted to predictable linear stiffness (2) by GTO inhibition (at Ⓐ)) and muscle spindle excitation (at Ⓑ)) of motoneurones.

disinhibiting motoneurones (arrows at Ⓑ). Thus the length/tension relationship becomes linear.

Descending motor commands probably determine the set-points of this system—the intercepts of the length/tension curve, i.e. the length of the muscle at constant tension and the tension of the muscle at constant length. If the load remains constant then a supraspinal signal shifting the length/tension curve to 3 in Fig. 14.9 causes the muscle to shorten by an amount equal to the change in intercept along the length axis (equal to l in Fig. 14.9) but if the load is unyielding and contraction is isometric, muscle tension would increase along the tension axis. It is a matter for conjecture whether the stiffness of the system itself (the slope of the length/tension curve) can also be varied by descending controls and, if so, under what circumstances. In general it seems to remain remarkably constant.

Long-loop (transcortical) stretch reflex

If a contracting muscle is suddenly stretched, one can record not only a short-latency electrical response in the e.m.g. occurring at about 25 ms, but also a longer-latency response at about 50 ms. This is not a voluntary reaction, as the shortest time in which a subject can react voluntarily to such a stretch is around 100ms. In view of the rapid lemniscal sensory pathway from spinal cord to motor cortex and the equally rapid pyramidal tract pathway back down to motoneurones, and since this later e.m.g. component is delayed after stretching leg muscles compared with arm muscles by an interval proportional to the distance between lumbar and cervical spinal segments, Marsden and colleagues suggested that the 50 ms e.m.g. response was probably mediated by a 'long-loop' trans-cortical pathway, travelling via sensorimotor cortex. This con-clusion was supported by the observation that patients with lesions in the dorsal columns, sensorimotor cortex or pyramidal tract often lack the long-latency muscle response to stretch, and that pyramidal tract neurones recorded in trained monkeys show responses to muscle stretch at the appropriate time to mediate such a trans-cortical reflex. However, under certain circumstances it is possible to show that decerebrate animals lacking cerebral cortex entirely may exhibit e.m.g. responses to stretch with this latency. Accordingly, the transcortical route may not be the only pathway underlying such longer-latency e.m.g. responses.

Although the long-loop stretch reflex is not a voluntary reaction, the question of whether or not its magnitude is affected by the prior intention of the subject to resist stretch of the muscle is of great interest since this may indicate how reflex sensitivities are 'tuned' by the central nervous system to anticipate actions. The instructions given to a subject can clearly affect the size of both short-latency and long-loop cortical stretch reflex components in the e.m.g., but the effect seems to be small.

Indeed although e.m.g. signs of the transcortical stretch reflex are in general clear, it is still not certain that the long loop produces any more worthwhile mechanical effect than the spinal stretch reflex. These e.m.g. responses are probably simply not large enough to explain phenomena such as load compensation. Alterations in long-loop reflexes occur in a variety of disorders. It seems that the chief reason for studying them at present is because they serve as a model of how somaesthetic pathways may control motocortical neurones directly, in health and disease. Their real contribution to motor control is still unclear.

FLEXION REFLEX

In spinal or decerebrate preparations a wide variety of powerful stimuli, particularly those exciting pain receptors, can cause the withdrawal of a whole limb from the site of stimulation—this is the nociceptor, withdrawal or flexion reflex (Fig. 14.10). It is a more complicated reaction than those we have so far considered because it may be elicited from a wide area of skin or deep tissues rather than from a single muscle, as in the myotatic or tension reflexes. Furthermore it is an open loop, eliciting a coordinated sequence of contraction and relaxations of many muscles. Thus it must have

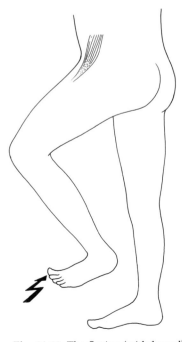

Fig. 14.10. The flexion (withdrawal) reflex.

access to a complete programme for the orderly sequencing of motoneuronal discharges within the spinal cord, which unfold largely independently of peripheral feedback. The precise direction of withdrawal depends on the site of the stimulus; the reflex therefore has local sign. It involves large numbers of interneurones and connections (propriospinal) extending through many segments of the spinal cord, providing features not developed in simpler reflexes.

In order to effect flexion at a joint, contraction of flexors must be accompanied by complete relaxation of extensors. Reciprocal inhibition is therefore more powerful in this reflex; in fact inhibition of antagonists often precedes excitation of agonists.

Temporal and spatial summation

Further features of the flexion reflex which are not highly developed in simpler reflexes are *temporal* and *spatial summation*. The magnitude of the reflex can be increased by repeated stimulation at the same site (temporal summation) or by applying stimuli simultaneously at different sites (spatial summation). Often 'subliminal' stimuli (dotted lines in Fig. 14.11b) which by themselves are insufficient to yield any reflex response can elicit the reflex when summed in these ways (α' and β' in Fig. 14.11b). The strength of the flexion reflex is seldom simply the algebraic sum of the responses to each of two separate stimuli, however, but rather shows *facilitation*

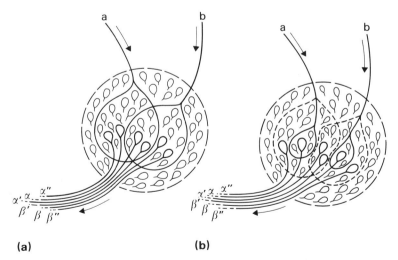

(a)   **(b)**

Fig. 14.11. (a) Occlusion. Stimulus a recruits α, α', α'' and β'. Hence stimulus b applied simultaneously can only recruit β' and β'' in addition, whereas alone it can recruit α', β, β' and β''. (b) Facilitation. Stimulus a alone fires only α but facilitates α', α'' and β'. If b is applied simultaneously or shortly after, α, β, α' and β' are brought to firing threshold. (After Creed R.S. *et al.* (1932) *Reflex Activity of the Spinal Cord.* Oxford University Press, Oxford.)

or *occlusion*. In the former, stimulation at two sites causes a reflex response which is greater than the algebraic sum of stimulating each separately; whilst the latter results in the response being smaller than that sum.

Motoneurone pool

Sherrington's explanation of occlusion was that there is a finite 'pool' of motoneurones engaged by the reflex. If one powerful stimulus excites most of them, then a second can only engage in addition the few members of the pool which are left (β' and β'' in Fig. 14.11a).

The biophysical basis of many of these summation phenomena can now be explained by considering the nature of postsynaptic potentials. EPSPs following one stimulus take some time to die away and they spread, diminishing, to other parts of the neuronal membrane. Thus temporal summation can be explained by the interaction of postsynaptic potentials—a second stimulus, riding on the remnants of the first, brings the motoneurone to firing threshold. Spatial summation similarly represents the summation of attenuating EPSPs arriving at different sites on a motoneurone. Facilitation in excess of the response to each input singly may be explained by the recruitment of further excitatory interneurones by the two stimuli.

After-discharge

The recruitment of interneurones probably also accounts for a third important characteristic of the flexion reflex, 'after-discharge'. This is the tendency of the reflex to outlast its original stimulus by several hundred milliseconds. It is likely that interneurones which are initially excited contact others, which then feed back excitation to form self-reexciting chains whose discharge can persist for long periods of time. Prolongation of this *central excitatory state* is essential to elaborate a sequence of muscle contractions such as that involved in withdrawing a limb in response to such a brief stimulus as a pinprick, or to elicit in sequence the series of flexions and extensions found in the scratch reflex or in spinal locomotion. The duration of after-discharge depends very much on the strength of a stimulus. Stimuli exciting only low-threshold A fibres yield virtually no after-discharge; those involving high-threshold C fibres give rise to prolonged after-discharge.

Fatigue and habituation

A fourth characteristic of complex reflexes is that they *fatigue*. The magnitude of the flexor contraction wanes after only a few seconds even when the strength of stimulation is held constant. This is not a result of the receptors themselves adapting, as it occurs over a much longer time course. It has been shown to be predominantly a central nervous phenomenon, rather than simply a result of a biochemical 'tiring' of the muscle. Habituation, the tendency of the power of the reflex to diminish when the stimulus is regularly repeated, is a related phenomenon, but neither is well understood.

The crossed extensor reflex

The flexor reflex may involve segments of the cord far removed from the site of entry of the original stimulus eliciting it. Stimulation of the flexion reflex also causes extension of the opposite limb, as if to bear the increased weight (the crossed extension reflex), approximately 250 ms after the onset of the flexion. This represents a very long time for the recruitment of interneurones and for setting up self-reexciting reverberatory chains, so it is not surprising to find that the crossed extensor reflex is often more powerful and longer-lasting than the flexor reflex giving rise to it.

CONCLUSIONS

Successful analysis of spinal cord reflexes has enabled us to understand many types of neuronal mechanism whose importance is by no means confined to the artificial conditions found in the decerebrate animal, but may be applied with profit to higher centres. These include static and dynamic responses, temporal and spatial summation, central excitatory states and so on. However, the general concept of servo-action is the one which many people find the most useful to characterize spinal cord operations. To regard reflex mechanisms as negative feedback control mechanisms clearly helps us to understand one of the ways in which sensory information may be used to control motor apparatus. However, this view is perhaps a little misleading, because it diverts attention away from the equally important role of open-loop control—of the importance of *central programmes* in the control of movement. The stretch reflex can only serve to return a muscle to its regulated length. The state of the spinal cord and brainstem centres determines what that regulated length is programmed to be, and in the intact animal it is usually the central programme, not peripheral feedback, which is more important in controlling the length of a muscle and in determining most of the features of reflex actions.

Chapter 15
The Motor Cortex

A motor map

In 1870, Fritz and Hitzig discovered that electrical stimulation of a region of the canine cerebral cortex just in front of the central sulcus causes well-coordinated movements of the contralateral extremities. Ferrier, a practising physician who contributed notably to the more humane treatment of the insane, confirmed this in monkeys; stimulation of the precentral gyrus in these animals also causes contralateral finger movements.

In fact Hughlings Jackson, another practising physician of great genius, had already predicted such a representation of limb movements somewhere in the brain by inspired deduction from his observations on the 'march' of convulsions in patients suffering from focal epilepsy. Often an epileptic discharge commences with twitching of, for example, the mouth, and then recruits convulsive movements in a characteristic sequence: mouth, thumb, forearm, shoulder, ankle, knee, hip, etc., always in the same stereotyped order. The epileptic discharge seems to 'march' over topographically organized areas responsible for movements of each of these parts. This was confirmed by the electrical stimulation experiments in animals.

Later the same pattern was demonstrated directly in man by Penfield (1937). He made a virtue of the necessity of stimulating cortical areas in epileptic patients coming to surgery—in order to localize epileptic foci prior to removing them it is necessary to stimulate adjacent areas of cortex.

These results represented the first unequivocal triumph of the theory of localization of function in the nervous system which has been so important to the progress of the neurosciences. It must have been very exciting at the time because it showed not only that the brain was, after all, accessible to experimental investigation, but it also seemed to promise a key to the understanding of much more basic questions such as how we conceive and command movements, and even where we might find a 'centre' for Free Will.

However, reality has been rather more prosaic. The discovery of the motor cortex raised many more questions than it settled. What precisely is represented in the motor cortex? Is it the conception of a movement, a plan for its execution, or merely a cortical map of the muscles to be employed? Are ideas, movements or muscles mapped there? None of these concepts is as clearly definable as the words we use to describe them suggest. Very often the arguments about them reduce merely to the meanings of these words rather than to matters of fact which can be settled by experiment.

Initiation of movement?

It is now clear that the motor cortex is not the seat of Free Will, the Wish to move, or the Conception or Idea of movement (whatever these words mean in physiological terms). All these things survive vascular accidents which can destroy the whole motor cortex leaving behind nothing more than fibrous tissue. The area is unfortunately a very common site for strokes, which are caused by cortical haemorrhage or thrombosis. Patients with such lesions can conceive the movement they wish to make and 'will' it, just in the same way as they did before their stroke, but nothing happens—no movement occurs. Equally striking is the fact that as they recover (which does not mean that the motor cortex regenerates, but rather that other motor systems take over many of its functions) the patients begin to be able to make many movements again, even though they now have no precentral area at all. The motor cortex, then, is not essential for making voluntary movements, as would be the case if it alone were responsible for their initiation. Furthermore, when the precentral gyrus is stimulated in unanaesthetized patients, they observe the resultant movements of their limbs with the utmost surprise, and invariably deny any knowledge that they were about to move or that they had experienced any 'desire' to do so. We can thus conclude that the motor cortex is not responsible for the initiation of movements in the sense of conceiving, commanding or deciding to move.

Supplementary motor cortex

Recent evidence suggests that the supplementary motor cortex is responsible for planning movements. When a subject is asked to think about making movements of the fingers without actually making them, blood flow to the supplementary motor areas in both hemispheres (measured using radioactive tracers injected into the blood stream) increases markedly. No changes occur in the motor cortex proper unless the subject does move, in which case contra-lateral finger-area blood flow increases just before the movement is made.

Movements or muscles?

These observations do not settle what is in fact represented in the motor cortex. Hughlings Jackson suggested that the CNS represents 'movements' rather than muscles. He noted that victims of a stroke are unable to make voluntary movements with their affected limbs, yet if these same muscles are called into play as part of an automatic postural reaction they contract quite normally. Furthermore, complete, coordinated movements of a limb, not isolated twitches of single muscles, are the consequence of stimulating the motor cortex. He therefore thought the motor cortical map must represent not simply the action of individual muscles but blueprints for their combined contractions, accomplishing complete and coordinated movements. According to Jackson the expansion of the motor cortical representation of particular regions—the face, hands and feet—corresponds not merely to the number of muscles acting on these regions but rather to the number, variety and complexity of the different movements they can make.

Representation of muscles?

An alternative view is that individual muscles are represented in the motor cortical map. Such cortical maps are usually constructed from the results of experiments in which the surface of the cortex is stimulated electrically. Much has been made of the problem of both physical and physiological current spread in such studies. However, physical spread of current can be kept to very low levels by taking appropriate precautions. On the other hand, physiological spread (i.e. the transmission of signals from one cortical neurone to the next by normal physiological processes) is probably reasonably similar after well-controlled electrical stimulation to what would happen during normal activation of the motor cortex; as such, therefore, it should not be avoided, because it is of real interest. In fact, the idea that a mosaic of individual muscle representations is laid out in the motor cortex was the outcome of using very weak electrical stimuli in deeply anaesthetized animals. In such preparations normal physiological mechanisms helping to integrate co-ordinated movements are profoundly depressed, and only the densest projections from a cortical area to one or a few finger muscles remain functional.

It is very doubtful whether such observations illuminate the normal function of the motor cortex, however. As there is already a complete map of individual muscles provided by the layout of motoneurones in the spinal cord, it seems unlikely that it would be duplicated all over again in the motor cortex. The striate visual cortex does not slavishly map the ganglion cells of the retina. Its orientation detectors commence analysis of the direction of lines and edges in the visual world; its binocular cells commence integration of inputs from the two eyes, and so on. Similarly, we may expect that the motor cortex does something much more sophisticated than merely mapping the muscles of the body. One of our challenges is to find out exactly what this is. What, to the motor cortex, is the equivalent of an orientated edge to the visual cortex? Many lines of evidence suggest that the motor cortex does not consist of patches of neurones projecting separately to each individual muscle of the body. Rather, programmes for complete, coordinated movements are somehow constructed there during its normal operation.

Movements?

It is very difficult to specify precisely what we mean by 'complete movements' in this context. A movement has a beginning and end point, a trajectory, rate, velocity, force, etc, and even the simplest movement of an extremity involves preparatory postural adjustments and contractions of muscles not directly involved in the movement. It seems most unlikely that the motor cortex alone could be responsible for calculating and regulating all these variables. Similarly, we did not expect the primary visual cortex, acting by itself, to be able to perform all the processes necessary for recognizing the Mona Lisa. The main function of successive stages of analysis by the sensory pathways is to detect and enhance discontinuities in space and time of sensory energies received from the environment. These indicate the edges, contours and shapes of objects, their movements, etc. Is there anything to correspond to such discontinuities in the motor sphere?

As a result of the reflex machinery of the spinal cord, a given degree of descending excitation of a muscle's motoneurones probably results in it producing a predictable amount of force, or if it is allowed to move, a standard-sized movement of the limb in one direction. If the group of motoneurones which is activated is changed, the muscle units which contract will change. Hence the space/time discontinuities with which the motor systems have to deal are changes in the amount of discharge required of individual muscle units, and changes in the motoneurones called into play. These alterations are necessary for the correct sequencing and coordination of movements. The motor system must itself generate them, rather than merely responding to changes in the outside world as the sensory systems are able to do; this makes understanding them that much more difficult.

The motocortical neuronal unit

The unit of motor cortex analogous to the orientated line of ganglion cells which excites a single neurone in the visual cortex is, therefore, probably an anatomically related group of motoneurones in the spinal cord, receiving input directly and indirectly from a single motocortical neurone (Fig. 15.1). This may be termed a motocortical unit. Such a system probably supplies all the muscles acting around one joint. It may well be employed during many different movements if they all require the participation of the particular set of muscle fibres influenced by the motocortical cell under consideration. In the same way, a particular striate neurone may be employed in the analysis of many different visual scenes if they all contain a line orientated at the angle to which it is tuned.

Pyramidal tract

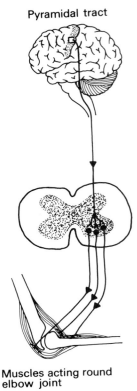

Muscles acting round
elbow joint

Fig. 15.1. Motoneurones supplying muscles acting around one joint receive signals from motocortical neurone either directly, via the pyramidal tract, or indirectly, via extrapyramidal pathways.

Thus it is likely that neither individual muscles nor complete limb movements are controlled by single motocortical neurones, but rather they regulate sets of spinal cord motoneurones, each set acting around a joint. Even weak electrical stimulation of the motor cortex would activate many such neurones and under light anaesthesia these would influence many of their neighbours by normal physiological processes. Coordinated movements of a whole limb may, therefore, follow electrical stimulation of a whole region of motor cortex, because many joint sets are thus excited.

Internal anatomy of motor cortex

So far, this argument has been developed only by analogy with sensory systems. However, there is powerful evidence to support it. The intimate anatomy of the motor cortex, its inputs and its connections with motoneurones are all consistent with the idea that components of a movement around a single joint, rather than movements of a whole limb or a single muscle, are represented by single neurones in the motor cortex.

Like other regions of the cerebral cortex, the motor area consists of six horizontal layers of neurones organized by predominantly radial connections into functional columns. All the neurones in a column mainly project to the same small group of spinal cord motoneurones.

The motor area, like the rest of the neocortex, contains two types of interneurone mediating lateral transactions—stellate and basket cells. The former are probably excitatory and the latter inhibitory, so that both inhibition and excitation of neighbouring columns is possible. The deeper interneurones ramify more widely than the more superficial ones, well beyond the confines of a single column. The length of the stellate dendrites is greater posteriorly than anteriorly, so that signals tend to spread back towards the central sulcus, where the representation of the most distal joints of the limbs is found. Although the detailed significance of these arrangements escapes us at the moment, it is clear that motocortical interneurones could provide a service similar to lateral inhibition in sensory systems by enhancing the sites of high activity in the motor cortex and extinguishing activity in more weakly excited areas, with a tendency for this process to be exerted more strongly nearer the central sulcus. Here, where the distal musculature is represented, finer 'fractionation' of control is necessary.

Projections from peripheral and subcortical motor centres are clearly important in determining which particular cortical sites are chosen for such peaks of activity; while diffuse non-specific inputs from thalamic intralaminar nuclei, locus coeruleus and ventral tegmentum are thought to control the general level of facilitation of the cortex (arousal) upon which the specific patterns play. The degree of this facilitation probably follows a judgement made by the limbic system about the necessity of doing anything at all.

Inputs to motor cortex

Since we have substantially downgraded the motor cortex from its classical role of initiating voluntary movement, we will have to pay more attention to its inputs than has been conventional. The inputs to motocortical columns are of four main types (Fig. 15.2).

(1) Local interneuronal connections from neighbouring columns (intracortical connections); these connect all layers.

(2) Corticocortical and callosal 'intercortical' fibres which pass chiefly to layer 3.

(3) Specific thalamic inputs from N. ventroposterolateralis pars oralis, ventralis lateralis and ventralis anterioris; these project to layer 4 and relay signals from cutaneous and proprioceptive receptors, and from cerebellum and basal ganglia.

(4) 'Nonspecific' inputs arising from the thalamus, the locus coeruleus (noradrenergic) and from the ventral tegmentum beneath the substantia nigra (dopaminergic). These probably supply rather diffuse input to superficial layers of the whole cortex.

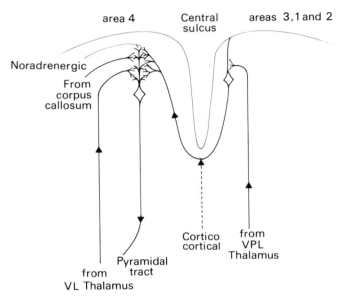

Fig. 15.2. Inputs to motocortical neurones.

Somaesthetic input

As discussed earlier, the motor cortex evolved alongside the dorsal column/lemniscal system, so it is not surprising to find that the most prominent sensory input to the motor cortex is from the somaesthetic system. Some signals pass there directly from the thalamus (VPL pars oralis) though most arrive indirectly via the sensory cortex (areas 3a, 2 and 1) which projects to the motor cortex just in front by means of 'U' fibres. A motocortical neurone receives short-latency inputs from receptors in the joints and muscles it employs, and also from the area of skin affected by contraction of these muscles (Fig. 15.3). Columns of motoneurones serving the same joint have similar sensory territories. Such somaesthetic inputs to motocortical neurones clearly underly tactile control of palpation,

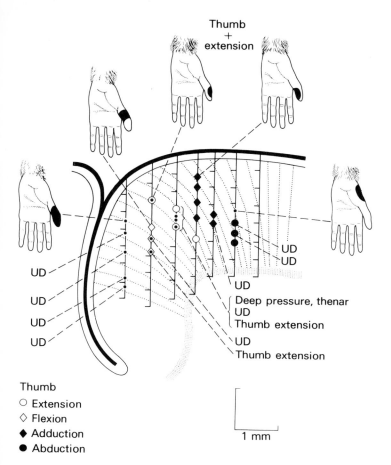

Thumb
+
extension

UD
UD

UD
UD
UD
UD

UD
UD

UD
Deep pressure, thenar
UD
Thumb extension
UD
Thumb extension

Thumb
○ Extension
◇ Flexion
◆ Adduction
● Abduction

1 mm

Fig. 15.3. Columns of motocortical neurones can serve one direction of movement around joints and receive sensory input from relevant skin and proprioceptors. UD, ulnar deviation. (After Asanuma H. & Rosén I. (1972) *Exp. Br. Res.,* **14,** 243.)

the placing and grasp reflexes and 'long-loop' transcortical stretch reflexes.

Corticocortical input

Further inputs to the motor cortex from other cortical areas include those from the supplementary motor area which lies medially to it and from the premotor cortex just in front of it, and callosal connections with the motor cortex on the other side. These commissural linkages are organized homotopically, i.e. mirror-image points on the two sides are linked together. Thus the cortical representation of the right arm is connected to the homologous area in the right cortex representing the left arm. Such linkages may explain why mirror-image movements of the fingers are so much easier to make than the identical ones required, for example, to play scales and five-finger exercises on the piano.

Thalamic input

'Specific' input from the ventrolateral nucleus of the thalamus conveys highly processed signals from the cerebellum and basal ganglia to the motor cortex. They are responsible for initiating and guiding the progress of movements; they also provide the main routes by which teleceptive signals from the eyes and ears can affect the motor cortex. In fact the cerebellum and basal ganglia are able to engage brainstem motor centres without involving the motor cortex at all, but in the normal animal precentral neurones are activated during almost every voluntary limb movement.

Touch, not vision or hearing, is the chief sensory input necessary for controlling the fingers, whose precise movements are the prime responsibility of the motor cortex. However, vision is more important early in a movement to activate proximal muscles of a limb, which are necessary for moving the whole arm to a target in order to touch it with the fingers. Thus in the visual control of the limbs the routes whereby vision may directly affect brainstem movement centres are probably just as important as those influencing the motor cortex.

Efferent projections

The efferent connections of the motor cortex are of three main types: local corticocortical (intracortical) connections, projecting via inter-neurones to neighbouring columns; long-distance corticocortical and callosal (intercortical) fibres; and corticofugal axons, which leave the cortex entirely and project to the brainstem and contra-lateral half of the spinal cord (Fig. 15.4). They arise from both large and small *pyramidal* cells. *Cortical* pyramidal cells are named thus because of their shape, but they can only be termed *pyramidal tract neurones (PTNs)* if their axons pass through the medullary pyramids in the medulla oblongata on their way to the spinal cord. Only 20% of axons leaving the motor cortex reach as far as the spinal cord. Most corticofugal pyramidal cells, including those which project to the spinal cord along the pyramidal tract, provide collaterals not only to neighbouring columns in the motor cortex itself but also to most subcortical motor structures, i.e. the basal ganglia, pontine nuclei, inferior olive, cerebellum, red nucleus, cranial-nerve motor nuclei and reticular formation. Many of these structures are organized topographically, and project also to the spinal cord; hence the final destination of indirect 'extrapyramidal' pathways from motor cortex (cortically originating extrapyramidal system (COEPS)) is often the same as that of the direct pyramidal projection.

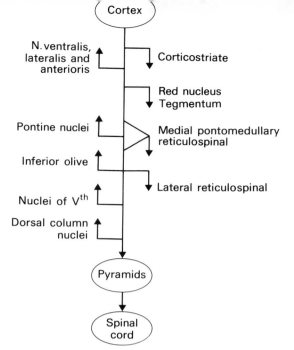

Fig. 15.4. Corticofugal outputs of sensorimotor cortex. 'Descending' pathways are shown on the right and centrifugal control of some ascending pathways on the left.

Pyramidal tract (Fig. 15.5)

Although the terms 'motor cortex' and 'pyramidal tract' are often treated as if they were almost synonymous, it must be remembered that only some 20% of axons leaving the motor cortex project as far as the spinal cord. Moreover, only some 40% of pyramidal tract fibres originate in the motor cortex proper, in area 4; a further 20% derive from the frontal cortex further forward; and 40% from the parietal lobe behind. Virtually none comes from temporal or occipital lobes. Only 3% of fibres in the pyramidal tract are derived from the large *Betz cells*, which were once thought to provide all the fibres of the pyramidal tract. In fact, only 10% of fibres in the tract are over 3 μm in size (having a conduction velocity of > 15 ms^{-1}). The rest are smaller myelinated (50%) or unmyelinated fibres (40%), conducting as slowly as 0.1 ms^{-1}, which cannot be of much use for rapid adjustment of muscular contractions in the feet! These small fibres probably fire tonically and help to set the general level of excitability of spinal interneurones, whilst the large fibres are responsible for moment-to-moment, phasic adjustments necessary for precise movement control.

Most pyramidal tract axons then make synapses with contra-lateral spinal cord interneurones. Some, especially those supplying

Motor cortex

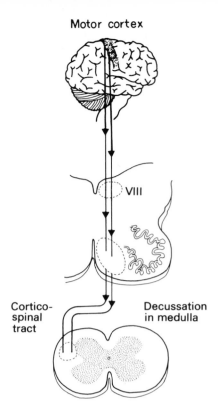

VIII

Cortico-
spinal
tract

Decussation
in medulla

Fig. 15.5. The pyramidal tract.

the distal muscles of the upper limb, make direct monosynaptic contacts with contralateral α- and γ-motoneurones. Phillips found that in the baboon each hand muscle motoneurone receives convergent pyramidal tract input, both directly and via interneurones, from a 5–10 mm diameter 'colony' of motocortical neurones (Fig. 15.1), and that each motoneurone probably receives indirect input from the same areas of motor cortex via indirect extrapyramidal pathways involving basal ganglia, cerebellum, red nucleus or brain stem reticular formation. Furthermore, each pyramidal tract or other descending axon diverges at its termination in the spinal cord to supply many interneurones and motoneurones. These motoneurones are not confined to a single muscle but often supply muscles innervated from different segments, even supplying antagonists as well. Nevertheless, most of the muscles supplied by a single large PTN appear to act primarily at one joint.

Thus the anatomical organization of columns in the motor cortex and of their connections with the brainstem and spinal cord suggests that they do not control only one motor unit or one muscle, but rather that they control a set of motoneurones whose combined actions around a joint are often required. Thus a motocortical column probably organizes neither the contraction of an individual muscle nor the execution of a complete movement, but rather an 'elemental' component of movement at one joint which might be employed for many different actions. As suggested by Hughlings Jackson, the large number of cortical motoneurones supplying, for example, the muscles of a finger reflects the large number of different movements the fingers can make.

Pyramidotomy

Lesions of the pyramidal tract are less damaging than lesions of motor cortex itself, since after pyramidotomy several indirect pathways survive by which the motor cortex can influence the spinal cord. On cutting one pyramidal tract in the medulla oblongata, paralysis of the contralateral side of the body lasts for only a few hours. It is difficult to determine how far this is merely the result of local oedema, etc. resolving shortly after surgery, and how far it is the result of withdrawal of tonic pyramidal influences on spinal motoneurones, which presumably take some time to adjust to the new situation. After the acute stage, animals recover remarkably. Stimulation of motor cortex is then almost as effective at eliciting movements as before pyramidotomy, although the pathway has a longer latency because it is entirely extrapyramidal and indirect. Posture and locomotion appear normal, though cats occasionally drag the affected leg and always find difficulty with complex locomotor problems, such as walking along a ladder.

The only permanent deficiency suffered by monkeys with chronic pyramidal tract lesions is that they cannot move their digits independently, as is required, for instance, in the *precision grip* of the thumb and index finger. They reach out hesitantly; they cannot accurately adapt hand and wrist movements to the shape of a stimulus under either visual control before they touch it, or cutaneous control when they begin feeling it; and they cannot easily relinquish a grip once formed. Their *power grip,* used for grasping and holding when climbing and swinging from branches, is totally unaffected, as are gross movements of limb and trunk. Thus it seems that the only motor skills in monkeys which never return after pyramidal tract lesions are those requiring accurately controlled hand and finger movements, whereas other extrapyramidal motor systems can take over other functions entirely.

'Pyramidal tract' signs in humans

We do not have much information about the effect of lesions confined to the pyramidal tract in man because they are not very common, but it seems that humans too are not greatly affected by losing pyramidal tract fibres. Following strokes and brainstem or spinal cord lesions, however, patients often present 'pyramidal tract signs'. These include weakness, spasticity (increased muscle stiffness supported by hyperactive stretch reflexes, as in decerebrate rigidity) and a positive 'Babinski' response (where the toes turn upwards and fan outwards on stimulation of the sole of the foot—it is thought to be a result of the spinal flexion reflex being released by the lesion). However, all three 'pyramidal tract signs' are probably the result of damage which deprives extrapyramidal systems of cortical control, and probably have little to do with the pyramidal tract as such.

The unimpressive consequences of pyramidotomy do not mean that the pyramidal tract normally does very little. Lesion experiments can only indicate functions that other regions cannot take over; they do not necessarily tell us what the normal functions of an ablated area are. The pyramidal tract and dorsal column systems evolved together to service precision control of the tactile surfaces important to animals—in primates particularly the fingers. Although this is the only function for which the intact pyramidal tract is essential, in order to provide control over the fingers, the system has also gained control of the shoulder, elbow and wrist. Thus there is a representation in the pyramidal tract not only of the fingers but also of more proximal joints, and pyramidal tract neurones may be activated during movements which do necessarily not involve precise finger control. Under normal circumstances, therefore, the motor cortex and pyramidal tract are active in most types of limb movement, not only those involving the hand, but after damage to the pyramidal tract surviving pathways can take over control of most movements apart from those of the fingers.

Motor cortex lesions

Recent findings about motocortical neuronal connections help to explain why ablation of small parts of the motor cortex does not eliminate the ability to make particular movements, contrary to what would be predicted if single neurones represent complete limb movements. Rather, such lesions reduce the dexterity of a whole variety of movements which employ the joint concerned, suggesting that they remove an element of the control necessary for all those actions. Even this deficit does not last, however. Because of the numerous parallel motor pathways which may take over many of the functions of the motor cortex, the effects of even quite large lesions become greatly reduced with time, particularly in younger subjects. The only permanent deficits which remain long after ablation of the arm area in young animals are not much worse than the chronic effects of pyramidotomy, namely unwillingness to use the arm, clumsy independent finger movements and slowness in releasing a grip.

Recording in conscious animals

Recent evidence derived by recording from conscious monkeys further supports the view that the overall function of patches of motor cortex is to execute whole movements. Murphy found that pyramidal tract neurones projecting to the muscles acting round the shoulder joint are organized in columns arranged in a semicircular band extending around the circumference of the arm area of the motor cortex. Inside this band is a similar one, containing neurones projecting to the muscles acting on the elbow. Nesting within this are circular areas projecting to the wrist and fingers (Fig. 15.6). Thus the motor cortical territory for the arm seems to consist of concentric rings of 'joint' columns, arranged as though the fingers had been collapsed telescopically inside the wrist representation, which lies within the elbow, and so on. The shoulder representation merges with the 'premotor cortex' where postural muscles are represented. Since the short, horizontal connections between columns are directed mainly posteriorly, activation of the shoulder area tends to

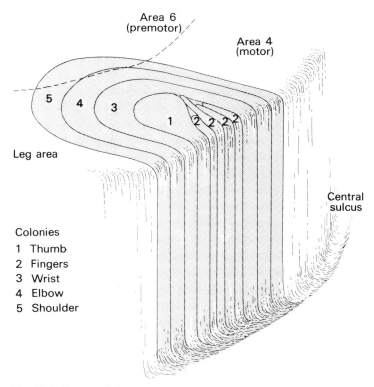

Fig. 15.6. Concentric 'nesting' of finger colonies surrounded by wrist, then elbow, then shoulder colonies in the arm area of motor cortex.

excite the elbow area, which subsequently engages the wrist, etc. Thus, whilst individual neurones project to the set of muscles surrounding a particular joint, the nesting of local intracortical connections in the motor cortex ensures that a coordinated movement of the whole limb follows stimulation of a motor cortical region.

Recording from motocortical neurones in conscious animals trained to make fairly simple, stereotyped movements has revealed, not unexpectedly, that many motoneurones discharge with a large phasic burst before movement commences, in order to get the sluggish muscles moving fast; they then maintain a higher, tonic level of firing to keep the muscle in its new position (cf. the pulse-and-step neurones of the oculomotor system, Chapter 20). In situations where the force demanded of the movement is dissociated from the position of the limb required, some, but not all, pyramidal tract neurones code for force rather than for position. Neighbouring pyramidal tract neurones may have totally different patterns of activity during the same movement, implying that they project to separate muscles which contract differently during the same movement.

While colonies of such neurones control the movements at a joint, Fetz has shown that animals can be trained to suppress the discharge of a cortical neurone during a movement in which it previously was active, and to facilitate its discharge during a movement in which it was previously silent. Thus the discharge of a single neurone is neither a necessary nor a sufficient condition for a given movement to occur. Clearly, many neurones have to cooperate to perform a movement and the loss of one is hardly noticeable.

Prefrontal cortex

In primates and humans the prefrontal association area, the region of the frontal lobe in front of motor and premotor cortices, is hugely expanded. Paradoxically, however, removal of this area by prefrontal leucotomy seems to make little or no difference to a person's intellectual or perceptual powers, but only to the relations between his emotions and behaviour. Leucotomized patients worry less, are less inhibited and in general less civilized; as a result, the operation is now seldom performed.

It is likely that different areas of the prefrontal region have different functions. Jacobsen found that prefrontal lesions produce a severe impairment of a monkey's ability to make accurate movements in response to a cue given some time earlier (delayed-response tasks). If a banana is placed under one of two cups in full view of a normal monkey, which is then made to wait for 10 seconds before being allowed to reach out for them, the animal will turn over the correct cup as soon as he can get at it. After lesions to the sulcus principalis, however, the monkey is unable to reach reliably for the correct cup. It has been demonstrated convincingly that this is not because the monkey fails to remember which cup covers the banana, but rather because after the delay it is unable to choose the movement with the appropriate spatial characteristics when presented with two or more alternatives. Passingham has shown that prefrontal lesions also prevent performance of the correct sequence of movements following a cue; in these experiments the monkey again has to choose the correct sequence from among a number of alternatives. Thus the prefrontal cortex appears to be responsible for selecting strategies of movement according to appropriate cues.

Jacobsen also showed that prefrontal lesions result in a reduction in the emotional responses of monkeys. This observation prompted Monez to introduce the operation of prefrontal leucotomy. The area responsible is the medial orbital cortex; stimulation there leads to EEG arousal and increases in heart rate, blood pressure and respiration. Hence this region may integrate behavioural and autonomic responses ready for action. One can incorporate this observation into a general view of prefrontal function by noting that drive-induced cues, with their autonomic correlates, are the most important of all forces. Together with more conventional sensory cues, they help to select one particular strategy or sequence of movements, rather than the alternatives.

Chapter 16
The Extrapyramidal System (EPS)

Because the pyramidal tract is so easy to identify and because some of its fibres pass monosynaptically from the motor cortex to motoneurones in the spinal cord, the motor cortex and pyramidal tract have attracted much more than their fair share of attention. Even those who emphasize the great size of the cerebellum and basal ganglia usually end up by pointing to the pathway to the motor cortex, via N. ventralis lateralis of the thalamus, common to both those structures. However, one should not forget that in fact only 20% of fibres leaving the motor cortex end up in the pyramidal tract, entering the spinal cord. Most of these fibres also give off collaterals to 'extrapyramidal' structures, to which the other 80% of fibres project. Furthermore, as we have seen, lesions of the motor cortex or pyramidal tract can be almost totally compensated for by the extrapyramidal system (EPS).

The extrapyramidal system has been likened to the 'terra incognita' of mediaeval map makers—tyger country which is too difficult and dangerous to explore. Logically, any motor pathway other than the pyramidal tracts, defined as the bundles of fibres which form the medullary pyramids, must be considered 'extrapyramidal'. The term is therefore far too vague to correspond to any single functional system. Until recently the extrapyramidal system was thought to play an entirely subsidiary role to the pyramidal tract. The latter was believed to define the goal of movements and to initiate them, while the EPS provided postural support and played some part in the coordination of different elements of a movement. However, as we concluded from considering the consequences of pyramidotomy, the EPS is capable of doing much more than this. Indeed, it can take over most of the functions that were originally ascribed to the pyramidal tract, as well as dealing with posture and coordination.

The list of extrapyramidal structures is very long. It includes the basal ganglia (caudate nucleus, putamen, globus pallidus, subthalamic nucleus and substantia nigra); associated thalamic nuclei (N. ventralis lateralis and N. ventralis anterioris); the red nucleus; parts of the brainstem reticular formation; vestibular nuclei; the cerebellum, together with the nuclei relaying to it (inferior olive, lateral reticular nucleus, external cuneate nucleus and pontine nuclei); and all the afferent and efferent projections to each of these structures. Most regions of the cerebral cortex project to the EPS via 'private lines' or collaterals of pyramidal tract fibres. Spinal cord afferents pass particularly to the cerebellum, reticular formation and red nucleus. The cerebellum also benefits from occipital (visual) and temporal (auditory) cortical afferents. Furthermore, it receives auditory and visual information directly from the superior and inferior colliculi, bypassing the cortex. The extrapyramidal system exerts its control over the spinal cord via reticulospinal, vestibulospinal and rubrospinal fibres; it influences the motor cortex (and, to a lesser extent, the frontal cortex in front and the parietal cortex behind) by the convergence of signals from both basal ganglia (globus pallidus) and cerebellum (dentate and interpositus nuclei) onto neurones of the N. ventralis lateralis and N. ventralis anterioris thalami.

It is highly unlikely that all these different structures have similar functions. There is probably a division of labour within the extra-pyramidal system, as there are divisions among sensory systems—somaesthetic, auditory and visual. As we saw in Chapter 13 a promising way to attempt a classification of motor structures is to consider the types of movement which each of them controls. The motor analogies to the different sensory systems would then be the different types of movements we can make: postural, locomotor, voluntary ballistic and voluntary pursuit. Though we cannot fully do this as yet, we hope that in the future we shall be able to classify different regions of the extrapyramidal system in terms of the types of movement they help to control. In the pages which follow we deal with the red nucleus, vestibulospinal and reticulospinal systems. The basal ganglia and cerebellum demand their own chapters.

RED NUCLEUS

One of the most important of extrapyramidal structures is the red nucleus. It is organized topographically, the forelimb being represented dorsomedially and the hindlimb ventrolaterally. Its main afferent inputs come from two sources: from the cerebral cortex, by collaterals and private lines from small pyramidal neurones found in the regions which give rise to the pyramidal tract, and from the cerebellum, chiefly via N. interpositus but also via collaterals of the dentate output which is passing to N. ventralis lateralis thalami on the way to the motor cortex. It also receives projections from the globus pallidus (the main output nucleus of the basal ganglia), from the mesencephalic reticular formation and from the spinal cord.

Its chief outputs are the *rubrospinal tract* (which is derived from both large and small cells in the nucleus) and projections to the surrounding lateral reticular formation. The rubrospinal fibres decussate, then travel alongside corticospinal fibres (Fig. 16.1), and terminate in approximately the same positions in the lateral part of the grey matter of the spinal cord as corticospinal terminals. Few, if any, make monosynaptic connections on ventral horn moto-neurones themselves, however. They mostly end on interneurones

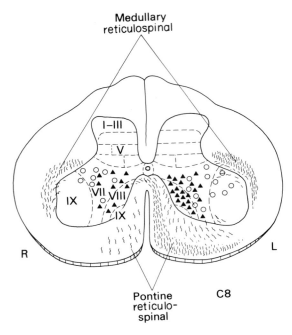

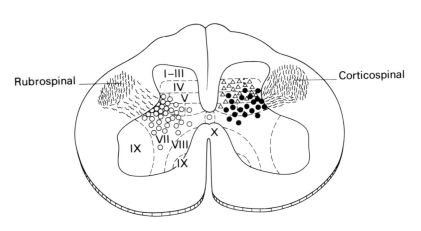

Fig. 16.1. Reticulospinal, rubrospinal and corticospinal tracts in the spinal cord.
Above:
  ▲ pontine reticulospinal terminals
  O medullary reticulospinal terminals
Below:
  O rubrospinal terminals
  △ corticospinal terminals (from somaesthetic cortex controlling dorsal horn transmission)
  ● motor corticospinal terminals.

in laminae VI and VII which excite flexor, and inhibit extensor, α- and γ-motoneurones supplying contralateral limb muscles. Lawrence and Kuypers found that the acute effects of ablating the red nucleus and surrounding reticular formation to a large extent mimic the effects of pyramidotomy. The only major difference was that pyramidotomy led to a lasting disturbance of accurate positioning of contralateral digits, whereas this ability was recovered following ablation of the red nucleus. Combined lesions permanently abolished the ability to make voluntary limb movements, although posture was remarkably undisturbed. Thus the rubrospinal system seems able to account to a large extent for the ability of the extrapyramidal system to take over the functions of the pyramidal tract.

By contrast, lesions of the *medial reticular formation* and *vestibulospinal system* (which make contact with medially placed interneurones and motoneurones on both sides of the spinal grey matter) permanently destroy the ability to maintain a normal erect posture but allow relatively normal limb movements—a very curious spectacle.

Thus the red nucleus and rubrospinal tract mirror the pyramidal system remarkably. The two appear to act synergistically. Like PTNs, red nucleus neurones receive indirect sensory feedback from the limbs and they discharge before movements of the arm, wrist or hand. It is almost as if some of the cells of the red nucleus are transferred to the motor cortex to form the pyramidal tract system.

VESTIBULOSPINAL SYSTEM

The vestibulospinal and reticulospinal systems are as important to the control of posture as the rubrospinal tract is to the control of limb movement.

Deiter's nucleus

The *lateral vestibulospinal tract* originates in the large and small neurones of the lateral vestibular nucleus (known also as *Deiter's nucleus*). The giant neurones found here are the largest neurones in the body. Deiter's nucleus receives input to its rostroventral section from the utricle of the vestibular apparatus (Chapter 10), to its caudodorsal section from the spinal cord, and to both sections from the flocculus, nodulus and fastigial nucleus of the cerebellum. Many ascending *spinovestibular* fibres are, in fact, collaterals of spinocerebellar axons. Deiter's nucleus projects to the other vestibular nuclei, and also back to the cerebellum, chiefly via the lateral reticular nucleus. However, its main output is to the spinal cord via the lateral vestibulospinal tract (Fig. 16.2). These fibres terminate bilaterally in the medial part of Rexed's laminae VII, VIII and IX.

Some connect monosynaptically with extensor motoneurones supplying trunk and proximal limb girdle muscles. Through their contacts with mid-line inhibitory interneurones, they can also bring about inhibition of flexor muscles. They often share common inhibitory interneurones with corticospinal and reticulospinal axons and with the reflex machinery which effects reciprocal inhibition.

Medial vestibulospinal tract

The medial vestibulospinal tract (Fig. 16.2), which is a continuation of the medial longitudinal fasciculus of the brainstem, is a more

Fig. 16.2. Connections of the vestibular system.

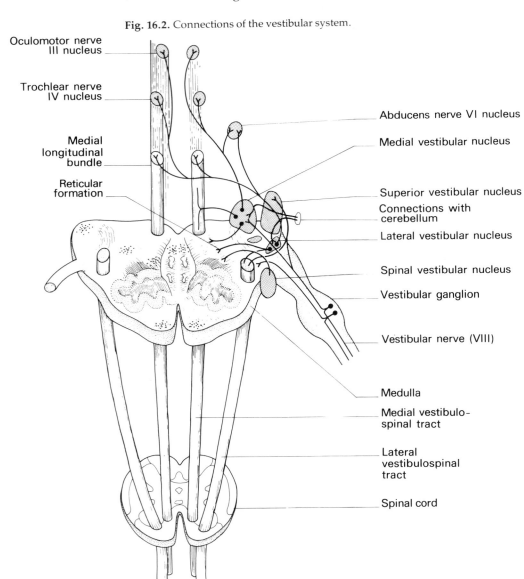

modest affair, petering out in the cervical part of the spinal cord. It originates from the medial vestibular nucleus, which receives its main input from the semicircular canals, and it terminates bilaterally in a similar way to the lateral vestibulospinal tract in the medial part of the ventral horn but only in the upper segments of the spinal cord which supply neck muscles. As the semicircular canals detect angular acceleration of the head, it is not surprising to find that the medial vestibulospinal system is concerned mostly with the control of neck muscles in relation to movements of the head.

In summary, the vestibulospinal system controls mid-line muscles in relation to the direction of gravity as perceived by the vestibular apparatus, i.e. it helps to regulate posture. It is striking how few influences from higher centres affect it. There are no known direct projections to the vestibular system from cerebral cortex or basal ganglia although, since the vestibular nuclei do project to the cerebral cortex (to an area just lateral to the face region of Brodmann's area 2), it is possible that there are, as usual, reciprocal projections from there to the vestibular nuclei. The main route by which the cerebral cortex can influence the postural control exercised by the vestibular system is indirect, via its connections with the cerebellum and basal ganglia.

RETICULOSPINAL SYSTEM

As outlined in Chapter 22, the reticulospinal system is a particularly difficult one to deal with because of difficulties with the whole concept of 'reticular formation' (RF). Ever since Moruzzi and Magoun's discovery of facilitatory and inhibitory influences on the EEG and spinal cord which follow stimulation of the RF, the identity of the pathways mediating these effects has been in doubt. Both of the myelinated *reticulospinal* tracts, which have been known to neuroanatomists for many years, originate in the medial, inhibitory part of the reticular formation (Fig. 16.3). However, some of the fibres originating more dorsolaterally in the pons are excitatory; these travel in the ipsilateral ventral column and terminate ventromedially in the spinal grey matter on both sides, some even making monosynaptic excitatory contacts with ventral horn motoneurones. The other pontine reticulospinal fibres travelling in the ventral column are inhibitory, as are the medullary reticulo-spinal axons that travel in the lateral column ventral to the corticospinal tract and terminate bilaterally amongst inhibitory interneurones in the intermediate part of the spinal grey matter. Thus, part of the pontine reticulospinal tract is excitatory but the majority of reticulospinal fibres are inhibitory. Stimulation of the dorsolateral reticular formation causes facilitation, as a result of the size principle, first of static and dynamic γ-motoneurones, then of α-motoneurones, whilst stimulation of the medial RF causes their inhibition.

Aminergic descending pathways

Since the introduction of methods for staining unmyelinated amin-ergic axons, much more has been learnt about other descending pathways which cannot be seen in sections stained only for myelin. It has been found that many *noradrenergic* fibres, derived from the region of locus coeroleus of the midbrain, pass as far as the spinal cord, whilst *serotonergic* fibres arise in the dorsal and ventral mid-line raphe nuclei and pass to all parts of the grey matter of the spinal cord.

Noradrenergic fibres have been implicated in functions as differ-ent as modulation of locomotion, the control of sympathetic outflow from the spinal cord, and suppression of sleep. They may well also play a part in the modulation of spinal cord excitability following stimulation of the dorsolateral facilitatory RF.

Likewise serotoninergic (5HT) fibres arising in the mid-line raphe nuclei have been implicated in the inhibitory effects of stimulating the caudoventral suppressor area of the reticular formation. This is the area which, if it is locally anaesthetized, causes a sleeping cat to wake up. Stimulation of these raphe neurones sends an animal to sleep, suppresses reflex activity of the spinal cord, and depresses C-fibre pain-signal output from the spinal cord, probably by activating a system of encephalinergic interneurones there. Thus serotoninergic axons probably play an important role in inhibitory effects of the reticular formation on the cerebral cortex and spinal cord. Their relation to the large myelinated inhibitory fibres of the medullary reticulospinal tract is not clear. It is likely that the latter can control the activity of spinal cord inter- and motoneurones phasically, since they conduct so much faster. They may therefore effect fine moment-to-moment adjustments, particularly those of extensor muscles defending a stable posture, whilst the noradrenergic and serotoninergic pathways may modulate activity, not millisecond by millisecond, but over a longer time-scale, setting background levels of facilitation of motoneurones, etc. Clearly, however, there is much more to be learnt about reticulospinal systems.

Chapter 17
The Cerebellum

The cerebellum is the largest motor structure in the human brain and its unfolded surface area approaches that of the cerebral cortex. Its inputs, internal arrangements and outputs are known in great detail (Fig. 17.1); yet despite all this information, its actual function is far from perfectly understood.

The cerebellum lies over the pons and medulla and below the overhanging occipital lobe, separated from it by a deep fold of dura mater, the tentorium. It is attached to the brainstem by fibres running in the superior, middle and inferior cerebellar peduncles on each side. These are also known, rather confusingly, as the 'brachium conjunctivum', 'brachium pontis' and 'restiform body', respectively. The cortex of the cerebellum is subdivided into anterior and posterior lobes by the primary fissure, and further

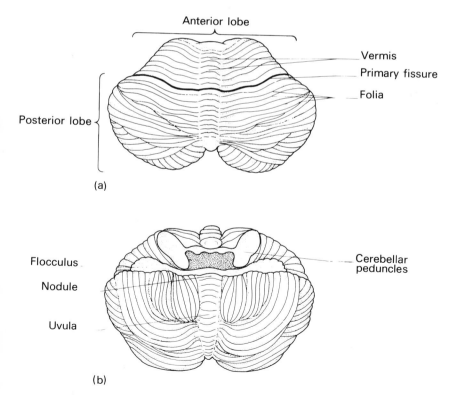

Fig. 17.1. Cerebellum seen from (a) above (b) below.

253

divided into ten transversely orientated lobules. Each of these is again extensively folded along the transverse plane into 'folia' (Fig. 17.1).

Deep within the substance of the cerebellum are the three *cerebellar nuclei* on each side. The most medial, the *fastigial* nucleus, receives fibres from the Purkinje cells of the most medial part of the cortex, known as the *vermis* on account of its worm-like appearance, and helps to control balance and posture by connections with axial muscles. Next comes the *interpositus* nucleus (in humans this is divided into two—the globose and embelliform nuclei). This serves the *intermediate, paravermal,* part of the cerebellar cortex and the *paramedian lobe,* and projects indirectly to ipsilateral limb muscles. The most lateral cerebellar nucleus is the *dentate,* which deals with the lateral cerebellar cortex, the *cerebellar hemispheres.* These are known as Crus I and II in most mammals, but as the superior and inferior semilunar lobules in man. The dentate nucleus projects to the contralateral motor cortex via the ventrolateral thalamic nucleus. The *flocculus* and *nodulus* which lie below the rest of the cerebellum send fibres out of the cerebellum altogether, to the *lateral vestibular* (Deiter's) nucleus; this part of the vestibular nuclear complex may therefore be considered as a displaced cerebellar nucleus.

'Longitudinal' organization (Fig. 17.2)

Mediolateral division of the cerebellum into vermis and paravermal and lateral regions makes it more comprehensible.

In evolution the flocculonodular part was the first to appear, in association with the developing vestibular system, and is known as the *archicerebellum.* The vermis (*paleocerebellum*) emerged later, in association with further development of the vestibular system as a sense organ, to control axial musculature via vestibulospinal and medial reticulospinal projections. It reaches greatest prominence in electric fish, which use their vestibular systems not only for balance but also for navigation, and in bats, which use their closely associated auditory system similarly.

The *paravermal* regions of the cerebellum (*neocerebellum* in evolutionary terms) are most highly developed in mammals with independent limb control. The *spinocerebellar* tracts, which relay signals from the limbs, project mainly to this region; descending cerebellar controls passing to ipsilateral limb motoneurones via the red nucleus and reticular formation originate here.

The *lateral hemispheres* (also neocerebellar), receiving from and projecting back to the contralateral cerebral hemisphere, dominate everything else in primates. This domination reflects the development in primates of the use of distance receptors and 'cognitive processes' for elaborating long-term strategies with which they can achieve complex goals; these usually involve skilled movements of the extremities perfected over long periods of time. Hence development of the lateral hemispheres is related to a huge expansion of the *teleceptive* and *association* areas of the cerebral cortex in these species.

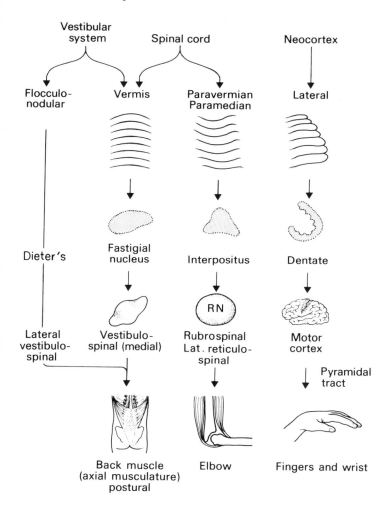

Fig. 17.2. Mediolateral organisation of the cerebellum.

In summary, the flocculonodular lobe and the vermis are responsible for balance and for the regulation of axial or postural muscles; the paravermal region of the cerebellum helps to control postural and proximal limb musculature, whilst the lateral lobes are probably essential for skilled movements of distal musculature. Note that, unlike the cerebral cortex, each half of the cerebellum receives from and controls muscles on the same side of the body.

INPUTS TO THE CEREBELLUM

One of the most remarkable features of the cerebellum is the multiplicity of its sources of input (Fig. 17.3). It receives *mossy fibres* from all the main sensory systems, all the main motor pathways and all the integrating centres in between. In addition, it receives a separate system of *climbing fibre* input, mainly from the inferior olive. These also pass on signals from the spinal cord and cerebral cortex.

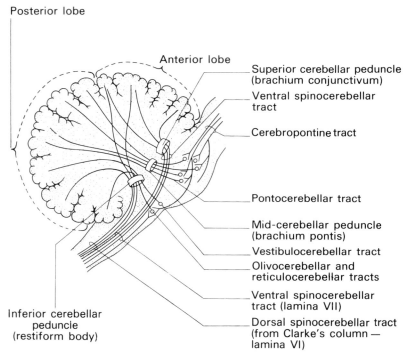

Posterior lobe

Anterior lobe

Superior cerebellar peduncle (brachium conjunctivum)

Ventral spinocerebellar tract

Cerebropontine tract

Pontocerebellar tract

Mid-cerebellar peduncle (brachium pontis)

Vestibulocerebellar tract

Olivocerebellar and reticulocerebellar tracts

Ventral spinocerebellar tract (lamina VII)

Inferior cerebellar peduncle (restiform body)

Dorsal spinocerebellar tract (from Clarke's column — lamina VI)

Fig. 17.3. Inputs to the cerebellum.

Pontine nuclei

Mossy fibre inputs from the cerebral cortex and superior and inferior colliculi are relayed via the *pontine nuclei,* which are situated in the ventral part of the pons, encircling axons travelling via the cerebral peduncles, some of which go on to form the pyramidal tract in the medulla. Those pontine neurones closest to pyramidal tract fibres receive collaterals from them, but around 80% of corticofugal fibres passing through the cerebral peduncles terminate in the pontine nuclei and do not proceed onwards to the spinal cord at all; the cerebellum thus receives by far the largest projection from the cerebral cortex of any subcortical structure.

The pontine nuclei send mossy fibres mainly to the contralateral cerebellar hemispheres via the middle cerebellar peduncle, though some of the most medial and most lateral pontine neurones also project bilaterally to both sides of the vermis. Pontine fibres also send collaterals to the appropriate cerebellar nuclei (the dentate and fastigial). The intermediate (paravermal) part of cerebellar cortex and N. interpositus thus receive fewer cortically originating signals via the pontine nuclei than the vermal or lateral parts, which receive from most parts of the cerebral cortex. Each cerebral cortical area projects to rostrocaudally aligned rows of pontine neurones. The axons of these neurones divide below the cerebellar surface and often project to quite widely separated strips of cerebellar cortex. Nevertheless, corticocerebellar projections show an overall topographical organization.

Inferior olive

Similarly, neurones in the inferior olive which receive from sensorimotor cortex, the pretectal region and the spino-olivary tracts project *climbing fibres* which divide some distance below the surface. They too supply collaterals to the cerebellar nuclei, as well as projecting to as many as ten Purkinje cells in two or more separate longitudinal strips of cortex. Olivo-cerebellar projections are also topographically organized.

Spinocerebellar tracts

Signals from the hindlimb segments of the spinal cord reach the cerebellum via the dorsal and ventral spinocerebellar tracts; the cuneocerebellar and rostral cerebellar tracts serve forelimb segments. Two indirect pathways—the spino-olivary-cerebellar and spino-reticular-cerebellar routes—deliver further information from the spinal cord to the cerebellum.

Dorsal spinocerebellar tract (DSCT)

The dorsal spinocerebellar and cuneocerebellar tracts are made up of the axons of neurones lying at the base of the dorsal horn, in the dorsomedial region of Rexed's lamina VIII (Clarke's column), and of neurones in the external cuneate nucleus, which is a rostral extension of Clarke's column in the medulla. These axons transmit cutaneous and proprioceptive information with a very high degree of fidelity from small, well-localized receptive fields situated on the hind and forelimbs respectively. They pass into the lateral columns of the spinal cord and enter the cerebellum via the inferior cerebellar peduncle; they are distributed in a somatotopical pattern to the vermis and paravermal parts of the cerebellar cortex. This disposition broadly matches that of the fibres relayed to the vermis from the sensorimotor cortex by the pontine nuclei. The tracts also supply collaterals to fastigial and interpositus nuclei. Thus, the dorsal spinocerebellar tracts carry topographically organized cutaneous and proprioceptive information to the vermal and intermediate parts of the cerebellum, but not to the lateral hemispheres.

Ventral spinocerebellar tract (VSCT)

The ventral spinocerebellar tract and its forelimb equivalent, the rostral spinocerebellar tract, pass less specific information to wider areas of cerebellar cortex. The cells from which these axons originate are rather smaller and are placed closer to the projection neurones of the somaesthetic spinothalamic system, lying more dorsally in Rexed's laminae V and VI. These cells are excited particularly by tendon organs, but also by a wide variety of high-threshold (nociceptive) afferents which give rise to the flexor reflex (they are therefore often known as 'flexor reflex afferents'—FRAs). Thus, ventral spinocerebellar axons cannot be said to have well-defined receptive fields. Rather, they seem to sample the activity of interneurones involved in the mediation of many of the reflex activities of the spinal cord. The mossy fibres in which they terminate branch much more widely than those of the dorsal spinocerebellar tracts, but lie in the same regions of vermal and paravermal cerebellar cortex. They may therefore contribute to the crude somatotopic maps found there, and by providing the afferent part of an internal feedback loop controlling spinal cord inter-neurones, they may play a part in adjusting the parameters of reflex action, as discussed below.

Spino-olivary-cerebellar tract (SOCT)

Spinal projections to the inferior olive also arise in the smaller neurones of dorsal horn laminae V, VI and VII; they carry cutaneous, tendon organ and FRA signals and travel in the anterior column of the spinal cord, passing chiefly to the medial and dorsal accessory olives. They project topographically, particularly to the vermis and the intermediate parts of the cerebellum.

Lateral reticular nucleus (LRN)

The remaining indirect projection from the spinal cord, acting via the lateral reticular nucleus, is not even crudely topographically organized. The spinoreticular fibres which we have already discussed in connection with the somaesthetic anterolateral sensory system also provide collaterals to the LRN. This nucleus projects to all parts of the cerebellar cortex and also to the cerebellar nuclei. The receptive fields of LRN neurones are very large, sometimes involving all four limbs, so topographical organization is clearly not possible.

Vestibular inputs

Another very important projection to the cerebellum comes from the vestibular system. Some primary vestibular fibres from the semicircular canals project directly to the flocculonodular lobe and fastigial nucleus. Of all the inputs to the cerebellum, these are the only first-order sensory fibres which pass to it directly; they testify to the importance of the lateral line/vestibular system to the evolution of the cerebellum. However, the majority of vestibular projections to the cerebellum travel indirectly via the vestibular nuclei.

MICROPHYSIOLOGY (Fig. 17.4)

The cerebellar cortex has a deceptively simple and uniform three-layered structure, which has often prompted rather superficial analogy to a computer on the simple-minded grounds that a computer also has a uniform structure consisting of many repeating general-purpose processing units.

The Purkinje (P) cell

The main output neurones of the cerebellar cortex are large *Purkinje cells*, the somata of which are found in the second layer. Their dendrites pass into the most superficial 'molecular' or *parallel fibre* layer. Parallel fibres run in a plane at right angles to the transverse orientation of a folium. As many as 200 000 parallel fibres running along a folium may synapse with the flattened dendritic tree of each Purkinje cell. These parallel fibres are up to 7 mm long, and each may synapse with a sequence of 50–100 Purkinje cells. They are the axons of very small *granule cells* (1 μm in diameter) which lie in the deepest, 'granule cell' layer of the cerebellar cortex. There are an astronomical number of these cells—some 10^{11}. Granule cell dendrites receive, via mossy fibres, the greater part of the external input to the cerebellum. Their axons ascend alongside the P cell bodies without synapsing with them and reach the molecular layer, where they divide in a T junction to give rise to the parallel fibres which course to the left and right along the folia through P cell dendritic trees. The dendrites of P cells are so long that conduction to the cell body probably needs assistance. It appears that small

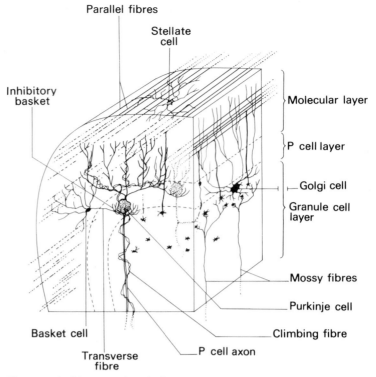

Fig. 17.4. Architecture of cerebellar cortex.

action potentials, mediated not by Na⁺ but by Ca²⁺, are generated at dendritic forks. Excitation of enough of the parallel fibres which make contact with a P cell cause it to discharge trains of *simple spikes* (Fig. 17.5).

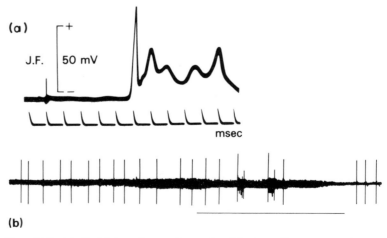

Fig. 17.5. (a) Purkinje cell complex spike (climbing fibre response) recorded intracellularly following stimulation of olivocerebellar fibres just by the fastigial nucleus (J.F.). (b) P cell simple spikes. Two complex spikes elicited by paw movement inhibit simple-spike activity for 100 ms.

The other excitatory input to a P cell is its climbing fibre. Most of these originate in the opposite inferior olive, though some may be derived from the surrounding reticular formation. Each region of the inferior olive projects to a separate longitudinal strip of cerebellar cortex. As mentioned earlier, most inferior olive axons divide deep in the cerebellar white matter and project climbing fibres to supply up to ten Purkinje cells as far apart as 10 mm. Once having gained the cortex, a climbing fibre makes several hundred synapses with each P cell dendritic tree. Thus, although the excitation of just a single parallel fibre has hardly any demonstrable effect on a Purkinje cell, the excitation of its climbing fibre always produces a large and prolonged discharge known as a *complex spike* (Fig. 17.5) or 'climbing fibre discharge' which is followed by a pause lasting some tens of milliseconds and then by depression of simple-spike activity for as long as a second. Nevertheless, activity of climbing fibres is essential to preserve the integrity of the spines on P cell dendritic trees upon which the parallel fibres make their synapses.

Inhibitory interneurones

All the other cell types in the cerebellar cortex are inhibitory. *Golgi cells* have dendrites which spread in all directions among the parallel fibres of the molecular layer, unlike the flattened P cell dendritic tree; they receive mainly from parallel fibres and inhibit granule cells. *Basket cells* also receive from parallel fibres but their axon terminals form baskets of inhibitory synapses clustering densely around P cell bodies and proximal dendrites. Their axons, known as transverse fibres, run at right angles to the parallel fibres as far as 300 μm across the folium, contacting 20 or more P cells. Thus they supply inhibitory baskets to a transversely orientated patch of P cells, some 20 cells long by ten or so wide. Similarly, *stellate cells* receive from parallel fibres but inhibit the superficial distal portions of P cell dendrites and do not extend as far along the folium.

Cerebellar nuclei

Each P cell axon ends in an extensive, bushy network within the deep cerebellar nuclei and there *inhibits* target neurones. The terminals contact nuclear cell bodies as well as their dendrites, thus inhibiting a fairly large group. Nuclear cells also receive excitatory collaterals from most mossy and climbing fibre inputs on their way to the cerebellar cortex, as we have seen. Thus the final output of the cerebellum relayed by these nuclei is the result of the interaction of their excitatory inputs with P cell inhibitory activity returning from the cerebellar cortex. One must assume, since nature has gone to the trouble of developing such complicated circuitry in the cortex, that the P cell is the most important influence on the final output of the cerebellar nuclei.

OUTPUTS FROM THE CEREBELLUM

Crude maps of the peripheral musculature exist in the cerebellar nuclei. The *dentate* nucleus projects (via N. ventralis lateralis of the thalamus) predominantly to the contralateral motor cortex, which is accurately topographically mapped, and shares many target neurones in the ventrolateral nucleus with the globus pallidus of the basal ganglia. The major output of N. interpositus is to the contralateral red nucleus (also topographically mapped) which gives rise to the descending rubrospinal tract; this is almost as important as the corticospinal tract in the control of limb musculature. Part of N. interpositus also projects to motor cortex via N. ventralis lateralis. The fastigial nucleus projects to the vestibular nuclei, particularly Deiter's nucleus which gives rise to the lateral vestibulospinal tract, and also to the pontine and medullary reticular formation, where the myelinated descending reticulo-spinal tracts arise.

Purkinje cell functional unit

Intimate examination of the cerebellum reveals an essentially rather simple functional unit repeated, in humans, some 15 million times. Mossy fibre activity from a very wide diversity of sources and sites together with a single climbing fibre excites each Purkinje cell. This in turn inhibits a group of nuclear cells. The selection of which P cells are maximally excited at any moment is determined by the interplay of the parallel and climbing fibres which happen to be active at the time and the 'sculpturing' achieved by surrounding inhibitory interneurones. These probably play a role similar to that of the neurones which effect lateral inhibition in sensory systems. They search out peaks of activity and inhibit less active spots, thus delineating specific patches of cerebellar cortex to be active under particular circumstances. It is possible that the special function of the climbing fibre input is to 'imprint' upon a P cell in some way a particular set of its parallel fibre inputs to which it becomes especially sensitive in the future; thus, when their combined discharge recurs, that P cell is preferentially selected.

Topographical mapping

The cerebellum is a motor organ indirectly connected to moto-neurones via corticospinal, rubrospinal, vestibulospinal and reticulospinal pathways, which are all to a greater or less extent topographically organized. Thus one might expect to be able to find 'motor maps' in the cerebellum. However, although stimulation in the cerebellar nuclei reveals a crude map of the peripheral musculature, stimulation of the cortex does not elicit any movements at all; presumably this is because the main output neurone, the P cell, is inhibitory.

Sensory maps (Fig. 17.6)

In fact, the topographical maps which have been discovered on the cerebellar surface are sensory ones. They have been obtained either by stimulating the periphery in order to map the termination of the spinocerebellar tracts and visual and auditory inputs, or by stimulating the cerebral cortex directly in order to delineate connections between the cerebral and cerebellar cortices.

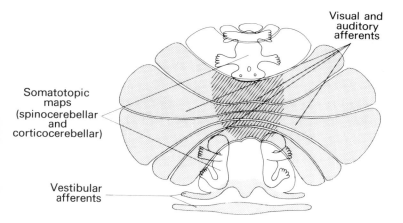

Visual and
auditory
afferents

Somatotopic
maps
(spinocerebellar
and
corticocerebellar)

Vestibular
afferents

Fig. 17.6. Widespread projections of visual, auditory, vestibular, proprioceptive and somaesthetic afferents to cerebellar cortex.

These sensory maps are very crude in comparison with those in the cerebral cortex. The degree of divergence of the main inputs and the convergence of thousands of parallel fibres on to single Purkinje cells makes any greater precision impossible. Indeed such precision would be undesirable, because as the cerebellum is a motor control organ it must be able to disseminate sensory control information widely. One might need the same visual information to control fingers, toes and even postural muscles (since these have to anticipate shifts in the centre of gravity caused by limb movements), so there should be a mechanism for routing it to wherever it is needed.

However, cutaneous and proprioceptive information from the fingers is most important in controlling the arm. Thus we find that teleceptive projections to the cerebellum are diffuse, whereas somaesthetic mapping is rather more precise. One can record visually evoked potentials over practically all parts of the cerebellum. There is little trace of retinotopic mapping in mammals, though its existence has been claimed in birds, in which vision may be used in a more stereotyped way in order to control flying and head movements, rather than controlling placement of all four limbs. Somaesthetic mapping in the cerebellum is rather more localized, however, as can be seen in Fig. 17.6.

Cerebellar disease

The traditional methods used in experimental neurology—neuro-anatomical tracing of pathways, stimulation, recording and ablation—have been rather unhelpful in unravelling the functions of the cerebellum. For all the wealth of knowledge we possess about its connections and intimate circuitry, we still have only the crudest idea of how it actually contributes to the control of movement. What ideas we have all pre-date by a long time the detailed information about its neuroanatomy and electrophysiology which we now possess. They derive from clinical observation, particularly of man's own unfortunate experiments on man during the First World War. In 1914, shrapnel velocities were high enough to ablate parts of the cerebellum but not high enough always to kill. In 1945, survivors of cerebellar wounds were rarer.

Although Flourens first showed that a pigeon deprived of its cerebellum could no longer balance effectively or move or fly in a coordinated way, it was Gordon Holms' meticulous correlation of injuries to the cerebellum incurred by soldiers during the 1914–18 war with the clinical symptoms to which they gave rise which contributed most to our present understanding of the functions of the cerebellum. He described a 'triad' of symptoms which have since become diagnostic of cerebellar disease—namely 'hypotonia', 'ataxia' and 'intention tremor'. All three may be ascribed to disruption of control of the site, timing and magnitude of muscular contractions.

Ataxia

'Ataxia' refers to unsteadiness, clumsiness and incoordination of movements; as such it covers a multitude of sins. Lesions of the flocculonodular region (vestibular cerebellum) lead to disturbances of balance; lesions of the vermis to unregulated contractions of the axial muscles of the trunk; and lesions of the paravermal cerebellum to uncoordinated contractions of the ipsilateral limb muscles.

Damage to the lateral lobes interferes with smooth and appropriately timed sequencing of skilled movements of the ipsilateral extremities, particularly those controlled by vision.

Intention tremor

'Intention tremor' really describes the effect of cerebellar disease on voluntary movements of the limbs. It is therefore pathognomic of hemispheric disease. On attempting to reach a target the patient overshoots it and then overcompensates time and time again, 'hunting' around the desired position before finally finding it. Correction movements are inappropriately large ('dysmetric') and badly timed, as would occur in a maladjusted negative-feedback control system.

Hypotonia

Hypotonia is the result of reduced activity of muscles; these feel flaccid to the examiner and also fatigue rapidly. As one might expect, the ipsilateral limbs are affected following lesions of the posterior lobe if a hemisphere is involved, and the trunk is affected if the vermis alone is damaged. In fact, the opposite state, hypertonia, ensues if the anterior lobe is affected, as occurs for instance in some alcoholics. In lower animals, hypertonia is much more common after cerebellar lesions, a fact which is still largely unexplained.

THEORIES OF CEREBELLAR FUNCTION

This description of the results of lesions in the human cerebellum incorporates none of the wealth of anatomical and electrophysiological data so painstakingly garnered by neuroscientists. Can we do anything to relate gross clinical observations to our newer, detailed knowledge of cerebellar function at the cellular level?

The seductive simplicity of cerebellar structure has stimulated a myriad theories to bridge this gap. But it should be emphasized that, as yet, none is more than a theory. They reduce to four main types (but they are not at all mutually exclusive—they could all be correct or all be wrong!): the cerebellum has been seen as a comparator, a timing device, a parameter controller, and a machine for learning motor skills. Most of these theories have been deduced from work with anaesthetized animals correlated with clinical observations, but none can be confirmed without experiments on unanaesthetized animals, cunningly designed to watch the cerebellar machinery actually doing its work.

The cerebellum as a comparator

The idea that the cerebellum works like the comparator element of a negative-feedback control system derives from considering the nature of its anatomical connections, and from the 'hunting' behaviour, described above, which ensues on damaging it and is thought to be analogous to the instability of a badly adjusted servomechanism. Since the cerebellum receives information from the spinal cord about all aspects of the movement of a limb and may receive from the cerebral cortex the intended details of the original signal to move it, before feeding back information to the motor cortex and other descending motor systems (such as the red nucleus and reticular formation), it could clearly detect errors in movement performance and elaborate signals to correct them. However, direct evidence that it actually does this is rather scarce, and this theory does not explain why the elaborate circuitry of the cerebellar cortex playing upon the cerebellar nuclei is necessary. Cooling the cerebral nuclei alters the later (non-reflex) behaviour of motocortical neurones in the arm area when they are forced to compensate for a sudden jerk. This is consistent with the idea that their late discharge is influenced by a corrective signal computed by the cerebellum, but quite how this influence contributes to control of the movement is not at all clear. Similarly, some visually responsive neurones in the lateral cerebellum discharge at a rate proportional to the mismatch between a target and the limb trying to reach it, but again it is not known how this information may be used.

The cerebellum as a timing device

Another proposed function of the cerebellum is that it is a motor 'timing' device. Impressed by the geometric organization of parallel fibres passing through a series of Purkinje cell dendritic trees, Braitenberg postulated that as a volley courses along them it might excite a fixed sequence of P cells. These might serve as a template for the sequence of individual muscular contractions which combine to accomplish a complete movement. A great drawback of this hypothesis is that the time taken for a volley to propagate along even the thinnest parallel fibre from one end to the other is unlikely to be more than 50 ms or so, whereas most movements take hundreds of milliseconds. Thus the P cells contacted by a single parallel fibre could not easily control the sequence of all the components of such a movement. Furthermore, as the deeper parallel fibres are thicker and longer than more superficial ones, they conduct at different rates. Finally, it is difficult to see how such detailed pattern of inhibition of nuclear cells by P cells could be propagated faithfully in order to underly the sequence of contractions of a series of muscles which are at least three synapses away. Nevertheless, these objections are not insuperable and the idea retains its attractions for many people.

Cross-correlation

A variation on the comparator and timing themes is the idea that Purkinje cells perform a sort of 'spatial cross-correlation' between their inputs—for instance between motor commands emanating from the cerebral cortex and feedback from the moving limb. The motocortical signal would pass to a band of parallel fibres on one part of a folium and spinocerebellar feedback would be delivered to another intersecting band. These two signals would interact maximally at only one site, thereby exciting a unique set of P cells determined by the magnitude and timing of the two inputs and by the nature and number of inhibitory interneurones between them. The P cells positioned at that site would then, in effect, have performed a spatial cross-correlation between the two inputs. Again, quite how this information might be used to control movement is unclear.

The cerebellum as a parameter controller

It has been suggested that rather than controlling motor systems directly, the cerebellum operates indirectly by regulating reflex parameters (i.e. their gains, operating ranges, etc.). Motor physiologists have been accustomed to think of movement control as a hierarchy of ever more complex reflex systems piled one on top of another. However, stereotyped reflex responses to sensory stimuli are very inflexible, and may be totally inappropriate under many circumstances. Clearly, there must be some ready way of adjusting their characteristics.

Vestibulo-ocular reflex

The vestibulocular reflex is a much studied example. This reflex ensures that the visual axes remain fixed in space despite movements of the head, so that one can keep one's gaze fixed on an object of importance in the outside world—for instance watching a tiger whilst fleeing from it. However, if one wants to keep one's eyes fixed on a girlfriend sharing the same swing boat, one does not want one's visual axes to remain fixed in space, but to move with the swing. To do this, one must be able to use visual cues to suppress the vestibulo-ocular reflex; otherwise one would never be able to keep one's eyes on any object moving at the same time as one's head; neither would one be able to change the direction of one's gaze keeping the head stationary.

Recent evidence suggests that the flocculonodular part of the cerebellum performs this function; it may adjust the parameters of the vestibulo-ocular reflex to suit prevailing needs. Ablation of the flocculonodular lobe prevents animals from being able to change the 'gain' of the reflex or switch it off, so that the eyes move in the opposite direction to the head even when this is totally inappropriate. Floccular Purkinje cells monitor the impulse traffic from the vestibular and oculomotor systems and project back to the vestibulo-ocular pathway. Their discharge modulates most strongly in phase with vestibular stimuli only when the animal is engaged in visually suppressing the vestibulo-ocular reflex, suggesting that their major role under these circumstances is to mediate this suppression. It is probable that other parts of the cerebellum perform similar services for other reflexes—in short, they liberate an animal from its reflexes.

Thus, cerebellar 'comparator' neurones which record the discrepancy between desired and actual values of important variables may, in fact, elaborate control signals which set at an optimum level the parameters of motor systems directly engaged in the execution of a task. Of course, we still do not know how these signals are used to change such parameters, but using such relatively simple 'model' systems as the vestibulo-ocular reflex we may soon learn more.

The role of the cerebellum in motor skills

Currently, the most fashionable theories concerning cerebellar function postulate that it is responsible for our ability to perform skilled movements. Cerebellar damage undoubtedly does lead to poorly coordinated and unskilful movements, though the overall memory of what sort of movements must be made in order to solve a problem is certainly not lost. Thus, loss of skills following cerebellar lesions might merely indicate a failure of motor machinery to execute certain movements properly, and have nothing to do with learnt skills as such. In fact, the idea that the cerbellum is a 'learning machine' is very difficult to prove, and there is, as yet, little hard evidence in its favour. Nevertheless, it holds great attractions.

Probably only 25% or so of the 200 000 parallel fibres coursing through any Purkinje cell's dendritic tree need to be activated in order to elicit simple spikes. So what is the function of the other 150 000? A number of theorists have suggested that each P cell is in some way conditioned to respond preferentially to only a subset of all its parallel fibre inputs. These particular fibres might be tively excited by only one combination of sensory and motor inputs—sometimes called the 'context' of a movement. Even if circumstances vary only slightly, another P cell would be preferentially activated.

It has been postulated that the specific subset of parallel fibres to which a P cell responds preferentially is imprinted on it by the activity of its climbing fibre. Thus when a climbing fibre discharges it might facilitate the parallel fibre/P cell synapses which happen to be active at the time; so that when the same set of parallel fibres discharge in the future, that particular P cell would respond more vigorously than the rest, even without climbing fibre assistance. We know that climbing fibre activity is, in general, essential in order to maintain the integrity of P cell dendritic spines for parallel-fibre contact. It is but a small step to suppose that climbing fibre complex spikes select particular groups of parallel fibres for favoured access. Now if the discharge of the climbing fibre were in some way made contingent upon P cell simple-spike activity, managing to optimize the movement currently in progress, then subsequent firing under the same set of conditions would improve the skill with which the movement was made.

Despite its attractions, there is only a small amount of evidence in favour of this theory. In particular, it has not been shown experimentally that combined stimulation of parallel and climbing fibres has any effect on subsequent parallel fibre excitation of a P cell. However, electrical stimulation may be alogether too crude a method to reveal the postulated subtle changes in P cell dendritic spines. Other, indirect, lines of evidence are more promising. For instance, it has been shown that when a monkey learns a new task, climbing fibre activity almost doubles—this is at least consistent with their contributing to the learning process.

Plasticity of the vestibulo-ocular reflex

A most useful system in which to study the contribution of the cerebellum to motor learning is our old friend the vestibulo-ocular reflex. We saw how this may be suppressed when occasion demands it. However, it is possible also to achieve much longer lasting changes in the parameters of the reflex if its normal actions are made enduringly inappropriate, as, for instance, when wearing inverting spectacles. Stratton found that the world ceased to appear upside down after wearing inverting spectacles for about three days, but turned on its head again when they are removed. A lasting alteration in visual perception of space had occurred. Melville Jones showed that this perceptual adjustment has a parallel in the motor system. When subjects wear reversing spectacles, the normal action of the vestibulo-ocular reflex makes normal vision impossible, as the compensatory eye movements effected by the reflex are made in the same direction as the apparent movement of the world, and thus makes matters worse. However, after three days of wearing the glasses, the reflex can be made to reverse entirely, so that it again becomes effective in stabilizing the visual axes (see Fig. 11.4). Like the immediate suppression of the vestibulo-ocular reflex which can be achieved when necessary, this long-term, 'plastic' adaptation cannot take place if the flocculonodular lobe of the cerebellum is removed.

Destruction of the vestibular nucleus on one side causes a profound disturbance of balance; rats tend to fall towards the side of the lesion and circle when attempting to advance. Over the course of a few weeks, intact rats can compensate for this imbalance completely, but those in which the flocculonodular region of the cerebellum has been ablated cannot do so. Furthermore, if the inferior olive or cerebellum is removed after successful compensation has taken place, the rats revert to their previous unbalanced state. This suggests that continuing climbing fibre input is necessary for this adaptation; it seems to be necessary both to promote and also to maintain postural stability in the face of unbalanced vestibular input. Clearly, if this is a valid model for the acquisition of more subtle skills, then climbing fibre activity is implicated in motor learning.

Chapter 18
Basal Ganglia

CONNECTIONS

All parts of the cerebral cortex project to the *corpus striatum* of the basal ganglia, which consists of the *caudate nucleus* and *putamen* (Fig. 18.1). These connections are topographically organized and excitatory and probably employ glutamate as their transmitter. The other important inputs to the corpus striatum arise in the thalamus from the intralaminar nuclei. These are also excitatory, but are organized diffusely not topographically. They relay from the brain-stem reticular formation and the basal ganglia on the other side. The corpus striatum projects to the *globus pallidus,* predominantly causing inhibition—this is the main output from the basal ganglia (Fig. 18.2). It projects downwards to the reticular formation and also to N. ventralis lateralis and anterioris of the thalamus—the same nuclei and often the same neurones as those to which the dentate and interpositus nuclei of the cerebellum project. These nuclei pass in turn to frontal cortex (particularly the motor area). Thus there is a

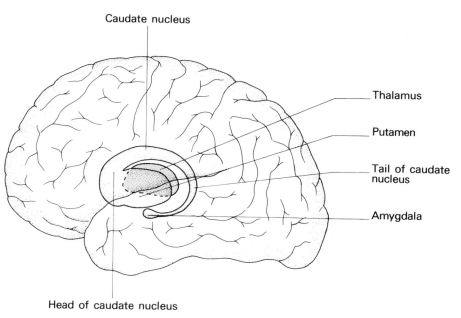

Caudate nucleus

Thalamus

Putamen

Tail of caudate nucleus

Amygdala

Head of caudate nucleus

Fig. 18.1. Arrangement of caudate/putamen (neostriatum) within cerebral hemisphere.

subcortical circuit joining all parts of the cerebral cortex to the basal ganglia and projecting back predominantly to the motor cortex. This is a very similar arrangement to the subcortical circuit linking the lateral cerebellum to the motor cortex, and suggests that the basal ganglia, like the cerebellum, contribute to the transformation of sensory input into movement.

The *substantia nigra* is linked to the other parts of the basal ganglia by reciprocal connections with the corpus striatum and globus pallidus. The pars reticulata of the substantia nigra is another

Fig. 18.2. Some connections of the basal ganglia.

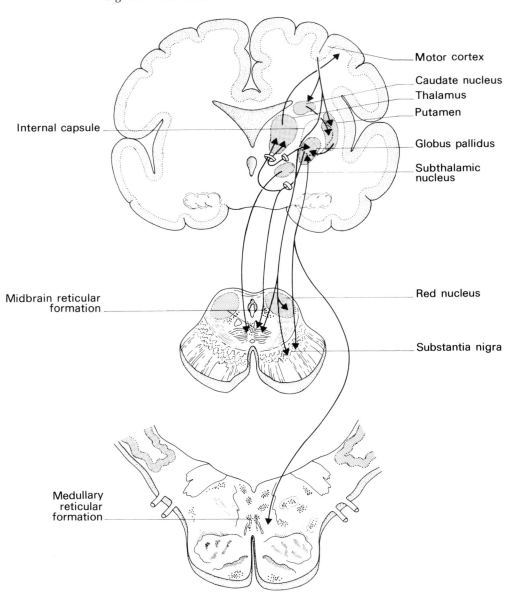

Motor cortex

Caudate nucleus

Thalamus

Putamen

Internal capsule

Globus pallidus

Subthalamic nucleus

Midbrain reticular formation

Red nucleus

Substantia nigra

Medullary reticular formation

important output of the basal ganglion. It projects downwards to the brainstem reticular formation and to the superior colliculus. The pathways linking the corpus striatum to the substantia nigra probably employ a peptide, *substance P,* as their excitatory transmitter and GABA as their inhibitor, whilst the pathway which travels back from the substantia nigra to the corpus striatum is dopaminergic (Fig. 18.3). Opinion is still divided as to whether dopamine is predominantly an inhibitory or an excitatory agent. However, it is the catecholamine that has achieved enormous importance since the discovery that the substantiae nigrae of patients with Parkinson's disease show degenerative changes associated with diminished dopamine content. Although dopamine itself will not cross from the blood into the c.s.f., treatment of these poor people with its metabolic precursor L-dopa has had a dramatic effect on the quality of their life, though unfortunately it does not affect the relentless progress of degeneration of substantia nigra cells which often leads to secondary damage in other parts of the basal ganglia.

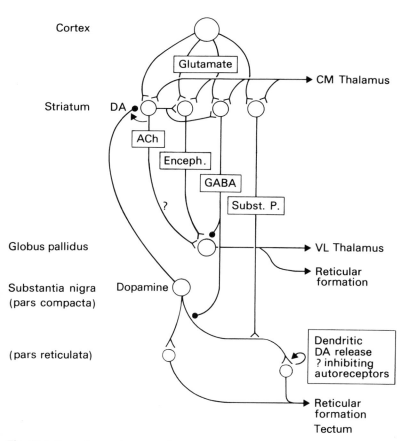

Fig. 18.3. Some transmitters employed by the basal ganglia.

Despite all that is known about the anatomical connections, electrophysiology and pharmacology of the basal ganglia, as with the cerebellum, very little is yet known about what precise function the basal ganglia fulfil in the control of movement. Nature has been very prolific with her own experiments here. The basal ganglia are afflicted by every possible type of pathological process, from genetically predetermined degenerations (as in Huntington's disease), deposition of metals such as copper (Wilson's disease), and mercury, through to accelerated ageing of the pigmented cells of the substantia nigra which may underly Parkinson's disease. The list of diseases which damage the basal ganglia reads like the contents of a textbook of pathology. Patients suffering from them have been studied very closely by neurologists, and their disabilities of movement documented minutely. This still forms the major source of our knowledge about the functions of the basal ganglia. However, the natural lesions these patients exhibit do not, of course, observe anatomists' boundaries, so that correlation of movement disorders with damaged structures is not easy.

The diseases of the basal ganglia in man cause two main types of disturbance:

(1) 'deficiency' (negative) symptoms, such as *bradykinesia* (slowing down of voluntary movements), which can be plausibly ascribed to elimination of some normal excitatory action; and

(2) 'release' (positive) symptoms such as *hypertonia, involuntary movements* and *tremor*; these may be the result of pathological processes ablating structures which normally restrain the performance of these movement patterns, hence they are displayed in the disease as involuntary movements.

The classical 'triad' of symptoms indicative of Parkinson's disease, for instance, consists of hypertonia, tremor and bradykinesia.

Hypertonia

Hypertonia is a release symptom in which excessive facilitation of motoneurones results in 'rigidity' of the limbs without overt distortion of posture. We know from studies of decerebrate rigidity that a balance of excitatory and inhibitory influences descends from the brainstem reticular formation to both α- and γ-motoneurones in the the spinal cord. Basal ganglia disease for some reason enhances excitatory and decreases inhibitory outflows to the spinal cord, but in a rather selective way. Gamma-motoneurones are not greatly stimulated, whilst the balance of ascending reticular influences to the cerebral cortex also remains unaffected as the state of arousal and the EEG are but little changed.

Thus the limb rigidity encountered in basal ganglia disease is rather different from that found in decerebrate animals. The latter is spastic, highly dependent on an overactive stretch reflex increasing reflex stiffness; it is much diminished if the dorsal roots are cut. Parkinsonian hypertonia, on the other hand, does not depend on the stretch reflex; it is often described as 'plastic' or 'lead-pipe' rigidity. The limb is much more difficult to move, but once moved it retains its new position and does not spring back like a spastic limb. This suggests that in basal ganglia disease it is not reflex stiffness which has increased, but rather reflex tension. It may be that alteration of the balance of descending excitatory and inhibitory influences brings about a specific enhancement of the Golgi tendon organ tension reflex.

Involuntary movements

Chorea

Chorea is named from the Greek word for 'dance'. It is a series of rapid, random, uncontrolled movements of muscles all over the body. The patient may perform a normal pattern of movements for a few seconds, then suddenly break into another inappropriate series of relatively normal actions, and then into a third phase of wild gyrations. The commonest cause of this used to be a streptococcal infection in childhood. It was known in mediaeval times as St Vitus' dance, after the saint at whose shrine in Germany sufferers were said to be cured (which was probably often true because the disease was usually self-limiting, and many were probably not suffering from chorea at all but indulging in a little epidemic hysteria). Later, it received the more prosaic title of Sydenham's chorea, after Thomas Sydenham who first correctly described it. The commonest cause of chorea nowadays, though fortunately still rare, is Huntington's disease, a dreadful hereditary condition appearing at around the age of 40, which progresses to complete incapacity, imbecility and death. Both Sydenham's and Huntington's chorea are probably caused by lesions of the corpus striatum. The latter has recently been shown to be associated with a deficiency of GABA and its synthesizing enzyme, glutamic decarboxylase, in the corpus striatum.

Athetosis

Athetosis is the name given to involuntary, slow, writhing movements of one or more limb—particularly the hands. This sinuous, worm-like activity seems a grotesque parody of normal movement. It is enhanced by emotion and naturally interferes a great deal with voluntary activity. The lesion responsible is usually to be found in the outer part of the globus pallidus and neighbouring parts of the putamen.

Hemiballismus

Hemiballismus means literally 'throwing half the body', and this striking event is just what happens. The entire arm or leg suddenly shoots uncontrollably outwards or the body twists sideways explosively. This is the sort of movement which might be released normally under voluntary control or to protect oneself when falling over. The lesion responsible for this is usually situated in the subthalamic nucleus, known also as the corpus luysii.

Tremor

The most common release symptom of basal ganglia disease, however, is tremor. The tremor of Parkinson's disease is an alternating contraction of agonist and antagonist muscles occurring about five times per second. In the hands this takes the form of 'pill rolling' (alternate flexion of the fingers and opposition of the thumb). Sometimes the whole trunk and head can be seen jiggling from side to side, or up and down, at this frequency. It is as if the normal actions of gripping and releasing the hand or nodding the head are endlessly repeated. In mild cases the agitation is arrested during voluntary movements, but in severe cases it persists throughout the movement. Even in very mild cases with no apparent tremor, intermittent tensing of muscles occurring four to five times per second can be felt as 'cogwheel' rigidity when the rigid limbs are flexed passively.

Nature of involuntary movements

Many of the involuntary movements which make their appearance in basal ganglia disease may be viewed as fairly normal patterns of movement which are released inappropriately and repeatedly by the disease process. Thus the movements seen in chorea and athetosis are often employed in normal behaviour, but are useless here. Similarly, ballistic flinging of the arms seen in hemiballismus would be perfectly normal when protecting oneself from falling or even when catching a cricket ball, but not when lying in bed in the middle of the night. It is as if the basal ganglia contain a store of these programmes for crude 'prototype' movements which are run through inappropriately when the structures are diseased.

Parkinsonian tremor is slower than normal 'physiological' tremor, which everyone exhibits to a greater or lesser degree, so that it is probably not just an exaggeration of pre-existing oscillations. Rather, one should view it as repeated activation of an essentially normal pattern of movement. Finger flexion, then opposition of thumb (as in normal grasping) is performed over and over again in the endless pill-rolling of Parkinsonism. Likewise, patients repeat the essentially normal movement of nodding the head over and over again without respite.

In Parkinson's disease and other basal ganglia diseases the tremor is probably the result not only of the basal ganglia replaying programmes for normal movement over and over again, but also involves imbalanced actions of the cerebellum. One of the prime symptoms of cerebellar disease is also a tremor—'intention tremor'. This is exacerbated by voluntary movement, unlike basal ganglia tremor which occurs at rest and is often improved during voluntary movement. Cerebellar and basal ganglia tremors are normally considered, therefore, to be quite different from each other. However, neurosurgeons have discovered that both may be alleviated not only by ablating N. ventralis lateralis thalami, to which both globus pallidus and the cerebellar dentate nucleus project, but also by severing the superior cerebellar peduncle, which contains only fibres coming from the cerebellum. Lesions of the globus pallidus alone seldom alleviate Parkinsonian tremor, although they may improve rigidity. Thus Parkinsonian tremor may be abolished by lesions placed entirely outside the basal ganglia, suggesting that the tremorogenic mechanism is at least partly the result of imbalance between the actions of basal ganglia and cerebellum.

Bradykinesia

The third important symptom found in basal ganglia disease is slowness in initiating and executing voluntary movements—a most incapacitating disability. To some extent bradykinesia can be explained by the obvious difficulty of making rapid movements with rigid limbs, but this is seldom the whole story. Bradykinesia is often a presenting symptom of Parkinson's disease long before hypertonia becomes evident. It is quite clear in many patients that they have lost the ability to make movements altogether. They simply cannot smile or stretch out their hands, however slowly. Surgical lesions of the ventral thalamus may alleviate rigidity and tremor, but they leave this bradykinesia totally unaffected.

Such deficiency symptoms are, unfortunately, only to be expected. If prototype movements can be released involuntarily following the liberation of one region from the restraining influences provided by another region, then further damage to the basal ganglia must be expected to eliminate such movement programmes altogether, thus impeding both voluntary and involuntary movement. This is precisely what is found.

EXPERIMENTAL NEUROLOGY

The reader will have noted that we have had to abandon neurophysiology in favour of clinical neurology over the last few pages. This is because results of the classical physiological techniques of stimulation, ablation and recording have not been able to match the wealth of useful detail about the basal ganglia that generations of painstaking neurologists have amassed.

Stimulation of the basal ganglia arrests the progress of a movement already in progress and 'freezes' an animal in a particular postural attitude, but rarely causes movements *de novo*. Though there may be a somatotopic map in the globus pallidus, stimulation does not easily reveal it. It is probable that the normal pattern of movement control by the basal ganglia is completely scrambled by gross electrical stimulation, providing us therefore with highly misleading information.

Ablation experiments have also proved disappointing. Small lesions do not seem to cause clear movement deficits at all, whilst large lesions render animals almost completely immobile, in 'flexion dystonia'. However, it is likely that ablation studies in trained animals will reveal much more in the future. Experiments with freely moving animals are unable to detect the subtle deficits to which small lesions of the basal ganglia may lead, though experiments with trained animals have begun to suggest that small lesions in the corpus striatum may prevent animals from using sensory cues to trigger movements correctly, as if they interrupt appropriate association of these cues with movement programmes.

Similarly, recording experiments have so far been rather uninformative. Those in anaesthetized animals suffer, of course, from the fact that such animals cannot make voluntary movements; whilst recording in conscious trained animals is still in its infancy. It is known, however, that neurones in the corpus striatum receive complex sensory inputs which are enhanced if the animal subsequently makes a movement in relation to them, and that neurones in the globus pallidus fire well in advance of movements, whether voluntary or involuntary, fast or slow (Fig. 18.5). These observations are consistent with the view that the basal ganglia contain elements of the internal programmes necessary for movement, as discussed in Chapter 13.

The pharmacology of 'circling'

Major advances in understanding the basal ganglia have come not from physiology but from pharmacology. Following the discovery that patients suffering from Parkinson's disease have pale substantiae nigrae (SN) lacking the usual amount of dopamine, a model of Parkinson's disease was developed in animals by administering 6-hydroxy-dopamine (6-OHDA). This is taken up preferentially by dopaminergic neurones in the substantia nigra and kills the cells which absorb it. If 6-OHDA is injected into the SN on one side, the experimental animal tends to deviate towards that side when moving around, because loss of one SN leads to postural asymmetry. If dopamine or, more conveniently, an agonist such as apomorphine which crosses the blood–brain barrier is now administered, the animal circles ceaselessly in the opposite direction, towards the intact SN. If rats prepared in this way are held up by their tails they rotate spontaneously away from the side of the lesion. This is because denervated striatal neurones on this side attempt to compensate for loss of their dopamine afferents from the SN by becoming hypersensitive to dopamine. When stimulated by apomorphine they therefore outperform the neurones on the other side. Hence, more powerful locomotor programmes pass to the ipsilateral side of the spinal cord, the other side remaining less activated, and the animals spin contralaterally.

The mechanism of circling is more complicated than it first appears. Circling occurs towards the side of an ablated SN, or away from supersensitized corpus striatum. Yet the ascending projections of the SN pass to the corpus striatum and pallidum on the same side, and these in turn project to the ipsilateral motor cortex. Thus if the motocortical route is employed, SN lesions should reduce the activity of the spinal cord on the opposite side rather than the same side, by the crossed corticospinal route. Therefore circling is probably not mediated by the projections of globus pallidus to thalamus and motor cortex, and indeed survives destruction of the latter. Circling probably depends on fibres linking SN and globus pallidus to the ipsilateral reticular formation and ipsilateral spinal cord.

Using this model together with appropriate biochemical techniques, a vast quantity of pharmacological data about the basal ganglia has been amassed over the last ten years. The area has turned out to be a treasure trove for the pharmacologist, since the basal ganglia contain large quantities not only of dopamine but also of GABA, substance P, enkephalin, cholecysokinin and, curiously, in the substantia nigra, acetylcholinesterase without associated choline acetylase or acetylcholine. Indeed, the dopamine-containing cells of the SN and neurones in the corpus striatum contain some of the highest concentrations of acetylcholinesterase found in the brain, and it is released when they are activated. The significance of this is unknown, but it obviously demands an explanation.

CONCLUSION

At present, a synthesis of basal ganglia functions can only be tentative. The general impression which emerges is that they are involved in very basic patterns of movement. Basal ganglia do not receive direct connections from sensory systems, unlike the cerebellum, and therefore they are unlikely to be involved in moment-to-moment feedback control over movement, or in the acquisition of motor skills. On the other hand, the release symptoms of disease suggest that they elaborate crude prototype movement 'programmes'. These are revealed by their release during various involuntary movements, by their imbalance in muscular rigidity and circling, and by their absence in akinetic patients. In normal subjects the appropriate programme may be selected by the corpus striatum in response to cues arriving from cortical association areas and are then released from the globus pallidus and substantia nigra, employing both rostral projections to the motor cortex and caudal connections to the brainstem reticular formation and spinal cord.

As explained in Chapter 13, most actions, whether automatic or voluntary, require not only regulation by feedback from the moving part and from distance receptors but also an internal 'central programme' of signals to provide the basic structure of the movement. Feedback control may then be superimposed on this basic pattern to confer finesse and precision. It seems as though the basal ganglia may contain these innate central programmes. The fundamental impetus for most movements may be provided by the basal ganglia, whilst the cerebellum may modify the programme afterwards in the light of past or current feedback from the periphery.

Chapter 19
The Control of Posture and Locomotion

Maintenance of a stable posture is a highly active process. When we stand up, our muscles must make continuous adjustments in order to keep us upright. Flexors and extensors must contract synergistically and at the correct times, converting limbs into compliant pillars able to withstand unexpected knocks, gusts of wind, etc. and to compensate for shifts in the centre of gravity during walking, turning and so on. Furthermore, for every voluntary movement a corresponding postural adjustment must be made beforehand to fix the base of the moving limb and to compensate for the changes in the centre of gravity which the movement causes.

In the normal human this is all done automatically, so that we do not have to attend to it. The extent of our release from having to oversee these functions consciously is exhibited in the agonized concentration which is essential for those unfortunate patients who have been deprived by disease of automatic postural control.

The problem of postural control may be divided into three parts. First, how is a particular postural 'set' selected? Secondly, how is it effected? Thirdly, how is it maintained?

Choice of posture is either a separate voluntary act or it is an automatic and essential accompaniment of a voluntary movement. In either case postural set is probably dictated by the cerebral cortex—particularly the anterior part of motor cortex, the premotor cortex, where axial (postural) muscles are represented.

How we effect a particular posture and maintain it reflects the important distinction, which we have emphasized repeatedly, between internally generated central programmes for action and control by peripheral feedback. The 'command' setting a selected posture in an intact animal is assembled entirely within the CNS, particularly in the basal ganglia, brainstem and spinal cord reticular formation, whilst feedback from sense organs such as the vestibular system and limb proprioceptors is used, with the help of the cerebellum, to maintain it. The so-called postural reflexes display these internal programmes (simplified by procedures such as decerebration), together with their regulation by peripheral feedback.

Passive aids to upright posture

Most of the reflexes we will discuss have been studied in experimental animals, but may be demonstrated in man under appropriate conditions. However, because we stand in an upright position some of our postural problems and their solutions are different. The centre of gravity in a standing man lies above a very small base; it runs behind the axis of the hip joints, so that the hips are extended. Thus a major part of the stress is taken by the ligaments of the hip joint, particularly the fascia lata, rather than by muscles. Similarly, when standing the centre of gravity lies in front of the knee joints, hence they are also extended; the tibia and fibula twist in relation to the femur and this tightens the very tough cruciate ligaments which pass between them. Thus, much of the work of actually supporting a human against gravity is performed by passive ligaments, leaving to the muscles the much more difficult task of maintaining dynamic equilibrium when unexpected displacements occur. However, it is likely that the basic neural mechanisms by which this is achieved are the same in man as in other animals. These mechanisms are usually shrouded by our rich repertoire of voluntary movements, but may be revealed in patients with neurological lesions—for instance, after a stroke.

Postural reflexes

Stretch and tendon organ reflexes

The stretch reflex is often seen as the basic building block of the postural system. It tends to fix antigravity muscles at constant lengths and to regulate the tension they produce when external forces disturb them. In principle, therefore, the stretch reflex alone could maintain the body in a fixed position, as long as its responses were quick and powerful enough. The dynamic endings of the muscle spindles ensure the former but, as we have seen, there are some grave doubts about the strength of the stretch reflex. The isolated stretch reflex has a low gain (force of contraction/unit increase in length), even in the extensor muscles of decerebrate preparations where it is relatively powerful. In flexor muscles of unanaesthetized, intact preparations it is difficult to demonstrate any worthwhile tonic stretch reflex at all. Thus, to rest a theory of posture entirely on the stretch reflex is to build it on shifting sand.

Nevertheless, we do normally manage to remain upright, so there must be some mechanism regulating muscle length which keeps us so. Studies of isolated reflexes in the decerebrate preparation neglect the importance of the 'central command' descending from higher levels, which prescribes required muscle length. Furthermore, as discussed in Chapter 14, we cannot view the stretch reflex in isolation from tension control by the Golgi tendon organs.

Together they set the relation between length and tension on which supraspinal mechanisms can act and ensure that limbs behave as compliant pillars. This is the first line of defence for maintenance of posture.

Crossed extensor reflex and magnet reflexes

When an animal withdraws a limb from a noxious stimulus (the flexion reflex) the opposite limb extends (the crossed extensor reflex); this helps to support its changed centre of gravity. Clearly, this is another reflex important to the maintenance of posture. Likewise we should include the *positive supporting reaction* of the spinal animal. This is a response to slight pressure on the footpads— the limb automatically extends against the pressure, as if to support the weight of the body. This reflex shows such a pronounced local sign that it has been called the 'magnet' reflex. If pressure is applied on one side of the foot, the foot moves by reflex in that direction; if it is applied at the front, the foot moves forward, and so on.

Spinal righting reflexes

When a spinal animal is laid on its side it will make crudely co-ordinated movements of all four limbs and the head, aimed at righting itself. These depend upon cutaneous sensation of unequal pressures on the two sides of the body, and can therefore be prevented by placing a weighted board on the upper surface. These spinal cord 'righting reflexes' involve long 'propriospinal' con-nections linking fore- and hindlimb segments of the spinal cord, as well as a complex array of interneurones which are necessary for the required movements to appear in the correct sequence. In the intact animal, neck, vestibular, basal ganglia and visual elements are superimposed on crude spinal cord righting to accomplish marvellous feats such as a cat's ability always to fall on its feet when dropped.

Neck reflexes

Proprioceptors in the joints and muscles of the neck are particularly important in the regulation of posture. On account of the flexibility of the neck, the position of the head is almost independent of that of the body. Furthermore, the head has its own systems for preserving a constant position in space, the vestibular and visual systems. Some mechanism for informing the head of the position of the body and vice versa is therefore essential. This is the function of neck proprioceptors.

In a high spinal, as in the intact animal, when the body is moved with the head kept immobilized, or when the head is moved after ablation of the vestibular apparatus, movements of limbs are instituted which help to compensate for consequent shifts in the centre of gravity. If the head is moved to the left, the left limbs extend and the right limbs flex; if it is deflected to the right, the right limbs extend. If the head is raised, the forelimbs extend and the hind limbs flex, as if the animal were looking up towards a shelf; but if the head is lowered, the forelimbs flex and the hind limbs extend, as when bending down to lap a bowl of milk (Fig. 19.1). All these reflexes help the basic stretch and tension reflexes to stabilize the appropriate muscles. In fact when the neck reflexes are temporarily eliminated by locally anaesthetizing the appropriate dorsal roots (C_1–C_3), monkeys lose their balance almost as badly as after labyrinthectomy.

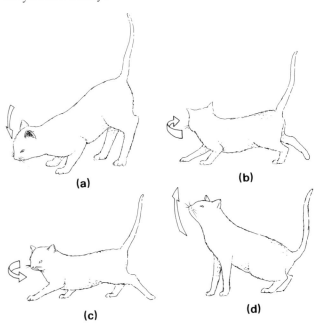

Fig. 19.1. Static postural reflexes. Placing head to left or right, or up or down, causes extension of appropriate limbs, mediated by the neck muscle spindles, the utricle and the saccule.

Vestibular role in posture

Static reflexes

When the head is moved, hair cells in the utricle, saccule and semicircular canals of the vestibular apparatus are stimulated (see Chapter 10). These structures initiate adjustments similar to those effected by the neck reflexes. That is, if an animal falls to the right, the right limbs extend automatically under vestibular control. If it falls forward, the extensors of the front limb contract, and so on. Interestingly, these reactions can also be seen in anencephalic babies, or adults rendered effectively anencephalic by a severe stroke. On turning the head to the left, the left leg and arm extend; on pulling the head back the upper limbs extend and the lower limbs flex (Fig. 19.1). In normal human subjects these signs of vestibular regulation are submerged and can only be discerned by careful analysis of e.m.g. and oculomotor records.

Dynamic reflexes

If a blindfolded cat is suddenly lowered head down, its forelimbs extend in preparation for landing. This response to linear accelera-tion is mediated by the otoliths of the utricle and saccule employing their connections with the lateral vestibulospinal tract which, as we have seen, makes monosynaptic connections with extensor α-motoneurones.

However, the way in which the vestibular system is most com-monly stimulated is by rotation. Angular acceleration is detected by the semicircular canals, and these institute a series of reactions of the eyes, neck, limbs and trunk. The vestibulo-ocular reflex (Chapters 10 and 17) allows the gaze to remain fixed in space, until interrupted by a return flick when the limits of the orbit are reached. This is *vestibular nystagmus*.

The dynamic effects of the vestibular system on the neck and limbs are most easily deduced from the consequences of removing the labyrinth on one side. Until the animal adapts to the new situation (a matter of some days or weeks) all its movements deviate towards the side of the lesion; thus under normal circumstances the two sides must inhibit each other powerfully. The intact side, which is normally kept in check by the other side, overstimulates postural muscles after the lesion, causing head turning, scoliosis (deviation of the spine) and flexion of the limbs on the damaged side, together with extension on the contralateral side.

These same influences can be examined, though with some difficulty, during rotation of intact animals and humans. E.m.g. records show that during rotation to the right, the right leg ex-tensors are facilitated in humans (as indeed one knows from one's own experience of turning suddenly, when the inner leg stiffens automatically). In fact, in humans the right arm also extends slightly; this is shown by the smaller circle it describes when we swing round to the right. In quadrupeds the pattern is slightly different; the forelimb on the side of rotation extends but the hindlimb on that side flexes and the opposite hindlimb extends, perhaps to help compensate for the centrifugal force of the turn.

Cortical role in posture

Contact placing

If any part of the body of a blindfolded animal is brought into contact with a surface, it will adjust the position of its paws to try to make contact, and adjust the disposition of the pads to allow for any unevenness. 'Contact placing' of this sophistication requires the integrity of somatosensory and motor cortices, together with the dorsal columns and pyramidal tract; it will survive ablation of all the rest of the cerebral cortex (Fig. 19.2). As described in Chapters 8 and 15, it is likely that the highly specialized dorsal column/sensorimotor cortex/pyramidal tract system evolved specifically to control the extremities. In comparison, its spinal counterpart, the positive supporting reaction, is a crude mechanism. A similar cortical reflex in humans is the grasp reflex found in babies. It is submerged in adults but maybe released again following prefrontal lesions.

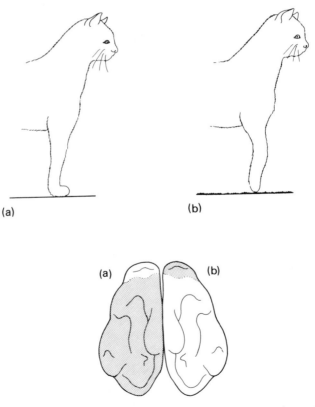

Fig. 19.2. Contact placing and hopping reaction survive destruction of all parts of cerebral cortex apart from sensorimotor cortex (a), but not ablation of sensorimotor cortex alone (b).

The sensorimotor cortex is also essential for another important postural mechanism, the hopping reaction. If an animal is held so that only one limb touches the ground, and the body is moved forwards, backwards or laterally, the leg hops in the direction of the displacement, so that the foot is kept directly under the appropriate shoulder or hip. First the extensor tone in the limb is reduced and flexion intervenes, then extension returns to support the body in the new position. If the sensorimotor cortex is destroyed this hopping reaction disappears, but it survives ablation of all the rest of the cerebral cortex.

Visual placing

The intact animal can tell from inspection of itself in relation to its surroundings whether its body is in an appropriate position, and make necessary postural adjustments if it is not. A 'model' for this reaction which has been much studied is the 'visual placing' reflex. If an animal is brought towards a surface, its limbs will extend and adapt themselves to the surface under visual control, even before they touch it. This reaction survives ablation of all the cerebral cortex apart from prestriate areas and posterior parietal area 7. Notice that neither primary motor nor visual (striate) cortex is essential.

In the cat there is a separate projection from the lateral geniculate nucleus to prestriate area 18, but in the monkey there probably is not, so that survival of the visual placing reaction in the monkey after removal of the striate cortex must depend on the tecto–pulvinar/prestriate/'second' visual system.

On the efferent side, the dense projection of prestriate areas to the cerebellum and basal ganglia and the contribution of area 7 to the pyramidal tract presumably explain the survival of visual placing after ablation of the motor cortex. These observations also help us to understand some aspects of the control of movement in general; they begin to show why animals can survive motor cortical ablation to such a remarkable degree.

A hierarchy of reflexes?

It is easy to become so impressed by reflex action as to conclude that the whole of postural control can be explained by more and more reflexes piled on top of one another, but one must not forget that the very concept of a reflex is only a convenient abstraction. It is an excellent means of dissecting the components of a physiological control system, but no more. Destroying all nervous pathways apart from the one under consideration naturally disturbs normal operations, and it prescribes a highly prejudiced view of how the intact system usually works.

Since reflex behaviour is triggered by sensory stimuli, studying postural reflexes encourages one to overemphasize the importance of peripheral feedback from muscle proprioceptors, the skin, the vestibular and visual systems, etc., whereas in reality, feedback merely informs of when adjustments are necessary. The major output to muscles is not the result of sensory feedback at all, but derives from centrally generated signals relayed from the basal ganglia, brainstem and spinal cord reticular formation.

Basal ganglia

J. Purdon Martin showed that the basal ganglia are probably the most important higher centres effecting postural set. As discussed in Chapter 18, they seem to contain basic blueprints for the set of muscle contractions needed to achieve any particular posture or to adjust it—for standing still, stiffening the left side when turning left or flinging out the arm to break a fall. These central programmes are revealed by their release at inappropriate times in the involuntary movements characteristic of basal ganglia disease.

Reticular formation

As discussed in Chapter 18 when considering 'circling', the most important connections of the basal ganglia regulating posture and locomotion are probably not those directed towards the motor cortex, but are projections to the medial reticular formation of the pons and medulla and thence, via the reticulospinal system, to the medial part of the ventral horn on both sides, where axial-muscle motoneurones are situated. In the spinal reticular formation are found also the interneurones which contribute to polysynaptic spinal reflexes. It is the state of these which determines, for example, the 'gain' of the static stretch reflex, which we introduced as the basic building block of postural control. Thus the spinal reticular formation, like the brainstem reticular formation and the basal ganglia, makes an important contribution to the central programmes determining posture.

LOCOMOTION

In Chapter 13 we made an important distinction between open-loop (preprogrammed, ballistic or feedforward) and closed-loop (feedback or pursuit) modes of motor control, and we concluded that most movements require both kinds of assistance. The neural mechanisms controlling walking exemplify these problems very well.

Sherrington found that the rhythmic limb movements which can be obtained in spinal animals are very disturbed after cutting the sensory nerves coming from those limbs. Similarly, monkeys find it very difficult to make effective use of a limb that has been deafferentated. Sherrington concluded that locomotion depends upon a sequence of reflexes, each triggering the next—'reflex chaining'. Thus, stretch of ankle extensors in the stance phase of walking (when the foot is on the ground) would trigger flexion of the opposite hip to swing the other leg forward. Thus chains of reflexes could take care of all the details of locomotion.

However, in 1911 Graham Brown showed that reflex chaining could not explain locomotion completely. He found that he could induce deafferentated spinal cats to perform rhythmic walking movements. Given suitable support, such animals could even be made to 'walk' on a treadmill. Fifty years later, Orlovsky showed that continuous stimulation of a locomotor region in the mesencephalon just beneath the subthalamic nucleus of the basal ganglia induces walking in decerebrate, deafferentated animals. One important source of this locomotor facilitation turned out to be noradrenergic output from the locus coeroleus, so that its effects can be mimicked by applying the noradrenergic precursor L-dopa to the spinal cord.

These results show that the isolated spinal cord is able to generate the complete pattern of rhythmic neural activity required for locomotion, although it may be modified by descending influences and peripheral feedback. In fact, the spinal cord locomotor programme is remarkably precise, timing the contraction of appropriate muscles in exactly the correct sequence for coordinated walking. Each limb seems to be provided with its own pattern generator, so that even if one is stopped for some reason the others may continue normally.

The existence of such intrinsic central neural oscillators does not mean that afferent input from the moving limbs is ignored altogether, however. The timing of the oscillators is usually 'entrained' by sensory feedback so that, for example, the 'swing programme' is usually switched over to the 'stance programme' when muscle spindles in the ankle extensors signal that they have lengthened by the required amount. Furthermore, peripheral feedback enables the locomotor system to adjust to unexpected events in the outside world. Compensatory reflexes such as the stretch reflex are enhanced during appropriate phases of a walk to overcome an unexpected obstacle, for example, but they may be switched off altogether at other phases of the movement. This is probably a further function of the cerebellum, one of whose main duties is to adjust the characteristics of different reflexes to be at their most useful in widely varying circumstances. It is not surprising to find, therefore, that the cerebellum receives a full account of the progress of the central locomotor programme via the ventral spinocerebellar tract which persists even after deafferentation of the moving limbs, and that the cerebellum also receives profuse signals from peripheral receptors via the dorsal spinocerebellar tract in order to modify reflex actions.

Chapter 20
Eye Movements

As the movements of each eye are effected by only six muscles and the eyes constitute a constant load for them, oculomotor control is considerably simpler than that of the rest of the body. As a result much more is known about it.

When we inspect a stationary object, the extraordinarily fine detail which we can resolve is determined by the optics of the eye, the spacing of receptors and the overlap of the receptive fields at central analysing stations, as was discussed in Chapter 6. However, the temporal resolution of the visual system is nothing like as fine. Thus, as soon as an image begins to move on the retina, either as a result of movement of the object or movement of the head or eyes, visual acuity deteriorates precipitously. In fact, it has been calculated that the image of a target moving as slowly as $1°$ s^{-1} (which would take three minutes to cross the whole visual field) is degraded by an amount equivalent to three diopters of myopia. The poor temporal response of the visual system (an unavoidable consequence of its excellent static spatial resolving power, which necessitates multitudinous time-consuming stages of lateral inhibition) would seem to preclude eye movements altogether, since they would always lead to a deterioration in vision.

Vestibular optokinetic and pursuit movements

Paradoxically, therefore, the most primitive eye movements were not those developed to shift the visual axes to a new position, but those designed to keep the visual world stable whenever the head moves (vestibulo-ocular reflex) (Fig. 20.1) or to keep moving objects fixed in relation to the retinae, by matching the movement of the eyes to movements in the surroundings (optokinetic eye movements).

In animals with a high-acuity fovea, the 'pursuit' system is a further development of the optokinetic reflex, specialized to match the movement of the fovea to the velocity of a target so that the foveae may lock on to it and inspect it despite its movements (Fig. 20.1). One might ask why it is necessary to have both vestibular and optokinetic reflexes, since each system should be able to stabilize the visual world when the head is moved. Head movements activate the vestibular system and cause a relative movement of the surroundings, stimulating the optokinetic reflex. However, only the opto-kinetic reflex can compensate for movements of the surroundings when the head is stationary, as happens, for instance, when travelling in a train. When the head has been moving at a constant velocity for some time, the semicircular canals cease to be stimulated, while the endolymph within the vestibular organs 'catches up'; only the optokinetic system can therefore compensate for such continued head movement. Nevertheless, a major limitation of the optokinetic system is that the processing of retinal input is so slow.

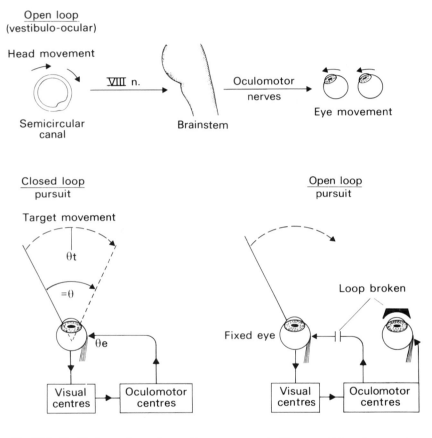

Fig. 20.1. Vestibulo-ocular and pursuit eye movements. The pursuit loop is opened by fixing the seeing eye and measuring movement of the blindfolded eye.

It takes about a quarter of a second for the visual system to respond to a sudden movement of head or object, whereas the vestibular system is much, much quicker. Hence you can see your finger clearly when you shake your head rapidly, but when you wave your finger rapidly and keep your head stationary it becomes very blurred (try it!).

The vestibulo-ocular and optokinetic reflexes tend to compensate for movements of the head or movements of an object, acting as a servo-system to effect velocity-matching. As we saw in Chapter 17, visual information can be used to alter the characteristics of the vestibulo-ocular reflex when necessary—for instance, suppressing it completely when one wishes to inspect something moving at the same speed as one's head.

Saccades

When the vestibulo-ocular reflex is elicited by rotating the head the eyes soon reach the limits of the orbits, hence they have to be repositioned repeatedly, by means of return flicks or 'saccades'. These movements are not velocity matching but enable the eyes to view new positions in space; they form the basis for a more recently evolved eye position or saccadic eye movement system. During saccadic movements, of course, nothing remains stationary on the retina; all images stream across it, so acuity is drastically reduced during repositioning movements. However, the enormous benefit of the saccadic system is that the fovea, which constitutes only a small part of the retina but has a resolving power many times greater than the periphery, can be used to inspect all parts of the visual world. By making saccades as quick as possible (often approaching velocities of $1000° \text{ s}^{-1}$), the price paid in terms of lowered visual acuity during a saccade is kept acceptably low.

Vergence movements

The most recently developed type of eye movement is 'vergence' change. In animals in which both eyes point towards the front there are obvious advantages in linking the two in parallel, so that they inspect corresponding points of the world. These are known as 'conjugate' movements. The slight differences of angle subtended on the two retinae by an object (retinal disparities) are used to reconstruct depth, as we saw in Chapter 6. However, whenever we wish to look at near objects with both eyes, we have to make them converge, so that the two fovea point at the object but from different angles. Probably only a few species have acquired this ability. Significantly, in man, vergence eye movements are the first to break down in disease. Diplopia (which follows failure of vergence movements) is one of the earliest symptoms of ocular motor disorder found in ophthalmic practice. Vergence signals are integrated with conjugate direction commands relatively late in the assembly of final oculomotor outflow. When you shift your gaze from a distant object to one closer to you and at a different angle, you first change the direction of conjugate gaze and then the eyes converge on the closer object. Interestingly, the vergence angle needed for any particular object depth varies with the distance apart of the eyes. This increases through growth, so vergence angle must adapt. Such adaptation has been demonstrated experimentally by diverting the visual axes with prisms. After wearing such prisms for some time, the vergence angles adopted show long-lasting modifications, probably mediated by the cerebellum.

CONTROL SYSTEM ANALYSIS

Optokinesis

Studying optokinetic movements of the eyes under 'closed-loop conditions' (i.e. when any mismatch between eye and target velocities is automatically corrected by the optokinetic feedback control system) is unlikely to be very helpful in determining what mechanisms are at work. We come to the unsurprising conclusion that they are very efficient. During optokinetic stimulation the eyes can follow at speeds up to about $30°\,s^{-1}$ (Fig. 20.2); they then begin to lag behind but the system only breaks down completely (the eyes no longer attempt to follow) at stimulus speeds greater than $100°\,s^{-1}$. If the lights are switched off during maximal optokinetic stimulation, effectively preventing the eyes from ever catching up with the target ('opening' the feedback loop), optokinesis after nystagmus (OKAN) continues for about 25 s. Opening of the loop can also be achieved experimentally by immobilizing the eye which is viewing the target, whilst occluding the other eye and recording its movements; or by moving the target by an equal amount whenever the eyes move, so that they can never catch up. What happens then is that eye velocity increases steadily, trying to overtake a target that it

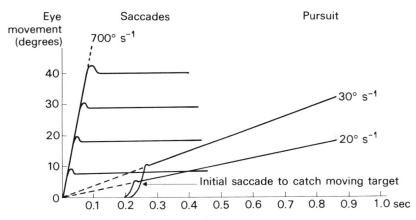

Fig. 20.2. The eyes achieve new positions at a standard $700°\,s^{-1}$ during saccades. Hence larger saccades take longer to perform. They eyes can lock on to targets moving at up to $30°\,s^{-1}$. Above this velocity the pursuit system can no longer keep up.

can never reach, until it is running at a high speed ($c.$ $100°\,s^{-1}$) (Fig. 20.2). However, this velocity is always well below the maximum velocity that can be attained during saccades.

Velocity v. position

This open-loop behaviour of optokinesis implies that when this control loop is closed the pursuit system makes use of 'velocity error' between fovea and target (sometimes known as retinal 'slip'), summing this over a few seconds (which is equivalent to the mathematical function of integration) and using the result to calculate required eye velocity. Notice that the system uses velocity, not positional, signals for control. Velocity signals may be derived by processing a small area of retinal output, for instance over the limited receptive field of a complex cell in the visual cortex, whereas positional information requires inspection of the whole retina in order to obtain the locus of a target in relation to the fovea. Thus positional signals can only be obtained much less rapidly than velocity signals. Furthermore, velocity information requires minimal recoding to regulate eye-muscle contraction, whereas positional information is coded spatially in retinotopic arrays of neurones. This positional information must be transformed radically in order to effect appropriate eye-muscle shortening.

The integrator

It turns out that a temporal integration stage is required for all types of eye movement—vestibular, pursuit or saccadic. The search for the location of this neural 'integrator' has become a classic oculomotor problem. We must not be too literal-minded about it however. Integration is a property of the whole oculomotor control system, hence it is not likely to be confined to any one anatomical site. Furthermore, if the integrator consists of self-reexciting loops of neurones, perhaps several in parallel, as seems likely, these would probably be very difficult to identify by conventional recording.

Saccadic pulse generator

The problems faced by the saccadic eye position system are difficult. Positional information is laid out topographically in retinotopic maps situated in various parts of the visual system. The locus of an object must be converted into a 'pulse' and then a 'step' of oculomotor nervous activity which will get the eyes moving fast, then hold them at precisely the right point (Fig. 20.3). The velocity of saccades is almost constant, whatever their size, so the amplitude of the pulses required is standardized and it is their duration which determines the magnitude of a saccade (Fig. 20.3). Hence a spatial neuronal array located in a visual map—probably that in the superior colliculus—has to be converted into a pulse of appropriate duration delivered to eye-muscle motoneurones. We saw in Chapter 17 how the cerebellum might contribute to the sequencing of muscle contractions using 'delay lines'. It is possible that the saccadic system may use a similar strategy, putting such a delay line into an oculomotor feedback loop. The spatial pattern generated by the delay line could then be compared with spatial input provided by the superior colliculus and the result of this comparison might then control the duration of the saccadic pulse and the magnitude of the step which is sent out to the eye muscles. Precise computation of pulse length is therefore probably the responsibility of the cerebellum, though crude saccadic movements, not well directed to their target, can be organized by the midbrain even after removal of the cerebellum.

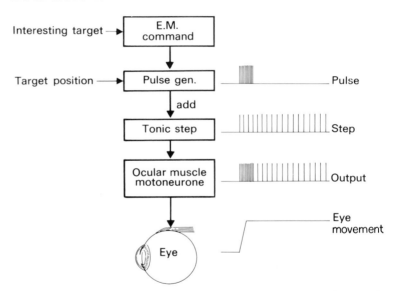

Fig. 20.3. Hypothetical generation of a 'pulse-and-step' signal for saccadic eye movement.

CNS ORGANIZATION

Figure 20.4 shows many of the CNS structures which have been implicated in the control of eye movements.

Brainstem mechanisms

We may take the vestibulo-ocular system as a starting point. There are three routes by which the VIIIth nucleus may affect ocular

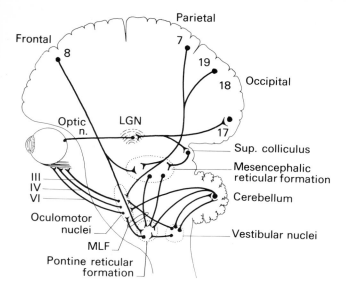

Fig. 20.4. CNS structures concerned with eye movement control.

motoneurones: (1) via the medial longitudinal fasciculus (MLF); (2) via the surrounding reticular formation; and (3) via the cerebellum. Since vestibular control over eye movements involves both smooth compensatory pursuit and saccadic return components it is reasonable to presume, and is abundantly confirmed by experiment, that later evolutionary modifications of the eye movement control system use the same basic circuitry. The MLF appears to be the main projection link between the vestibular system and ocular motoneurones. It is essential for horizontal and vertical eye movements in both pursuit and saccades.

Organization of vertical movements of the eye is to some extent segregated in the interstitial nucleus of Cajal (INC) situated just at the rostral tip of the oculomotor (IIIrd) nucleus. The INC receives from the MLF and surrounding reticular formation, and projects directly to vertical-eye-muscle motoneurones.

Separate processing of saccadic and pursuit signals probably occurs at stages prior to this. As we have seen, the saccadic system requires machinery to transform information about the locus of a stimulus, represented in retinotopic maps, to a 'pulse-and-step' signal delivered to the motoneurones in order to move the eyes to their new position quickly and hold them there. This involves both spatial and temporal integration. However, the pursuit system uses velocity information summed over time to match eye and object speeds. This needs temporal integration only; the signal can be derived from the velocity responses of single neurones. The temporal integrator is probably located in the paramedian pontine reticular formation (PPRF). Some systems of PPRF neurones probably perform velocity integration for the smooth pursuit system, and others transfer the results of precisely computed spatial integrations, which take place mainly in the cerebellum, to the saccadic system.

Higher control of eye movements

Five areas are considered important in the higher control of eye movements. These are the cerebellum, superior colliculus and basal ganglia subcortically, and the frontal eye fields and posterior parietal cortical areas.

Superior colliculus

As discussed in Chapter 6, the superior colliculus receives a full retinotopic hemifield map, chiefly supplied by collaterals of retinal Y ganglion cell axons passing to the LGN. Stimulation at any point on this map causes the eyes to move in such a way that the point in visual space represented at the site stimulated is then fixated. Clearly this could act as a 'template' for visually triggered saccades.

The superior colliculus organizes not only eye movements but head movements as well. One of its chief functions appears to be to keep all 'egocentric' spaces (visual, auditory, vestibular and somaesthetic) in register.

As might be expected, the superior colliculus does not project directly to oculomotor neurones, since its complete spatial map has to be transformed into appropriate pulse-and-step saccadic signals in single neurones. It projects to all the oculomotor regions which have been implicated in eye movement control: the vermis of the cerebellum (via the tectopontine tract), the medial longitudinal fasciculus, the interstitial nucleus of Cajal, and the pontine paramedian reticular formation. Similarly, signals from the frontal eye fields do not project directly to the oculomotoneurones but travel via the superior colliculus, cerebellum or reticular formation.

Basal ganglia

The basal ganglia are also implicated in saccadic eye movement control. In basal ganglia disease, eye movement initiation is delayed and saccade size is reduced, though saccade velocity is not usually diminished. Smooth pursuit movements, driven by continuous visual feedback, are not greatly impaired. Indeed, in some patients the tendency of the eyes to lock onto visual detail may be one of the things that slows down their eye movements, so that saccadic movement is, paradoxically, improved by shutting the eyes. These observations further support the proposition that the basal ganglia are especially important for ballistic, preprogrammed movements such as saccades, and are not concerned with continuous feedback control as in pursuit and optokinetic eye movements.

Frontal eye fields

The frontal eye fields (area 8) lie in front of motor and premotor cortex (areas 4 and 6) and anterior to the arcuate sulcus. Here, low-intensity stimulation causes contralateral conjugate deviation of the eyes. Combined ablation of both superior colliculus and frontal eye fields has a disastrous effect on voluntary saccadic eye movements, but lesions of either alone cause minor long-term changes. Thus, probably, both occipito-tectal and occipito-frontal routes are equally important for voluntary eye movement control. One puzzle is that neurones in area 8 related to saccades do not normally appear to discharge until after eye movements have begun, as if they merely register that the movement has taken place. Those in the superior colliculus and in posterior parietal area 7, on the other hand, fire well in advance of eye movements. However, some neurones in the frontal eye fields have clear visual receptive fields. If an animal is going to look at a target situated in the receptive field of one of these neurones, its response to the visual stimulus is enhanced well before the execution of the saccade. Hence discharge of a class of visually responsive cells in the frontal eye fields may trigger saccades, whilst a larger class of non-visual cells situated there registers when they are made.

Posterior parietal cortex

Low-intensity stimulation of area 7 also causes deviation of the eyes to the opposite side, whilst stimulation further back may cause convergence. These observations led David Ferrier into the mistake of thinking that the primary visual centres were in the posterior part of the parietal lobe. Neurones in area 7 are not retinotopically organized, but they receive visual input and have large (up to hemifield-sized) receptive fields. Their discharge is markedly enhanced when an object in their receptive field is about to be the target of an eye movement. Different classes respond before slow pursuit and saccadic eye movements. These neurones project to the frontal eye fields via the occipito-frontal bundle, probably providing neurones there with their visual responsiveness. They also project to the superior colliculus and to the cerebellum and basal ganglia. Bilateral ablations of area 7 leads to disturbance of visually guided or visually triggered eye movement. To achieve comparable disabilities, lesions in both frontal eye fields and superior colliculus must be made. Thus we should probably consider the posterior part of the parietal lobe (area 7) as the highest centre for visually controlled eye movements, whilst the frontal eye fields are more important in visual 'search'—random eye movements not motivated by any specific visual target but by curiosity, etc.

Chapter 21
Sleep, EEG, Reticular System

It is only possible to study sleep effectively by recording the *electro-encephalogram (EEG)*. Obvious signs of sleep, such as closed eyes, steady breathing, lack of response to stimuli, etc, are unreliable since they can all occur in circumstances other than sleep; moreover, they give no indication of the different stages within sleep which have been revealed by EEG recordings.

THE ELECTROENCEPHALOGRAM

The EEG is simply the fluctuating potential which can be recorded, after suitable amplification, from electrodes placed on the scalp. It was named and first analysed systematically by Hans Berger, a German psychiatrist, in the 1920s. Although it is widely accepted that these potentials are produced by the brain, there are still arguments about the origin of some of them. In fact, one theory proposes that the alpha wave seen in relaxed subjects with eyes closed is in fact derived from the eye muscles and not from the cerebral cortex at all!

Clearly the CSF, dura, bone and scalp must considerably attenuate any potentials produced by the brain. Hence the amplitude of the EEG is very small (usually less than 100 μV—though paradoxically it is larger over diseased areas). However, it is surprising that any potentials are recorded at all, since it would seem most unlikely that the activity of different parts of the brain, carrying out their separate sensory, perceptual, cognitive and motor functions, would ever be synchronized under normal circumstances. Nevertheless, even an alert subject performing strenuous mental arithmetic shows small (around 20 μV) randomly occurring potential fluctuations of the EEG, averaging between 15 and 30 per second, known as *beta* (β) waves (Fig. 21.1). These are said to be *desynchronized* by comparison with *alpha* (α) waves which occur when the subject relaxes and closes his eyes. This is a larger (*c.* 50 μV), more regular wave, synchronized at 8–10 Hz (Fig. 21.1).

Origin of the EEG

Fluctuations in EEG potential are probably not the result of action potentials developed by cortical neurones. The major source of

Excited

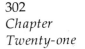

(1)

Relaxed

(2)

Drowsy

(3)

Asleep

(4)

Deep sleep

(5)

50 μV

1 sec

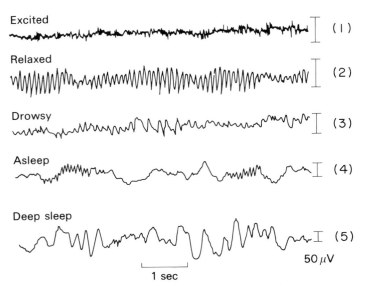

Fig. 21.1. EEG waves: (1) β (desynchronized) wave when alert and excited; (2) α (synchronized) wave when eyes are closed and subject relaxed; (3), (4), (5) successive stages of sleep. The EEG becomes more synchronized, slower and greater in amplitude.

spikes is not found on the surface but deep in the cortex at the axon hillocks of corticofugal neurones, most of which lie in cortical layer 5. Yet if the EEG is recorded directly from the exposed brain in animals or humans, it is found to be maximal in the superficial layers of cortex, not deep down in layer 5. Furthermore, if single unit activity in layer 4 is recorded simultaneously with the EEG at the surface, there is often little correspondence between the two.

Dipole model

The EEG probably represents the sum of the local currents flowing in the dendrites of superficial cortex. Despite their variable geometry with respect to electrodes on the scalp, these can successfully be modelled as 'dipoles'—that is, elongated elements with oppositely charged poles acting as sources and sinks of current, on average orientated at right angles to the cortical surface. Figure 21.2 shows how activation of such elements by an incoming sensory volley may lead to a surface negative wave followed by a positive wave. Despite the convolutions of the brain, recording disparate cortical elements altogether in this way seems to be valid; electrodes on the scalp can pick up the attentuated sum of the activity of thousands of such dipoles. These cause potential changes large enough to indicate the broad nature of local currents. The specialized activities of individual neurones, such as those detecting bars and edges in the visual world, are lost in the crude EEG; but the fact

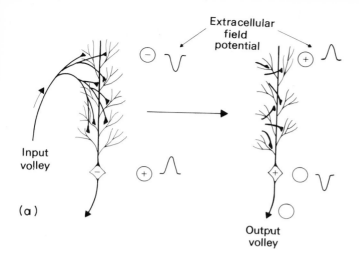

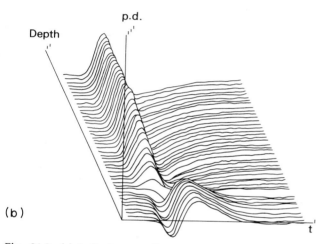

Fig. 21.2. (a) Left. Input volley depolarizes dendrites, causing negative wave extracellularly in superficial cortex whilst deeper in the cortex the pyramidal cell soma is still at resting potential (positive outside). Right. Later, the pyramidal cell body depolarizes and extracellular field potentials reverse. (b) Reversal of field potential with depth.

that anything at all is recorded implies an underlying synchrony of the local currents flowing in very large numbers of neurones.

Role of the thalamus

This synchrony is perhaps, to a small extent, the consequence of the proximity of neighbouring neurones. Current flowing in one nerve cell induces tiny currents in its neighbours. Much more important, however, is the effect of thalamic regulation of impulse traffic to the cerebral cortex. Circular islands of cerebral cortex isolated from adjacent areas, but still connected to the thalamus, preserve rhythmic activity; whereas large regions of cortex separated from the thalamus do not. Lesions of the reticular and intralaminar nuclei of the thalamus destroy the EEG rhythm, whilst stimulation of these nuclei at 8 p.p.s. elicits the 'recruiting response', which looks much like the waxing and waning of alpha rhythm (Fig. 21.3). However, the reticular and intralaminar nuclei project predominantly to other parts of the thalamus and basal ganglia, not directly to the cerebral cortex.

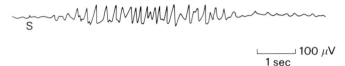

Fig. 21.3. Recruiting response following stimulation of intralaminar nuclei.

The thalamic projections probably achieve synchrony of cortical neurones as a result of negative feedback. The reticular and intra-laminar projections to specific thalamic relay nuclei give off re-current collaterals which impinge on a common inhibitory neurone; this synapses in turn with a large number of intralaminar cells both axosomatically and dendrodendritically. Hence recurrent excitation of this interneurone is followed by coordinated inhibition of all the cells affected by it, which thus removes the source of its own ex-citation. Therefore, intralaminar thalamic neurones tend to be synchronized themselves, and their projections to the thalamic relay nuclei and onwards to cerebral cortex tend to synchronize the cortical neurones to which they relay. This process predominates only when specific afferent systems are not engaged and cortical neurones are not performing their specialized functions. Thus the alpha rhythm, like slow-wave sleep (see below), is seen when the brain is doing nothing in particular, and is probably a secondary consequence of the synchronizing effect of non-specific intra-laminar thalamic neurones receiving from the basal ganglia and reticular formation.

STAGES OF SLEEP

As a person progresses from drowsiness to deep sleep, the EEG becomes more and more synchronized, becoming slower and stronger (slow-wave (S) sleep) under the influence of the ascending reticular formation. This is a gradual process, though four stages of sleep are commonly described on more or less arbitrary EEG criteria. *Rapid eye movement (REM)* sleep interrupts stage IV, and is a distinct physiological process.

The loss of consciousness which occurs when sleep supervenes on drowsiness is probably not a sudden event. If a subject is given a

motor task involving continuous effort, muscle tension and electro-
myographic activity gradually fall off as sleep overcomes him. The
EEG signs of sleep progress gradually at the same time.

Rapid eye movement (paradoxical) sleep

After about an hour and a half of slow-wave sleep (S-sleep), however, a new EEG pattern suddenly commences, known as 'paradoxical' or rapid eye movement (REM) sleep. The waves desyn-
chronize (D-sleep) as if the subject had woken up (which he does
not), whilst electro-oculographic recordings show very active eye
movements (Fig. 21.4), which can often be observed through the

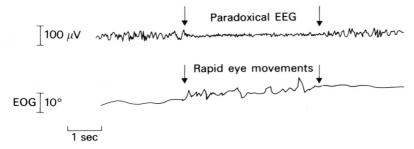

Fig. 21.4. Desynchronized EEG during slow-wave sleep, associated with rapid eye
movements shown on electro-oculogram (EOG).

subject's closed eyelids. As early as 1883, Hammond observed short
periods during normal sleep in which rapid eye movements
occurred. These are accompanied by intense cerebral activity, which
is revealed by increases in cerebral blood flow in patients who have
lost a good deal of their cranium. Close inspection of the rise and fall
of a baby's brain through the open fontanelle confirms that they too
go through periods of intense cerebral activity in REM sleep.
Cerebral blood flow, blood pressure and respiration all increase in
REM sleep but, paradoxically, muscle tone in the rest of the body
diminishes. D-sleep occurs for about 30 minutes in every two hours.
It seldom occurs more frequently, suggesting that some cyclical
process underlies it (Fig. 21.5).

Dreams

Dreaming is probably most common during D-sleep. The eye movements may correspond to visual events in the dream. D-sleep
dreams usually seem to tell a story of some curious sort, whereas
less-detailed 'feelings' are characteristic of S-sleep. In fact, the terri-
fying experience of the worst nightmares—being crushed, burnt,
suffocated or pushed over the edge of a precipice—probably occur
in S- not D-sleep.

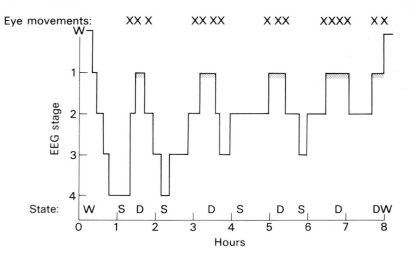

Fig. 21.5. Periodicity of REM sleep, accompanied by dreaming (D).

Functions of sleep

The foregoing pages of description of the physiology of sleep have not told us *why* we have to sleep. It must be admitted that we still do not know. We cannot really improve on classical ideas: (a) that repose is an adaptive response to the difficulty of finding food and the dangers from predators at night (if it's dangerous, do nothing!); and (b) that sleep has a restorative function.

However, what it is that we have to restore by sleeping is not at all clear. Sleep deprivation causes the frequency of error-making to increase throughout the duration of a task; hence longer, more complicated tasks are more disturbed by sleep deprivation. The psychotic effects of lack of sleep alleged from the evidence of early studies are likely to have been the result of stressing unstable subjects, rather than the result of sleep deprivation itself. In short, the only thing that is certain about sleep deprivation is that it makes subjects want to go to sleep. Why this is so, we still do not know.

D-sleep function

Nevertheless, something slightly more constructive can be said about selective D-sleep deprivation. Subjects can be woken up each time they begin rapid eye movements—a celebrated group of unfortunate cats was deprived of REM sleep by floating them on cork mats so that each time the tone in their neck muscles relaxed during REM sleep they woke up because their noses fell in the water! Such animals suffer a decline in learning ability, particularly so-called *latent* learning—the phenomenon whereby animals which have been free, for example, to explore a maze with no reward, later learn to run the maze for a food reward much faster than their colleagues which have never seen it.

Humans deprived of D-sleep show a rebound increase in REM sleep afterwards, suggesting some inner drive for this type of sleep. They also show learning disorders and subtle emotional changes which are difficult to categorize. The emotional implications of words and pictures are less accurately assessed at the time or remembered afterwards. Such subjects can view pictures of horrifying events involving blood, guts and genocide with complete equanimity, and barely remember later that they were even unpleasant. Also, patients with Korsakoff's syndrome, which is characterized by a specific deficit of long-term memory associated with confabulation to fill the gaps, have very few periods of REM sleep.

A speculative conclusion from this, admittedly fragmentary, evidence is that the special function of D-sleep is to help consolidate short-term memory traces, transforming them into long-term memories under the control of motivational state. Ultimately, long-term memory storage is only undertaken if the information so stored is likely to benefit an animal in some way, by enabling it to satisfy its drives more effectively. Emotions are the subjective corollaries of these drives. No doubt it will be possible to clarify this rather nebulous description of the function of D-sleep in the future.

Other applications of EEG recording

Cortical damage

Over a damaged area of cortex the EEG becomes larger and slower, as in the deepest stages of sleep, probably because cortical spike activity, and so the interneuronal processing which depends on this, are more vulnerable to pathological processes than the non-specific thalamic synchronizing circuit described earlier. The EEG may therefore be used to locate such damage, although modern techniques, such as the EMI computerized X-ray scanner, often allow more precise location.

Epilepsy

The main use of the EEG today, however, remains in the diagnosis of epilepsy. It is often impossible to demonstrate any macroscopic lesions in the brain of epileptics. For reasons unknown, a point in the brain can cease to be subservient to its normal inputs and becomes autonomous, producing characteristic spike and wave complexes which can then spread to involve the whole cortex in an epileptic attack. In 'grand mal' attacks generalized convulsions occur, whilst in *'petit mal'* the patient suffers from temporary loss of consciousness without convulsions. It is not at all clear why people develop epilepsy. A genetic predisposition often seems likely, while trauma to the cerebral cortex is sometimes followed by epilepsy. However, only in a small proportion of epileptics can a cause be found.

Evoked potentials

To clinicians and experimental psychologists much of what has been discovered by neurophysiologists is at present of little practical value because knowledge of the minutiae of a neurone's electrical behaviour contributes little to treating disease, understanding behaviour or explaining disordered mental activity. It is rewarding but rare for discoveries in neurophysiology to be applicable to treatment of disorders in man. It was hoped, of course, that the EEG might serve as a link between the neurophysiologist and the neurologist. However, apart from a few cases, such as sleep, cortical damage and epilepsy, the EEG has been remarkably unilluminating. For more subtle analysis of cerebral activities, the EEG has proved itself but a crude tool. A more promising approach has arisen however from further analysis of the EEG; this is the technique of averaging evoked potentials (AEPs).

Visual evoked potential (VEP)

Each time a light is flashed in the eyes, a synchronous wave of electrical activity occurs in the visual receiving areas of the occipital cortex. This is known from direct recording from the surface of the cortex in experimental animals and in humans at operation. This wave is superimposed on background EEG activity. With modern computers, the electrical activity evoked by the light can be detected through the head, even though it is attenuated 100-fold by the short-circuiting effects of the c.s.f., dura, skull and scalp. Since only the potential evoked by a stimulus is locked in time with it, whilst the fluctuations of the EEG occur randomly, a computer may be used to sum together EEG potentials at equal time intervals following repeated presentation of the stimulus. The size of the potential evoked by the stimulus is thus increased many times, whereas the background EEG, not being related in time to the stimulus, tends to cancel out completely. The advantage of this averaging process over simply amplifying EEG voltages following a stimulus is that only the signal which is of interest is enhanced, whilst background EEG is reduced. In communications jargon, the 'signal-to-noise ratio' is increased—in fact by the square root of the number of readings averaged.

This technique is now being exploited by psychologists and clinicians as well as neurophysiologists, because it can be used as an objective measure of the neuronal activity of specific sensory and motor systems under many different conditions. For example, when the intensity of a stimulus is just sufficient to be detectable subjectively, it is found that the amplitude of the cortical potential evoked by it may just be discriminated above the residual EEG noise level after averaging. Cortical potentials following different visual, auditory and somaesthetic stimuli (Fig. 21.6) have been used in all manner of ways, and even those preceding movements have been obtained by averaging the EEG over motor areas immediately before a movement. However, the problems of recording from large numbers of neurones simultaneously which we outlined in Chapter 2—namely the unknown geometrical relations between electrode and neurones and the number of different neurones contributing to the voltage fluctuations—make interpretation of EPs extremely difficult.

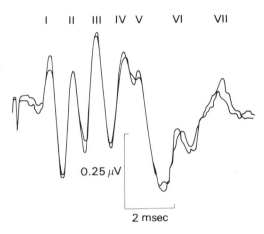

Fig. 21.6. Averaged auditory potentials in human subject evoked by a click, recorded from the mastoid processes on either side. Response in: I, VIIIth nerve; II, cochlear nucleus; III, IV, trapezoid body and lateral lemniscus; V, inferior colliculus and medial geniculate; VI, VII, temporal cortex.

RETICULAR SYSTEM AND AROUSAL

We have mentioned the reticular formation on many occasions, in connection with pain, movement control, sleep and the EEG. Like another unsatisfactory term, the 'extrapyramidal system', which describes those descending motor systems not running in the pyramidal tract, the term 'reticular formation' is a rag bag. The name describes the network (reticulum) of neurones and fibres which surrounds brainstem nuclei and fibre tracts. It contains small, large and very large neurones, some projecting locally, others stretching from top to bottom of the neuraxis. There are clear architectonic differences between different areas of the reticular formation which may reflect real functional differences, but as yet physiological techniques have not clarified these much. The largest cells lie in the medial two-thirds of the reticular formation. They give rise to the descending reticulospinal tracts and to fibres ascending to the reticular and intralaminar nuclei of the thalamus. The cells of origin of the long descending axons are concentrated (though not exclusively) in the rostral pons and rostral medulla, while the ascending fibres originate in the medial part of the reticular formation in caudal pons and caudal medulla.

Decerebrate rigidity

Interest in the reticular formation was aroused by Sherrington's studies of decerebrate rigidity—the rigidity of extensor muscles which follows midcollicular separation of the midbrain from the spinal cord (Fig. 21.7). It is supported by an overactive stretch reflex; the rigidity collapses when muscle spindle afferent signals are eliminated by cutting dorsal roots. Gamma-efferent neurones are facilitated by decerebration; this is what leads to the increased muscle spindle activity (Chapter 14). This facilitation was shown by Sherrington to originate in the upper brainstem; after midcollicular decerebration, further section of the brainstem at the upper border of the medulla oblongata abolishes decerebrate rigidity.

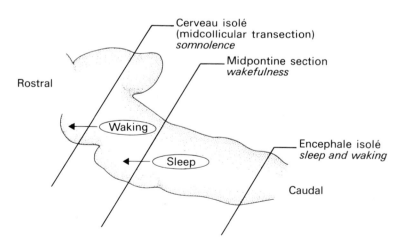

Fig. 21.7. (1) Midcollicular section causes decerebrate rigidity because it deprives the brainstem and spinal cord of cortical inhibition, whilst the cortex 'sleeps' because ascending facilitation from the reticular formation is removed. (2) Midpontine section abolishes decerebrate rigidity by removing midbrain facilitation. The cortex 'wakens' because medullary inhibitory centres are cut off. (3) High spinal section, encephale isolé, has full sleep/waking cycle, but spinal reflexes are depressed.

In 1937, Bremer observed corresponding effects on the EEG. Section of the brainstem at the midcollicular level, the cerveau isolé preparation (Fig. 21.7), causes the EEG to become slow, large, synchronized and sleep-like; while division below the pons (medullary or high spinal section) leads to low-amplitude, desynchronized EEG waves, as in wakefulness. Hence it is probable that midcollicular decerebration deprives the midbrain of inhibitory influences from the cortex which normally restrain it, and deprives the cortex of excitatory influences from the midbrain which normally facilitate it. Thus the midbrain and spinal cord overact, while the cortex 'sleeps'. Section of the brainstem at the level of the medulla prevents the midbrain RF over-exciting the spinal cord, but leaves the reticular activating system free to arouse the cortex. Hence a high spinal section (encephale isolé) leaves the isolated brain with a normal sleep/waking EEG cycle. However, it is possible to dissociate EEG and behavioural state pharmacologically, so one must not assume that EEG synchronization and sleep are always synonymous.

Reticular activating and inhibitory areas

These results from ablations were confirmed and extended in stimulation experiments by Moruzzi and Magoun. They defined reticular activating areas and inhibitory areas in the rostral dorsolateral and caudal ventromedial regions of the reticular formation, respectively (Fig. 21.8). Stimulation of these areas alters both the level of cortical arousal, as indicated by the EEG, and also the excitability of the spinal cord, assessed by the magnitude of the monosynaptic stretch reflex. They also alter the behaviour of cardiovascular, respiratory

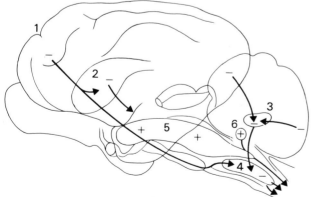

Fig. 21.8. Reticular activating and inhibiting areas. (1) Frontal cortex; (2) basal ganglia; (3) cerebellum; (4) ventromedial medullary RF; (5) rostral dorsolateral RF; (6) vestibular nuclei.

and other visceral systems, increasing or decreasing blood pressure, heart rate, respiratory frequency, tidal volume, etc.

Modern studies have advanced our knowledge of the reticular systems considerably. Reticular neurones receive convergent inputs both directly and via collaterals from practically all sensory and motor systems, with a particularly powerful input from the slowly conducting pain fibres of the archispinoreticular system. They project upwards, mainly to the hypothalamus but also to the reticular and intralaminar nuclei of the thalamus, which indirectly control transmission through the specific thalamic relays. These in turn project to all parts of the cortex; this explains the generalized effect on the EEG of all cortical areas of stimulating the reticular formation.

Reticulospinal tracts

The large myelinated descending reticulospinal pathways—the dorsal and ventral reticulospinal tracts (Fig. 15.4)—exert mainly inhibitory influence over the spinal cord. The dorsal tract originates in the medulla and depresses the activity of interneurones in Rexed's laminae V, VI and VII of the spinal grey matter, whilst the ventral pathway arises in the pontine reticular formation and inhibits motoneurones directly. A descending excitatory pathway arises in the dorsolateral facilitatory area of the brainstem reticular formation and travels to the motoneurones of axial muscles in the ventral funiculus of the spinal cord. All the descending reticulospinal neurones receive dense projections from motor cortex, basal ganglia and cerebellum.

Noradrenergic systems (Fig. 21.9)

Promising new information is now emerging about non-myelinated aminergic pathways originating in the reticular formation. Noradrenergic fibres arise in the region of the locus coeruleus in the midbrain and project via the dorsal noradrenergic bundle directly to the cortex without synapsing in the thalamus. Collaterals of these same fibres pass also to the cerebellum and to the spinal cord. Fibres in the ventral noradrenergic bundle originate in the ventral part of midbrain RF and pass to the hypothalamus and hippocampus. All these catecholaminergic fibres are small in number, thin and unmyelinated, so they were not recognized until special histochemical techniques for staining monoaminergic fibres had been developed.

Stimulation of dorsal and ventral noradrenergic bundles leads to EEG arousal, spinal cord facilitation and, in some circumstances, even locomotion. Their activity is essential for the proper maturation of synaptic interactions (e.g. ocular dominance arrangements in the visual cortex) during early development. Animals will work hard for electrical stimulation of these areas, so such stimulation is said to be rewarding. Thus despite its modest dimensions the nor-adrenergic system is probably a vital component of the reticular activating system.

Serotoninergic systems (Fig. 21.9)

Histochemical techniques have demonstrated not only diffuse nor-adrenergic projections in the brain and spinal cord, but also parallel systems of neurones containing serotonin (5HT) and dopamine (see Chapters 8 and 15). Serotonergic cell bodies are all found in the mid-line raphe nuclei of the caudoventral inhibitory part of the reticular formation. They project rostrally to the cortex and caudally to the spinal cord. Stimulation of this system sends an animal to sleep, diminishes the reflex and motoneuronal activity of the spinal

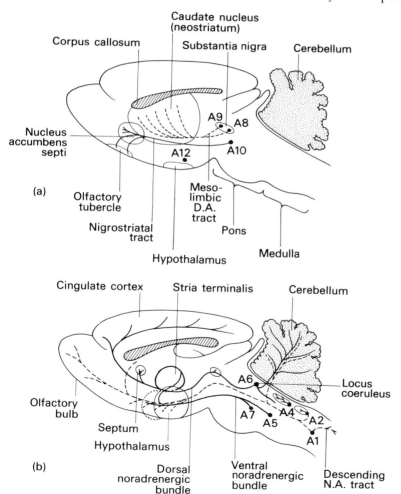

Fig. 21.9. (a) Dopaminergic pathways. (b) Noradrenergic pathways.

cord and depresses the transmission of painful stimuli from C-fibre skin afferents, probably by activating encephalinergic dorsal horn interneurones. The drug parachlorophenylanaline (PCPA), which depletes neurones of 5HT, curses the animal with temporary insomnia and unusual sensitivity to pain. Thus serotonergic fibres may well play an important role in the reticular inhibitory system.

CONCLUSION

Despite its diffuse anatomical structure, it is clear that the reticular formation plays a critical role in controlling 'arousal' in its broadest sense. Perhaps its true function is to coordinate total-body behaviour patterns, including cortex, brainstem, spinal cord and visceral mechanisms, under all conditions.

Chapter 22
Autonomic Nervous System

The part of the nervous system which controls the visceral functions of the body (the heart and circulation, lungs and respiration, kidneys, guts, etc.) is largely separate from the central nervous system (Fig. 22.1). It is called the autonomic nervous system, because it is almost completely autonomous and not usually subject to voluntary control. It has connections with the CNS via *brainstem*, *thoracolumbar* and *sacral* segments of the spinal cord (Fig. 22.1); ultimately, it is regulated by the hypothalamus, cerebellum and frontal lobes. However, it can, in fact, operate satisfactorily even if entirely separated from CNS control. As with the remainder of the CNS, a large part of our understanding of this system comes from studies on autononic reflexes, such as the baroreceptor, chemo-receptor and Hering–Breuer reflexes.

The autonomic nervous system is usually divided into two major subdivisions, known as the *sympathetic* and *parasympathetic* systems (Fig. 22.1)—so called because the sympathetic system was thought to act in sympathy with emotional reactions such as fear, anger, etc., whilst the parasympathetic system restrained the sympathetic system, promoting calm and repose.

Sympathetic system

The heart of the sympathetic system consists of a chain of *paravertebral ganglia* running down each side of the vertebral column. These are joined to spinal thoracolumbar nerves (segments T1–L2) by 'white' *rami communicantes,* which carry to the sympathetic ganglia the axons of sympathetic motoneurones situated in the lateral horn of the spinal grey matter (Fig. 22.2). The spinal cord possesses a lateral horn only at the level of the thoracolumbar sympathetic outflow and the sacral parasympathetic outflow. A 'grey' ramus communicans runs back from the sympathetic ganglia to each spinal nerve, carrying sympathetic fibres to be distributed to the muscles, skin, etc., via that nerve. Most peripheral nerves contain about 10% of such sympathetic fibres. Sympathetic ganglia also give rise to fibres passing to secondary, more peripheral ganglia situated closer to the visceral organs which they supply, such as the coeliac and hypogastric ganglia. All these nerves also carry afferent sensory fibres passing from the viscera to the paravertebral ganglia and onwards into the CNS.

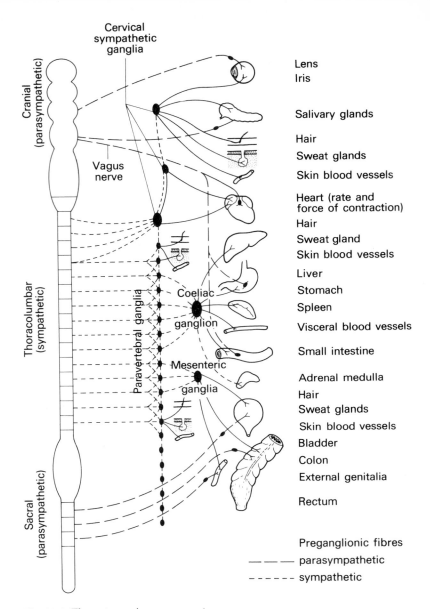

Fig. 22.1. The autonomic nervous system.

Pre- and postganglionic neurones

The neurones of the sympathetic system are basically of two sorts—*preganglionic* (with cell bodies lying in the lateral horn of the spinal cord and axons passing via white rami communicantes to the sympathetic ganglia) and *postganglionic* (whose axons supply target organs). In general, preganglionic fibres of the sympathetic system are short, since they only have to pass from the spinal cord to the paravertebral ganglia, whereas the postganglionic fibres are long,

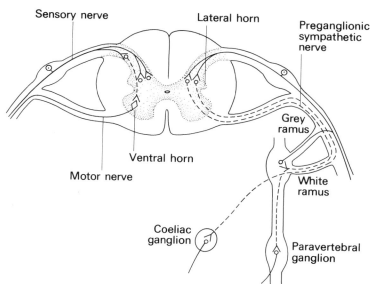

Fig. 22.2. Arrangement of the sympathetic nervous system.

since they have to run from the ganglia all the way to the periphery. In the parasympathetic system, on the other hand, preganglionic fibres are long and postganglionic fibres are short, since parasympathetic ganglia lie in the walls of the organs they supply (Fig. 22.3). Another important difference between sympathetic and parasympathetic systems is in the transmitters they employ. While the preganglionic fibres of both systems release acetylcholine, the catecholamine noradrenaline (known in the USA as norepinephrine) is released at the target organs by sympathetic postganglionic nerves; on the other hand postganglionic parasympathetic fibres release acetylcholine.

Adrenal medulla

The adrenal medulla merits special attention as it is derived embryologically from nervous tissue; it releases both adrenaline and noradrenaline into the bloodstream when the sympathetic nervous system is powerfully activated. It has therefore turned out to be a very convenient place to study neurosecretion of both hormones and neural transmitters. (There are grounds for believing that there is no fundamental distinction between these two, hormones being merely transmitters acting at a greater distance.) Sympathetic preganglionic fibres pass directly to the adrenal medulla in the splanchnic nerve without synapsing in the paravertebral ganglia. There they release acetylcholine when activated. This acts on modified postganglionic neurones, the chromaffin cells of the medulla, which may release large quantities of adrenaline and noradrenaline on demand.

Sympathetic tone

Normally, sympathetic nerves and the adrenal medulla release catecholamines continuously, establishing a certain basal level of sympathetic *tone*. This is sufficient, for instance, to keep arterioles normally constricted to about 50% of their fully dilated calibre. Adjustments to regional blood flow or overall blood pressure can then be effected by increasing or decreasing sympathetic activity. Sympathetic nervous activity is thought to be rather diffuse normally, affecting most blood vessels impartially when, for example, blood pressure is adjusted ('mass discharge'). However, the arterioles concerned with supplying the heart and brain are largely exempt from such mass discharge. The parasympathetic system, on the other hand, acts much more discretely, acting on organs individually.

Parasympathetic system

The parasympathetic division of the autonomic nervous system consists of axons of parasympathetic nuclei in the brainstem, travelling with the IIIrd, VIIth, IXth and Xth cranial nerves, and those of motoneurones in the lateral horn of the sacral enlargement of the spinal grey matter, travelling in the 2nd, 3rd and 4th sacral nerves. By far the greatest contribution is provided by N. ambiguus and N. motoris of the Xth cranial nerve, whose axons travel in the vagus and supply parasympathetic fibres to exocrine glands, lungs, heart, stomach, small intestine and most of the large intestine apart from the descending and pelvic colon, rectum and anal canal. The sacral parasympathetic fibres segregate from the sacral plexus, as the nervi erigentes, to supply the lower part of the large intestine, ureters, bladder, penis or uterus, clitoris and vagina.

Parasympathetic pre- and postganglionic fibres

The small ganglia of parasympathetic nerves are situated in the walls of each of the organs they supply, so that preganglionic fibres are long, passing from CNS to viscera, whereas postganglionic fibres are short, extending only locally. Both pre- and postganglionic parasympathetic fibres release acetylcholine, as mentioned earlier, but cholinergic receptors on parasympathetic postganglionic neurones are nicotinic, whilst those on their target organs are muscarinic (see Chapter 4).

In general, one can describe the overall actions of the sympathetic nervous system as preparing the animal for action—'the flight, fright or fight' reaction. Arterial pressure is increased because heart rate, cardiac muscle contraction and arterial and venous tone are increased. The blood flow to the brain, heart and exercising muscles increases, however, because sympathetic vasoconstriction is weaker in brain and heart, and brain and muscles are supplied with a separate vasodilator cholinergic supply which runs with the sympathetic nerves. One of the effects of adrenaline (which is released from the adrenal medulla) is to cause dilatation of blood vessels by acting on their β receptors, which are found predominantly in those supplying skeletal and cardiac muscle. Sympathetic activity also dilates the pupil and shuts down gut action by inhibiting its movements and constricting sphincters. Blood sugar is raised by increasing glycolysis, and metabolic rate is also increased. Mental activity accelerates, due to increased cerebral blood flow, increased blood glucose levels and partly, perhaps, because of activation of monoamine pathways in the CNS. All these changes clearly contribute to the preparation of an animal for intense exertion.

Stimulation of the parasympathetic system has opposite effects, however, returning the animal to a calm and placid state. Heart rate and blood pressure are reduced. The gut resumes its activity and the sphincters can open. The pupils constrict and the racing mind slows down.

CNS regulation of the autonomic nervous system

Little is known about the way in which the CNS exerts its control over the autonomic system. Like other functions of the CNS, autonomic control is thought to be organized at a series of hierarchical levels. Simple autonomic reflexes such as peristalsis—the travelling waves of constriction which propel food down the gut—are organized locally, so that the gut can still perform most of its functions even when entirely separated from the nervous system. Other autonomic reflexes, such as the local vasodilation which follows application of radiant heat to the skin, are organized at a spinal level (Fig. 22.3). (More intense heat, sufficient to cause damage to the skin, triggers the purely local reactions of the 'triple response', the first defence against injury.) Generalized sympathetic responses, for instance those involved in the continuous control of blood pressure, are integrated in the medulla and pons, whilst autonomic adjustments to cope with situations detected by teleceptors and analysed by the cerebral cortex are probably instigated by the frontal lobe and organized in the hypothalamus. For example, a large part of the increase in cardiac output which can be achieved during exercise can occur in preparation for it, before the exercise even starts. This suggests that cardiovascular adjustments during exercise are not merely slavish feedback responses to the conditions brought about by muscular activity, but rather they are executed by an autonomic 'programme' which can be brought into play in advance of anticipated exertion.

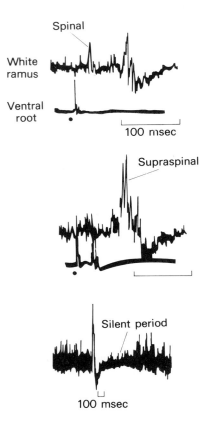

Fig. 22.3. Top: autonomic responses following sciatic nerve stimulation (at ●). Early spinal response in white ramus followed by later supraspinal responses travelling via brainstem. Somatic reflex response shown in ventral root.
Middle: increasing stimulus strength increases supraspinal response.
Bottom: the slower time-base shows a long silent period after autonomic response.

Hypothalamus

Stimulation of the posterior hypothalamus can to a large extent mimic the circulatory and respiratory changes which occur during exercise. Hence autonomic programmes are probably organized in the hypothalamus, although they can no doubt be triggered by higher centres.

Brainstem centres

Far more is known about the cardiovascular and respiratory centres in the brainstem than about those in the hypothalamus. Stimulation in appropriate parts of the reticular formation of the medulla and pons can cause hyperventilation, cardioacceleration and increases in blood pressure, together with facilitation of spinal reflexes and EEG desynchronization, denoting arousal. It is probable that the same, or closely adjacent, neurones in the medulla are involved in mediating all these effects (Fig. 22.4). Simply dropping the frequency of electrical stimulation may often reverse these responses, presumably because the change in stimulus parameters favours a new population of reticular neurones with opposite autonomic effects.

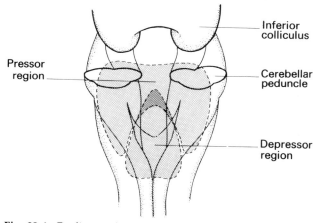

Fig. 22.4. Cardiovascular 'centres' in the medulla are coextensive with respiratory and reticular excitatory and inhibitory regions.

Shifting the site of a stimulating electrode while keeping stimulation parameters constant can also alter cardiovascular and respiratory responses. Hence particular sites in the reticular formation were originally thought to be specifically 'pressor', 'cardio-accelerator' or 'inspiratory' centres whilst others were termed 'depressor', 'cardioinhibitory' or 'expiratory'. It is now clear that such anatomical distinctions are oversimplified. Although we retain the term 'centre' for convenience, the respiratory and cardiovascular centres actually have rather loosely defined anatomical locations. Heart and lungs probably share many of the same brainstem reticular neurones, and the final effect of their activity is as much a consequence of peripheral connections as of a clear segregation in the brainstem.

Cardiovascular neurones in brainstem

Recording from neurones in the cardiovascular and respiratory areas of the brainstem reveals many with a respiratory rhythm but few, apart from the first relay neurones for baroreceptor inputs, with a clear cardiac rhythm. This is because autonomic neurones do not exert a beat-by-beat control over the cardiovascular system. The vagus can affect heart rate within one beat but its full effect takes several seconds to develop, whilst the sympathetic system requires even longer. Thus the autonomic system acts relatively slowly to modulate the activity of the heart and circulation. Unlike respiratory neurones, therefore, which discharge in phase with respiration, few brainstem cardiovascular neurones discharge with each heart beat; hence there is no easy way to decide whether they are anything to do with the cardiovascular system at all.

The discharge of sympathetic nerves supplying heart and blood vessels waxes and wanes with a 2–6 Hz rhythm. This rhythm is probably induced by pathways (many of them catecholaminergic) descending from the medullary reticular formation. Hence a promising way of identifying cardiovascular neurones in the RF is to cross-correlate their discharge with that of sympathetic efferent nerves. By this means and by observing their behaviour during procedures known to elicit cardiovascular reactions (such as lowering blood pressure or changing P_{CO_2}), much more information about brainstem mechanisms of cardiovascular control is now emerging. For example, the so-called 'A5' catecholaminergic neurones situated at the level of the superior olive project to the lateral horn cells of the thoracolumbar spinal cord sympathetic outflow; they exhibit rhythmic activity at 2–6 Hz and so probably drive sympathetic efferents. Their integrity is essential for 'pressor' reactions—the increases in blood pressure which follow brainstem stimulation or reduction in baroreceptor discharge (baroreceptor reflex). Such techniques have unexpectedly demonstrated that the vermal part of the cerebellum and rostral part of the fastigial nucleus are also highly important in cardiovascular control.

Respiratory centres

Respiratory neurones in the medulla are much more easily identified because they discharge synchronously with respiration. They continue to discharge phasically even if the medulla is entirely isolated from the rest of the nervous system, demonstrating that a basic respiratory pacemaker mechanism, the *respiratory oscillator*, lies there. Normally, however, the respiratory centres are greatly influenced by input from the pneumotaxic centre in the pons (considered by some to be merely part of the reticular inhibitory system with specialized respiratory functions) and from the apneustic centre of the upper medulla (again, perhaps merely a specialized region of the reticular activating system). Their most important sensory input is supplied by carotid and aortic body chemoreceptors in the periphery and central chemoceptors in the medulla, which adjust ventilation in accordance with the body's requirements for gas transport, and by powerful inputs from lung mechanoreceptors which discharge phasically via the vagus nerve and enable the system to respond to the mechanical condition of the lungs. The medullary respiratory centres are usually considered to consist of two 'half-centres'—inspiratory and expiratory. As with medullary regulation of the cardiovascular system, these are not distinct anatomically, although inspiratory neurones tend to be concentrated rostrally and expiratory neurones, caudally.

Inspiratory neurones fire before and during inspiration; their axons cross the mid-line and descend to cervical and thoracic motoneurones supplying the muscles which effect inspiration, the external intercostals and diaphragm. Expiratory neurones in the caudal medulla fire before and during expiration. They only actually influence expiratory muscles (the internal intercostals and the accessory muscles of respiration, such as the trapezius, scalenes and sternomastoid) during forced expirations, but they supply hyperpolarizing input to inspiratory motoneurones to ensure that they remain inactive during expiration, even during shallow breathing.

The respiratory oscillator

The spontaneous oscillations displayed by respiratory neurones in the medulla have attracted a great deal of interest because under-

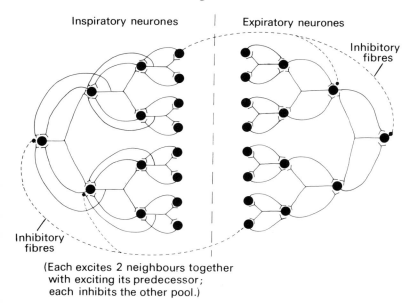

Inspiratory neurones | Expiratory neurones

Inhibitory fibres

Inhibitory fibres

(Each excites 2 neighbours together with exciting its predecessor; each inhibits the other pool.)

Fig. 22.5. Respiratory centres. Self-reexciting pools of neurones inhibit the other half-centre reciprocally.

standing their mechanism may not only elucidate the control of breathing, but may also provide insights into the nature of other rhythmic actions of the CNS, such as locomotion and the scratch reflex. Activity in inspiratory neurones builds up exponentially to a plateau, and then abruptly switches off; expiratory neurones then begin to discharge. Burns and Salmoirhagi postulated the existence of a neural network with three key features in order to explain this rhythmic activity: (1) self-exciting chains of neurones, (2) reciprocal inhibition and (3) fatigue (Fig. 22.5).

They suggested that exponential build-up of inspiratory activity is the result of progressive recruitment of self-reexciting circuits of neurones. If this were the case, neighbouring neurones would repeatedly excite one another by the same pathways during inspiration, so the discharge of one should be related in time to the discharge of a second. However, when this is examined experimentally, no temporal correlation between the firing of neighbouring inspiratory neurones is found, suggesting that reverberating loops are probably not responsible.

The second important feature of Burns and Salmoirhagi's model was the suggestion that inspiratory neurones restrain expiratory neurones and vice versa, because the two sets make reciprocal inhibitory connections. This implies that the stronger inhibitory activity is, the weaker expiratory activity should be, and vice versa. Such an inverse relationship, however, is seldom found in practice. Furthermore, there is normally a brief period at the end of inspiration when inspiratory and expiratory neurones fire simultaneously, which would be impossible if effective reciprocal inhibition existed between them. This overlap may be prolonged by appropriate manoeuvres.

Finally, Burns and Salmoirhagi suggested that the switch over from inspiration to expiration occurs, despite the inhibition of expiratory by inspiratory neurones, because the latter *fatigue*, so that when their activity wanes expiratory neurones are released from inhibition and may fire. However, it has not been possible to fatigue inspiratory neurones significantly by repeatedly stimulating them electrically. The theory thus appears to be discredited. It is likely that both the restraint of one type of neurone while the other type is firing and the switch over from one to the other are effected by an inhibitory system originating not in the classical respiratory centres at all but some way away, in the upper medulla.

The attractively simple model of respiratory-centre activity proposed by Burns and Salmoirhagi has unfortunately had to make way for much less explicit concepts involving neurochemicals as yet unidentified.

Chapter 23
Control of Body Weight, Fluid Balance and Temperature

APPETITE, FEEDING AND THE CONTROL OF BODY WEIGHT

The precision with which body weight is controlled is a very remarkable example of physiological regulation. For many animals in the wild, meal times are unpredictable, as is the quality and quantity of food at each meal, yet animals' weights remain extraordinarily constant. For humans, social convention prescribes three meals a day, regularly timed. Again, the amount and type of food varies widely, but on the whole our weights remain stable.

One of the central problems of understanding this is that there is usually a long delay (up to four hours) between the consumption of a meal and its absorption into the bloodstream. Hence eating must stop long before the food which has to be digested can restore blood and body fluids to their optimum chemical state. There must, in fact, be a *satiety* mechanism which operates in advance of restitution of glucose, fat and amino acid levels in the blood. This is known as the *cephalic phase* of feeding control. On the other hand, the initiation of eating (at least in animals other than man) is probably controlled by the state of the body fluids, sensed by glucose- fat- and amino-acid-sensitive chemoreceptors, which are found in the hypothalamus, stomach, intestine and (most important of all) the liver. This is the *intestinal phase* of eating control.

Hypothalamic half-centres

The classical theory of appetite control postulates the existence of two antagonistic half-centres. The *satiety centre* lies in the ventro-medial hypothalamus (VMH); ablation leads to hyperphagia and stimulation arrests eating. Pictures of extraordinarily fat rats are common in this literature. This is balanced by a *feeding centre* situated in the lateral hypothalamus, where ablation leads to aphagia and anorexia (and thin, emaciated rats) whilst its stimulation prompts feeding.

This scheme is probably too simple. Ablation of the VMH divides the 'ventral noradrenergic bundle', which runs from the pons to the forebrain through the ventral hypothalamus. Lesions of this system in the pons also disturb feeding, so the hypothalamus itself may not be as important as was originally thought. In the same way, lesions of the lateral hypothalamus have a profound effect on many aspects of behaviour besides eating, probably because they interrupt meso-limbic dopaminergic pathways. Similar effects on motor activity can be obtained by destroying the better-known nigrostriatal dopamine system in the basal ganglia. Nevertheless, the hypothalamus probably does play an important role in feeding control, because it is here that most of the afferent signals affecting appetite arrive. Regulation of the hormones affecting metabolic adjustments also occurs here.

Absorption and insulin

Two metabolic states may be identified in animals in the period between meals—*absorption* and *fasting*. Immediately after a meal is consumed, food is absorbed from the gut into the portal circulation (the gut's private vascular connection with the liver) and distri-bution of glucose, fatty acids and amino acids occurs throughout the body. This phase is mainly regulated by *insulin*, released under central nervous control in response to rising levels of glucose in the blood consequent upon eating; these are detected in the hypo-thalamus. Glucose and amino acid levels also have a direct effect on insulin secretion by the islets of Langerhans in the pancreas, where it is synthesized.

Insulin lowers the blood sugar level (Fig. 23.1) by facilitating the entry of glucose into cells (1); by speeding the conversion of glucose into glycogen (2) and fats (3); it also encourages the entry of amino acids into cells (4). Thus after a meal it restores blood sugar and amino acid levels to normal, and in so doing removes the stimulus for its own release.

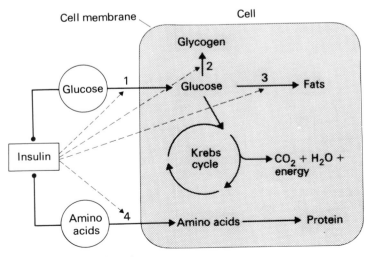

Fig. 23.1. Actions of insulin.

The next, fasting phase is therefore characterized by low insulin levels and by the release of substances which promote a rise in blood sugar level (glucagon, adrenaline and growth hormone). These promote the conversion of muscle and liver glycogen to glucose, and the release of energy-rich fatty acids from fats. Quite soon, of course, these readily available stores run down, blood sugar, fatty acid and amino acid levels in the blood fall and the aversive sensation of hunger drives the animal to search for food.

Hunger

It is not possible to identify a single factor which causes hunger, though at various times gastric stretch receptors, hypothalamic glucoreceptors and liver chemoreceptors have all been invoked. Almost certainly, the sensation of hunger depends upon the interaction of all these factors and many more. For some reason it is a recurrent obsession among physiologists that it ought to be possible to explain homeostatic control systems in terms of a single feedback pathway; it is recurrently proved a delusion.

BODY FLUID BALANCE

Not only the total volume of water in the body but also its mineral composition and overall osmotic pressure are precisely controlled. This is not the place to consider how K^+, Ca^{2+}, Mg^{2+}, H^+, Cl^-, etc. are regulated, which may be found in textbooks of general physiology, but water balance and osmotic pressure control are further important functions of the hypothalamus and should be outlined. Osmotic control is essential to preserve a precise balance of intracellular, interstitial and intravascular fluid volumes. The chief osmotically active crystalloid in the extracellular fluid (e.c.f.) is sodium, so the problems of body fluid volume and osmotic pressure control boil down to the control of salt and water balance.

Salt and water intake

Intake of salt is usually far in excess of the body's requirements, varying widely according to the nature of the food consumed. Although selective taste for salt-rich foods is found in salt-deficient animals and can help to compensate for lack of salt, the more usual problem is to regulate salt loss through urine and sweat. The availability of water, on the other hand, is often limited, hence both intake and output are closely regulated, the former by thirst and the latter by controlling reabsorption in the kidneys.

Osmotic pressure regulation

Two sorts of receptor monitor the concentration of solutes in the body fluids. The existence of central *osmoreceptors* was demonstrated by Verney, who injected hypertonic saline or sucrose into the carotid artery, whereupon the kidneys promptly secreted less urine. It has since been verified that these osmoreceptors are located in the hypothalamus. They help to control the production of *antidiuretic hormone (ADH)* by the posterior part of the pituitary (the neurohypophysis). This hormone adjusts the amount of salt-free water able to pass back from the kidney collecting ducts into the hypertonic renal papillae, thus controlling the amount of water which is reabsorbed and hence body fluid osmotic pressure. The osmoreceptors are probably not themselves the neurones which synthesize ADH; some osmoreceptors are probably situated in the heavily vascularized nucleus circularis which lies near the IIIrd ventricle, some distance from the supraoptic nuclei of the hypothalamus where ADH is synthesized. Increased osmotic pressure of hypothalamic blood causes increased discharge of osmoreceptors; this in turn increases synthesis of ADH in supraoptic neurones and causes its release from their axon terminals in the posterior pituitary.

It is likely that some osmoreceptors also lie in the stomach, intestine and liver; these appear to be more involved in the regulation of appetite and satiety than with body water control. Whether or not they have any effect on ADH production is not known, though it seems highly probable that they do, since osmotic conditions in the gastrointestinal tract must to some extent anticipate those in the blood reaching the hypothalamus. By analogy with peripheral temperature receptors helping to predict future core-temperature changes, or even with muscle spindle dynamic receptors giving advance warning to the postural system of dangers to one's equilibrium, one might expect the peripheral osmoreceptors to be able to provide advance warning, in order to facilitate ADH control.

Body fluid volume control

Osmotic pressure regulation is only one aspect of body fluid balance. Control of the total volume of the body fluids is another. Paradoxically, the chief effector of volume change is not water intake or loss, but the quantity of sodium in the body. Because water is able to move freely from one fluid compartment to another following osmotic gradients, wherever Na^+ moves, water follows.

The chief hormone regulating Na^+ balance is *aldosterone*, which is released from the adrenal cortex. This regulates reabsorption of Na^+

into the body from the proximal tubule of the kidney nephron and from sweat glands. Aldosterone secretion is directly affected by plasma Na^+ levels; it is also under sympathetic nervous control, and furthermore is influenced by blood levels of angiotensin. Angiotensin is split off plasma angiotensinogen when renin is secreted by the kidney in response to a fall in renal blood pressure or renal Na^+ levels, or following stimulation of the renal nerves. Thus whenever plasma volume drops, causing a fall in renal blood pressure or Na^+ level, renin is released causing the release of angiotensin and aldosterone. This helps to reverse the fall in blood volume by causing the kidneys to reabsorb more Na^+ and therefore to retain more water.

However, this is rather a slow and cumbersome response, taking at least 30 minutes. A much quicker reaction is needed to combat a dramatic volume change, such as a haemorrhage. The immediate effect of a sudden drop in blood volume is to cause a reduction in arterial blood pressure as the venous return to the heart diminishes. This drop is detected by stretch receptors (baroreceptors) in the walls of the arteries, which trigger the engagement by the medullary vasomotor centres of all inessential blood vessels in support of continued circulation to the heart and brain.

Volume receptors

Loss of blood volume also causes stretch receptors in the large veins to discharge less vigorously. Those on the venous side are more important in this context, since 80% of the systemic blood volume is in the veins at any instant. Hence in haemorrhage the veins are more strongly affected and venous stretch receptors (volume receptors) decrease their discharge more than arterial baroreceptors change theirs. When arterial and venous stretch receptor input to the hypothalamus is reduced, ADH output increases, as does traffic in sympathetic nerves to the adrenals and kidneys. This autonomic reflex causes increased release of aldosterone, both immediately and after a delay during which the renin–angiotensin mechanism is activated. Thus in a relatively short time, the kidney is able to increase salt and water reabsorption to compensate for the lowered blood volume. An inverse train of events follows overhydration.

Thirst

So far, we have only considered the output side of body water control. Although salt balance is almost entirely controlled by regulating its loss, thirst and drinking are probably as important as the kidneys in controlling body water volume. The same receptors, many of the same hormones and the same centres in the hypothalamus integrate the various incoming signals for thirst and renal control of water output. Impulses from volume receptors in the veins and atria inhibit drinking, whilst their reduced discharge following a reduction in blood volume stimulates it.

An increase in blood osmotic pressure, detected by the osmo-receptors in the hypothalamus, increases thirst; this is well known to sweating miners who, on emerging from their mines, make straight for the nearest bar and consume large quantities of beer. Beer has three advantages over water for this purpose: (1) it contains salt which replaces that lost in sweat, (2) it contains calories which replace the energy used up in mining, (3) it contains alcohol which restores morale, lost down the mine.

Angiotensin

A further important influence on thirst has recently been identified. This turns out, unsurprisingly, to be angiotensin, formed in the blood when the kidney releases renin. Injections of angiotensin into the hypothalamus elicit drinking in experimental animals. The site which it stimulates (the periventricular optic recess in the anterior hypothalamus) is separate from the region where drinking behaviour is thought, from the results of stimulation and ablation experiments, to be organized—the lateral hypothalamus and septal region. Lateral hypothalamic destruction leads to reduction in drinking (adipsia), whilst lesions in the septal region lead to thirst-induced excessive drinking (polydipsia). This polydipsia is not dependent on the kidneys, unlike diabetes insipidus which follows destruction of the ADH-synthesizing neurones in the supraoptic or paraventricular nuclei.

Gastrointestinal receptors

Finally, it is likely that a mechanism exists for metering the amount of water drunk, before it ever leaves the gastrointestinal tract and has had time to restore osmotic and volume conditions. This system is analogous to the cephalic influences on feeding behaviour. It is probably served by stretch receptors in the stomach and intestine and osmoreceptors in the mouth, stomach, intestine and liver.

TEMPERATURE CONTROL

The temperature of the core of the body of warm-blooded animals is kept relatively constant and independent of changes in the temperature of the environment. This is why they are called homeotherms (from the Greek for 'same temperature'). Preservation of this stability demands a very precise balancing operation between the body's activities, which produce heat, and the generally cooler environment, which steals heat. The control centres for thermo-regulation are also found in the hypothalamus.

Heat production

On the input side are the following.
(1) *Basal metabolism,* the continuous background of metabolic activity which takes place even at rest. This produces a minimum of 8.4 kJ/24 h.
(2) *Muscular exertion* (which of course varies a lot).
(3) The *specific dynamic action* (S.D.A.) of foods, particularly proteins, which often stimulate the body's chemical activity by a great amount in order to expedite their own metabolism. This phenomenon is also known as diet-induced thermogenesis (D.I.T.).

'Brown' fat

It used to be thought that only in infants was 'brown' fat an important source of heat. It is found in certain subcutaneous regions, such as between the scapulae and over the sternum. The fat cells are brown because they contain large numbers of mito-chondria, so that they can potentially achieve a very high metabolic rate. Brown fat is under the control of sympathetic nerves, with which it is liberally supplied. The system is a baby's physiological 'electrical blanket'. However, adults also have large amounts of brown fat and it is possible that one underlying genetic cause of obesity is replacement or inadequate mobilization of this brown fat, resulting in a lower than normal metabolic rate.

Hormonal and neural control of heat production

Basal metabolic rate can be increased by many hormones, for example thyroxine, growth hormone and adrenocorticoids; all these are also ultimately controlled by the hypothalamus. Thus in a cold environment, the hypothalamus is stimulated to release more thyrotropin releasing factor (TRF), the hormone which releases thyroid stimulating hormone (TSH) from the anterior pituitary. This in turn controls the production and release of thyroxine. Hence the basal metabolic rate may be raised for as long as is required. The hypothalamus probably also controls the activation of brown fat, via sympathetic nerves.

Following a fall in environmental temperature, muscular activity can also be increased, both voluntarily (putting on more clothes and jumping around to keep warm) and involuntarily (shivering). The execution of both shivering and behavioural responses is a further responsibility of the hypothalamus. Rats with thermodes cooling the hypothalamus will work, by pressing a lever, to obtain puffs of warm air; the rate of lever pressing is accurately related to the degree of cooling of the hypothalamus. The voluntary activity of lever pressing is regulated by hypothalamic assessment of the heat deficit.

Heat loss

Skin

Control over loss of heat is more flexible than control of heat gain. Apart from inevitable small amounts of heat lost in urine, faeces and breath, in man the main temperature-regulating organ is the skin. When the circulation to the skin is reduced to the bare minimum required to oxygenate the dermis (the superficial cells in the epidermis being dead anyway), the skin acts as an extremely efficient insulator, but when all the capillaries and arteriovenous anastomoses of the skin are fully dilated and the sweat glands are fully active, it acts as a highly efficient conductor, convector, radiator and evaporator of heat. The flow of blood can readily be altered between these two extremes. Thus the skin acts as a *variable insulator*; heat loss through it can be varied sensitively over an extremely wide range.

Neural control of heat loss

The thermoregulatory function of the skin is also controlled by the hypothalamus, employing sympathetic, noradrenergic, vaso-constrictor nerves to cutaneous blood vessels, and also a specialized cholinergic vasodilator supply to sweat glands travelling via sympathetic nerves. Little is known about pathways from the hypothalamus to the sympathetic outflows to the skin, and still less is known about vasodilator routes.

Bradykinin

An intriguing mechanism about which more is known is the control exerted by sweat glands over their own blood supply. When activated to secrete sweat they release an enzyme, kallikrein, which splits the octapeptide bradykinin from a longer-chain precursor in plasma. Bradykinin is one of the most potent vasodilator agents known, and it ensures a brisk blood supply to active sweat glands. Indeed, it is possible that release of kallikrein is the sole function of sudomotor fibres. Increased sweating may then follow automatically from the increased blood supply.

Thermoreceptors

The obvious candidates for the receptors supplying the information which the hypothalamus needs in order to control body temperature are the warm and cold receptors found in the skin which we have already considered under the heading of somaesthesia (Chapter 8). However, they are, in fact, not very well placed. The organs at the *core* of the body are the ones whose temperature control is ultimately the goal of hypothalamic thermoregulation; these are the brain, heart, liver, etc. It is the temperature of these organs which needs to be monitored, not that of the skin. Skin temperature varies as a result of the thermoregulatory reactions in progress and environmental temperature changes. During heat loss, skin temperature receptors relate a very different temperature to that signalled during heat retention, as we know subjectively from the contrast between our chilly first encounter with a freezing cold day and the feeling of warmth which follows a run on a frosty morning. Skin receptors, then, give an unreliable picture of both core temperature and environmental conditions. Nevertheless, as we shall see, they do play a very important subsidiary role, providing thermoregulatory centres with advance warning of impending temperature changes.

Hypothalamic temperature receptors

The temperature receptors most important for thermoregulation are situated in the hypothalamus itself. This was first suspected from ablation experiments, though destroying a headquarters can never prove that the spies were there. The existence of central temperature receptors was confirmed by injecting warm or cold saline into the carotid artery, which supplies the hypothalamus, and by altering the temperature of the hypothalamus directly, using thermodes implanted there. Alterations in hypothalamic temperature provoke powerful compensatory thermoregulatory responses.

Single temperature-sensitive neurones in the anterior hypo- have now been recorded. When hypothalamic temperature is raised, central warm receptors increase their discharge, whilst cold receptors (a smaller population) decrease their rate of firing. When hypothalamic temperature is decreased, cold receptors increase their discharge and warm receptors decrease theirs. The resultant thermoregulatory responses are heat loss through the skin when hypothalamic temperature rises, and heat production and retention when it falls.

The temperature 'set point' around which this system operates is not really fixed but varies throughout the sleep/waking cycle, with the amount of physical activity and with the stage of the female menstrual cycle. Furthermore, it is not a 'point' but a range of temperatures. For instance, heat loss following increased hypothalamic temperature may not commence until the body temperature reaches 40°C; whilst heat production may not start until body temperature falls to below 36°C (even though we think of normal body temperature as being precisely 37°C). When a thermoregulatory response commences, its sensitivity is proportional to the amount by which core temperature has departed from the middle of the set range. Thus, in our example the rate of heat loss in response to a core temperature which has risen to 40°C is greater than the rate of loss when the response starts at 38°C.

Role of skin thermoreceptors

The other important factor which determines thermoregulatory sensitivity is environmental temperature, sensed (albeit imperfectly) by skin receptors. Their signals must be 'calibrated' in relation to the prevailing skin circulation as increased blood flow warms them up. The exact route of the spinoreticular, spinothalamic or cortical projections of thermoreceptors to the hypothalamus is unknown. Their effect, however, is to alter the amount of heat loss or gain for a given core temperature deviation from the hypothalamic set point, and also to alter the threshold at which such responses commence, i.e. both the slope and the intercept of hypothalamic thermoregulatory curves are adjusted by input from skin thermoreceptors. Thus, shivering can start immediately on going outside into the cold, before hypothalamic temperature has been affected; the threshold for cold responses falls, whilst their sensitivity increases. Similarly in the sun, skin circulation increases long before core temperature rises. Cutaneous receptors are highly sensitive to the rate of change of skin temperature, as well as to its current level. Hence the hypothalamus can anticipate future changes in the thermal environment on the basis of rate of temperature change as well as static temperature level, and take appropriate action.

Hypothalamic centres

Little is known about the way in which all this is put together in the hypothalamus. Two half-centres have (as is usual for the hypothalamus) been described. A heat-loss centre in the anterior lobe is postulated from the evidence of ablation and stimulation experiments, whilst a heat-gain centre is found in the posteriomedial hypothalamus. The two regions are thought to employ different transmitters (5HT for heat gain, noradrenaline for heat loss). However, as noted earlier, autonomic 'centres' are functional rather than anatomical concepts. Heat control is not physically separable from the centres performing very different roles—controlling eating, drinking, fluid balance, etc. It is probable that, like the reticular formation of the medulla which controls blood pressure, heart rate, respiration and the gastrointestinal tract, so in the hypothalamus many systems share the same neural networks. It is probably the efferent connections of these which confer specificity upon their regulatory functions. Accordingly, if only the principles of the functioning of these neurones could be discovered, our general understanding of the control of these basic processes would be greatly enhanced.

Chapter 24
Hemispheric Specialization, Speech and Reading

At many points in this book the subject of hemispheric special-ization has cropped up. The most obvious outward and visible sign of its importance in everyday life is the fact that the great majority of us prefer to use our right hands for writing and our right feet for kicking, etc. The specialization of the left hemisphere for language-related motor tasks follows from the location of the *speech centres* on the left in most people. This has been shown directly by infusing a barbiturate, sodium amytal, into the left carotid artery; this operation depresses the left hemisphere, and reversibly dis-organizes speech in about 95% of people. It is easy to see why left-sided speech results in people writing with their right hands, since speech and writing may thus communicate with each other within the same hemisphere. However, using the right foot for kicking does not have such a clear rationale; indeed many people are almost equally good at kicking with their left foot.

A perplexing question is why speech is confined to only one hemisphere. A completely symmetrical animal would probably never be able to tell left from right since both sides of its body would be identical; the evolution of one hemisphere to be different from the other may thus have been necessary, simply to distinguish left from right. However, a more convincing explanation is derived from considering the complexity of the control problem presented by speaking. Speech demands minutely precise contractions of the vocal muscles. These are axial, and therefore bilaterally rep-resented. It is clear that to organize such accurate control by linking both hemispheres together would be much more difficult than to employ just one area to do the job. This is probably why Broca's area is found only in the left hemisphere. The siting of Wernicke's auditory language area and Dejerine's visual language area on the left side thus followed from the location of Broca's area (Fig. 24.1).

Broca's area

The location of language areas in the left hemisphere was originally deduced from the site of the lesions in humans which cause language deficits. One type results from damage to Broca's area, which is situated just in front of the mouth region of the motor cortex. These patients suffer from *motor aphasia;* they can only make

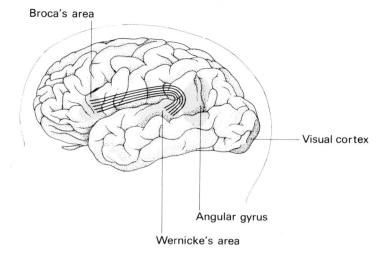

Broca's area

Visual cortex

Angular gyrus

Wernicke's area

Fig. 24.1. Language areas.

simple articulations such as 'da', 'ba' and 'cat', because precise control over vocal muscles is lost, and they simply cannot pronounce complicated, polysyllabic words. However their understanding of language, and often their writing, may be completely unimpaired.

Wernicke's area

On the other hand, damage to Wernicke's area, which lies in the superior temporal gyrus just behind the primary auditory receiving areas, leads to *sensory* or *receptive aphasia*, inability to name objects (such nominal aphasia is sometimes the only residual symptom of a resolved stroke), and inability to understand the meaning of words. In Wernicke's aphasia, however, motor production of speech (and so the speech sound itself) is normal. Of course the meaning of much of what the patient says is nonsense, due to the perceptual deficit. A most dramatic example of this is 'jargon aphasia', in which the patient emits a stream of utterly incomprehensible words, and is completely unaware that he is talking nonsense. However, since diseases of the nervous system are often diffuse and do not recognize the anatomical boundaries of functionally localized areas, the aphasias seen in normal clinical practice are seldom purely motor or purely receptive.

Angular gyrus

A further area in the left hemisphere important for reading and writing is the angular gyrus (Dejerine's area), which lies between posterior parietal visual association cortex and Wernicke's area in the superior temporal gyrus. Lesions here give rise to *specific alexia* (inability to read) because the visual patterns of written material are disconnected from Wernicke's area, and therefore cannot be associated with the stored memory of words and their meanings.

Planum temporale

It has recently become apparent that in man, and even in other primates, the anatomical complexity of the area at the back of the temporal lobe devoted to language, the planum temporale, is greater in the left hemisphere than in the right. This is true even in newborn babies, and it is therefore probably genetically endowed. In monkeys, the cross-modal association of different colours with different sounds is specifically disturbed by lesions in the posterior part of the left, but not the right, superior temporal gyrus. Even in birds, lesions of the left hyperstriatum ventrale (thought to be equivalent in many ways to mammalian cortex) disturbs the singing ability far more effectively than lesions to the right hand side.

Thus one can conclude that the left hemisphere (not only in humans) is specialized for the production and analysis of vocalizations and language, whether transmitted by sound, vision or, in fact, touch. One can generalize by saying that all human mental activities which depend on *encoding* experience in some abstract form (as language, numbers and algebraic or logical symbols) are mainly performed by the left hemisphere.

Split-brain studies

The prepotency of the left hemisphere for language has been shown most clearly by Sperry's studies of 'split-brain' patients. These are usually people who suffered from severe epilepsy, in whom the corpus callosum and anterior commissures were divided surgically to prevent the transfer of epileptic discharges from one half of the brain to the other (epileptic foci often lead to mirror-image damage on the opposite side). If the two hemispheres are disconnected from each other in this way, when visual information is presented in one half of the visual field the other hemisphere may not 'see' it at all (Fig. 24.2). A word flashed in the right hemifield can be correctly reported by the left hemisphere, since it reaches the left visual areas, and can pass via the left angular gyrus (Dejerine's area) to Wernicke's and Broca's areas. (The word is presented for less than 200 ms, so that the eyes can not have time to move and place it in the other hemifield.) However, if the word is flashed in the left hemifield, a split-brain subject cannot report what he has seen, since his right visual cortex is disconnected from the speech areas in the left hemisphere. Such patients are therefore unable to read ('alexic') in the left visual field. Subcortical connections, which could in principle effect the transfer, do not seem to be able to handle these complex cortical functions. By suitable tests, it is possible to show that the right hemisphere does actually see words and has some degree of reading ability, but cannot verbalize the experience as speech is wholly organized in Broca's area in the left hemisphere. If the word 'cat' or 'mouse' is flashed in the left hemifield, and the patient asked to point to the correct pictures of a cat or mouse with the left hand without speaking, he can usually get the answer right.

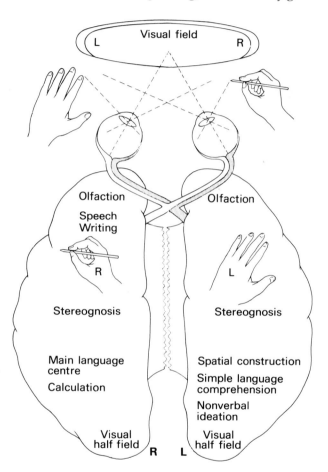

Fig. 24.2. In a 'split-brain' subject, visual signals from the right half of the visual field pass only to the left hemisphere and vice versa. Thus the functions of each hemisphere may be deduced. The left hemisphere is specialized for working with symbols (language), and the right hemisphere is specialized for 'holistic' functions (calculation, spatial construction, stereognosis, map reading, etc.).

However, the right hemisphere seems to be mainly specialized for 'spatial processing'—finding the way out of a maze, determining whether complex patterns flashed successively in the left hemisphere are the same or different, recognizing faces or pictures, and so on. It can perform these operations more efficiently than the left hemisphere; disease of the right hemisphere affects spatial performance far more than damage to the left. For example, 'dressing apraxia' (inability to dress oneself) is found following right- but not left-sided parietal-lobe lesions. Sometimes such lesions are accompanied by unilateral perceptual neglect, leading to bizarre situations such as the patient who, with difficulty, dresses the right side of himself perfectly, but leaves the left side completely undressed and does not realize it. Aprosopagnosia (inability to recognize faces) is another symptom found in right-hemisphere disease. Constructional apraxia is probably the most common however. The right hemisphere is probably also superior to the left in musical appreciation and imaginative thinking.

Left-handers

In about 50% of left-handed people, the speech centres are nevertheless found in the left hemisphere, whilst 40% have bilateral speech centres. Only 10% of left-handers (one per cent of the total population) have right-sided speech centres. Their rarity confirms an evolutionary pressure in favour of the left hemisphere; though why the left was chosen we do not know. The incidence of left-handedness may be increasing, though whether this is a real trend or a statistical aberration is not clear. If it is a real trend, it is unclear why it should occur.

Chapter 25
Reward, Learning and Memory

REWARD

One of the most interesting questions of all is *why* we behave as we do. We have eschewed metaphysical and religious answers to this question, though not denying that such answers might exist, by embarking upon the study of neurophysiology. What we are looking for are the mechanisms which impel us to behave in certain ways. Psychologists talk of instinctive *drives* (hunger, thirst, sex and so on) and *reinforcers* (rewards or punishments following particular actions). Drives are reduced by removing the deficits (e.g., lack of food) which stimulate them in the first place. The very process of reducing the drive is said to be pleasurable. For example, eating itself is rewarding if we are hungry, as we all know. In the case of behaviour only distantly related to instincts—such as the curiosity of an animal which prompts it to explore a new environment—this explanation is not very convincing. What drive is reduced by looking over the edge of a cage? Even in the case of clearly drive-induced behaviours it seems rather a sleight of hand. In effect, we say that to feed is itself a reward, so that we feed because we are rewarded—a circular argument. The real question is 'why is feeding pleasurable?'

The brain's 'reward' system

A clue to answering these conundrums came from the discovery of the 'reward' system of the brain. In the early 1950s James Olds, almost by accident, discovered the rewarding effect of stimulating certain parts of the brain. He was wondering whether stimulating the reticular activating system, recently described by Moruzzi and Magoun, would increase an animal's rate of learning. He found that animals would sometimes actually work very hard for the experience of being electrically stimulated. When electrodes placed at the lateral boundary of the hypothalamus were stimulated, rats would return again and again to the corner of the cage where they happened to be when they first experienced the stimulation, for all the world as if they had enjoyed the experience and were hoping to have it repeated. Such electrode sites became known as self-stimulation sites, because animals learn very quickly to press a lever in order to obtain their electrical 'reward' (Fig. 25.1). Other sites are *aversive*, in that an animal will do what it can to avoid stimulation. Most shocks are aversive if stimulus strength is high enough, and even potent self-stimulation sites are aversive if the stimulation is carried on for too long. For stimulation at a powerfully rewarding site, such as the medial forebrain bundle (MFB), animals will press the self-stimulation lever at rates as high as 100 times per minute. If supply of food is restricted to the time when self-stimulation is available they will starve themselves in favour of their 'fix' of self-stimulation.

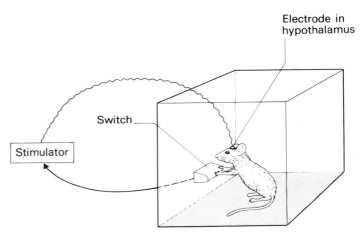

Fig. 25.1. A rat learns very quickly that switching on stimulation of lateral hypothalamus is pleasurable.

This discovery was greeted with exaggerated publicity. It was alleged that our 'pleasure centres' had been found, and that cures for all manner of problems such as drug addiction and schizophrenia (the latter alleged to be the result of actions losing their reward value) were just around the corner. Scares that unscrupulous dictators would radio into our pleasure centres were fomented. In fact, of course, matters are much less clear cut. First, the areas which support self-stimulation are ubiquitous, and include the dopaminergic MFB and its rostral connections with the entorhinal cortex, frontal cortex and hypothalamus, and also its caudal projections to the ventral pons. Secondly, the dopaminergic neurones found in the substantia nigra whose axons project upwards to the corpus striatum support self-stimulation. Thirdly, a totally separate noradrenergic system, centred around the locus coeruleus and giving rise to extensive diffuse projections to cortex, cerebellum and spinal cord, also supports self-stimulation.

Moreover, ablation of no single area will abolish self-stimulation altogether. It is likely that both dopaminergic and noradrenergic neuronal systems are involved. It is incorrect therefore to talk of a single pleasure centre. Furthermore, the satisfaction obtained from this system, which impels animals to seek more, is strikingly 'unnatural'. Human volunteers with electrodes implanted in the MFB express no more that mild curiosity about their sensations following stimulation. They certainly do not feel ecstasy or bliss. Experimental animals forget the joy of self-stimulation by bar-pressing much more quickly when the current is switched off than they lose their memory of how to obtain food by bar-pressing. Thus *extinction* of the memory of self-stimulation is much quicker than that of food rewards. Similarly, animals tend to forget the pleasurable qualities of self-stimulation after just one night, and have to be reminded of it the next morning by application of a few 'free' bursts; this is known as 'priming'.

Quite apart from these problems, the unitary reward concept meets great difficulties when applied to the major problem it was meant to explain—instinctive behaviour. Two different types of question arise in this connection. First, how does an animal manage to select among competing drives—whether to feed, drink, mate, run away or explore in the hope of finding food, water or a mate? Secondly, how does an instinctive drive activate the particular behavioural pattern that has been selected?

Selection of behavioural priorities

One hypothesis to explain why a particular behaviour is selected is that drives stimulate the reward system directly, in such a way that the stronger the drive (signalled by time elapsed since last meal, level of blood sugar, time since last mating, etc.), the greater is the reward value of reducing it (by eating, mating, etc.). The idea implies that a drive somehow stimulates the reward system to the degree to which it remains unsatisfied. Then, so the argument runs, the most important drive is satisfied first, because behaviour reducing that drive is the most rewarding. According to this hypothesis, selection among possible behaviour patterns results automatically from the relative strengths of drives controlling the magnitude of the rewarding effect of the behaviour. Consequently, the greater the drive (i.e. the size of the food, drink or sex deficit) the more strongly it stimulates the reward system.

There is some experimental support for this hypothesis. When an animal is hungry or loaded with insulin (both of which lower the level of blood sugar) it will of course eat; but it is also more likely to self-stimulate. Thus the generalized reward system appears to be sensitized by hunger, at least according to the criterion of rate of self-stimulation.

However, it has not been shown that this sensitization of the reward system is in any way specific for hunger. If the reward system is enhanced non-specifically by any deficit, then of course it could not serve to select among competing behaviours as postulated. The satisfaction of any drive would be equally rewarding. In fact, the rewarding effect seems to spread non-specifically, often facilitating inappropriate behaviour. For example, a hungry animal deprived of food will drink more, even when suffering no water deficit; this implies that it derives some satisfaction from performing even that irrelevant act. This may be explained by supposing that hunger sensitizes the reward system non-specifically in such a way that irrelevant act. This may be explained by supposing that hunger sensitizes the reward system non-specifically in such a way that any behaviour can tap into it. Of course, this does not account for the normal selection of behaviours—a hungry animal will always feed before drinking if both food and water are available.

Aversion

The concept of reward probably cannot by itself explain selection of behaviours. We have to invoke 'punishment' as well. A powerful drive, such as a low blood glucose level, probably does sensitize the entire reward system, but only sparingly, until after feeding begins. What induces feeding to commence is the specific *aversive* state of hunger caused by low blood glucose, etc. This is perhaps the unpleasant state that stimulating electrodes placed at sites which cause feeding without enhanced self-stimulation manage to mimic. Once feeding commences, however, the reward system is highly sensitized—a positive feedback mechanism operates to activate feeding and encourage it to continue because it engenders such a pleasurable sensation.

In conclusion (and executing summary justice to the immense literature which now surrounds the reward system), aversive states such as hunger, thirst and lust probably *select* the behaviour that an animal will perform, whilst the reward system supplies non-specific *activation* of the behaviour once it has been selected.

Anatomy of reward

The above theory helps to explain the multitude of sites and pharmacological agents which support self-stimulation. Self-stimulation 'is associated with both the noradrenergic and dopaminergic systems. The dorsal noradrenergic bundle originating in the locus coeruleus is a potent site for self-stimulation, but another noradrenergic system, the ventral noradrenergic bundle, is not. Complete destruction of the locus coeruleus, destroying all its projections, does not abolish self-stimulation in other areas however, so the dorsal noradrenergic bundle is not essential for self-stimulation, although it supports it.

MFB

Caudal lesions of the medial forebrain bundle considerably reduce the degree of an animal's self-stimulation by electrodes placed anywhere in the neuraxis. Part of the explanation for this is that such lesions may damage the dopaminergic projections from the substantia nigra to the rest of the basal ganglia, and thus reduce self-stimulation rates simply by causing motor impairment.

Mesolimbic DA system

Another dopaminergic pathway that is eliminated by an MFB lesion is the ventral dopaminergic 'mesolimbic' pathway from the ventral tegmentum (where self-stimulation can reach its highest levels) to the ventral part of the basal ganglia, the nucleus accumbens and entopeduncular nucleus, the hypothalamus, and the entorhinal and frontal cortex. This pathway may well be the most important component of all in the reward system, due to its connections with the limbic system.

It is clear that all these pathways are highly diffuse. As they are probably all activated during drive-reducing behaviours, such a widely distributed organization makes sense because all behavioural responses involve sensory, perceptual, associative, memory and motor systems, each of which needs to be facilitated if the reward process is going to optimize behaviour.

LEARNING AND MEMORY

This is not the place to enter into too much detail on a subject that demands a library of books in order to be understood even slightly. However, our considerations of sensory and motor systems, sleep and reward have brought us to the brink of the problem of memory, so a short section is in order.

Learning in Aplysia

Long-lasting changes which can be induced in the simple reflexes of invertebrates can serve as useful models of learning in higher animals. The advantage of choosing invertebrates for study is that their nervous systems are simple and are comprised of neurones which are large and easily identifiable. Kandell and his colleagues have studied habituation and sensitization in the gill-withdrawal reflex of *Aplysia* (a sea slug) with great success. On repeated application of a stimulus, the gill-withdrawal reflex is depressed (habituation), while the application of a novel stimulus enhances it (sensitization), even after habituation. Habituation leads to a decrease in transmitter release from sensory afferent terminals ending either directly on gill-muscle motoneurones or on reflex interneurones. This decrease is probably a result of Ca^{2+} channel inactivation, which in turn results from increased outward K^+ current. Sensitization causes enhanced transmitter release; K^+ current is depressed and this leads to increased Ca^{2+} influx. Both habituation and sensitization are associated with morphological changes at the synapse which may be detected with the electron microscope. One of the transmitters involved is serotonin (5HT); this activates a specific cyclic AMP which causes the inactivation of K^+ channels by phosphorylating a K^+ channel protein.

Subcortical learning

The simplest examples of mammalian 'learning' can be found in animals totally lacking any cerebral cortex. A spinal cat can be conditioned to withdraw its leg to avoid a shock at only the touch of an electrode, even before the shock is delivered; whilst a decorticate dog can be taught almost as fast as an intact control to withdraw following auditory, tactile or visual stimuli. These responses persist for a long time, implying that structural, plastic changes in the nervous system, analogous to those in *Aplysia*, have taken place. Whether or not we call these simple changes in experimental animals 'memories' is really only a matter of terminology. In humans, learning is the process by which material is committed to memory, and memories can be recalled to consciousness. The consciousness of animals, if it can be said to exist, is not accessible to us, so the word 'memory' should be restricted to the human context.

Pavlovian conditioning

Classical conditioning (discovered by Pavlov) is the simplest example of associative learning. An unconditioned stimulus (food) is paired with a conditioned stimulus (a bell which rings on every occasion food is presented). The dog's response (salivation) eventually occurs whenever the bell sounds and before food is presented. However, if food is then systematically withheld whenever the bell sounds, the conditioned reflex is extinguished and the bell no longer causes salivation.

Operant conditioning

Operant conditioning—the technique that Skinner introduced and with which experimental psychologists have made great strides in understanding animal behaviour—is now beginning to contribute to physiology as well. One may view it as an extension of classical conditioning. The animal is taught to operate on its environment in order to obtain an unconditioned stimulus (food or drink reward) or to avoid punishment. The conditioned stimulus is the cue which signals the animal to perform its task. Very complex, controlled behaviours can be obtained from animals trained in this way. This is the technique which physiologists have borrowed to allow the study of the activity of single neurones in conscious animals performing stereotyped actions.

However, whether what goes on at membrane level during conditioning in higher animals is similar to that in *Aplysia* is not known. clear that permanent structural changes in the nervous system can take place remarkably quickly. If half the cerebellum of a rat is removed, it develops an abnormal posture. If the spinal cord is then separated from the brain within 45 minutes, the unusual stance disappears; if more than 45 minutes elapse before the section is made the disturbed posture persists. Thus, in those 45 minutes a lasting change in the wiring arrangements of the spinal cord has taken place.

Structural modifications

That such transformations in vertebrates as well as *Aplysia* involve structural alterations of neuronal architecture is suggested by a great deal of evidence. For example, only when mice reared in darkness are transferred to daylight do dendritic spines appear and multiply in their visual cortical neurones. Rats reared in a visually enriched environment and trained in visually guided tasks have thicker occipital cortices than those brought up in monotonous and uniform surroundings.

Moreover, there is overwhelming evidence that during development not only genetic, but also environmental, factors affect the way in which neurones grow and make contact with each other. If such structural changes can occur as a result of an animal's experience at the hands of its environment during development, then similar processes could clearly operate during adult learning. Indeed, this is one of the chief reasons (apart from simple curiosity) why so many neuroscientists are now engaged in the study of the growth and development of the nervous system.

Biochemical changes

Another approach has been to investigate biochemical changes during learning, such as the phosphorylation of K^+ channel protein in *Aplysia*. The argument runs that since long-term memories involve structural changes, and all structural changes can ultimately be traced to changes in protein production, then learning may also result from synthesis of new protein. Unfortunately, it is very difficult to ensure that the changes in protein synthesis detected by the relatively crude techniques which are available have anything specific to do with learning. Nevertheless, there are now enough well-controlled observations of changes in RNA and protein metabolism in simple learning situations for us to be confident that they do occur. However, it is a long haul from this point to determining how these changes bring about the alterations in the intimate relationships between neurones which must underly memory.

Storage—the search for the engram

It is quite clear that memories are not stored separately in individual neurones. Lashley showed that the only way to rid rats of a visual memory altogether was to deprive them of sight by ablating both visual cortex and superior colliculus. Small ablations of any part of the visual system or visual association areas merely degraded the learnt habits in proportion to the amount of damage, and could not eliminate them completely. These observations were slightly misinterpreted by Lashley, who concluded that there was no localization of function in the cerebral cortex beyond the primary sensory areas when, in fact, all he had shown was that there was no localization of memory 'engrams' in individual neurones. Indeed, the past 100 years of neuroscience have abundantly demonstrated that there is clear localization of function in different parts of the brain.

Electrocortical conditioning

When a new stimulus is first encountered by an animal, it leads to arousal associated with diffuse desynchronization of the EEG—the orientating response. Habituation to the stimulus, with gradual reduction of the orientating response, occurs if the stimulus is associated with neither pain nor pleasure. However, if the animal is rewarded or punished in association with the stimulus, the orientating response does not habituate; instead the stimulus alone will soon reliably elicit desynchronization of the EEG (sometimes called α-block or electrocortical conditioning) (Fig. 25.2).

Motivation

Learning is thus intimately bound up with motivation. Only that which has some relevance to drive reduction, reward or punish-

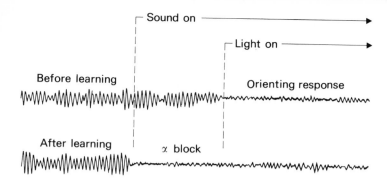

Fig. 25.2. Electrocortical conditioning. Before learning, the rhythm stops only when the light is switched on. After learning, α block occurs in response to a preceding sound.

ment is learnt, and EEG conditioning can serve as a model for this. Electrocortical conditioning is unaffected by ablation of the specific thalamic nuclei involved in relaying the stimulus, but disappears if the non-specific intralaminar nuclei are ablated, as might be expected from their role in EEG arousal. Extinction of electrocortical conditioning, which occurs if a stimulus is no longer reinforced, is associated with the development of extremely large, regular (hyper-synchronized) waves in the EEG. This suggests that unlearning (clearing the memory) may be as active a process as learning itself.

Human memory

We assume that the learning of relatively simple things by animals may be taken as indicative of the presumably much more complex processes taking place in human memory. There are three essential stages that we have to consider: selection of what is to be remembered, storage and retrieval.

Selection

First we need a system for selecting those sensory events and experiences which we need to memorize. Unfortunately, this stage is not entirely under voluntary control, as we all know to our cost! It is this stage of selection which is most obviously under emotional or drive-related, involuntary control. The evolutionary advantage to an animal of being able to learn is derived from the fact that it can thereby profit from its past experience in the struggle for food, protection, a mate, and so on. Therefore only those things that have a bearing on these drives are worth learning, so it is not surprising to find that the limbic system, which orchestrates our emotions, also selects our memories.

Storage

Not only is the limbic system involved in the selection of what we wish to remember but it is clearly also involved in the storage of memories. *Short-term memory,* which is what we rely on for temporarily remembering things like seven-digit telephone numbers and the beginning of a sentence when we reach its end, is under more voluntary control. It probably depends on the setting-up of reverberating circuits—self-reexciting chains of neurones in the appropriate sensory, association and motor areas. We suspect that this is so because short-term memory is very susceptible to anything which temporarily disrupts the electrical activity of the brain, such as blows on the head, electroconvulsive therapy and epilepsy.

Long-term memory, however, depends on structural changes such as those discussed in relation to animal learning. The limbic system's function is probably to select those short-term memories which need to be consolidated as long-term memories. This process can be interrupted using inhibitors of protein synthesis. Memory traces are probably not usually stored in the limbic system itself, but in the sensory, association and motor areas to which they relate.

Papez circuit

The important areas of the limbic system in this respect are the elements of the *Papez circuit* (Fig. 25.3). This consists of the hippo-

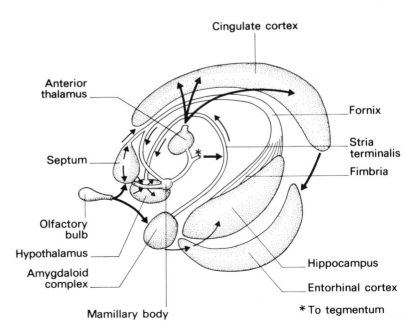

Fig. 25.3. The Papez circuit.

campus and its projections to the mamillary bodies and septum via the fornix, the mamillothalamic tract to the anterior thalamic nucleus and its projections to cingulate cortex, and the pathway from there back to the hippocampus. Bilateral damage to any part of this circuit, particularly common in the mamillary bodies of chronic alcoholics, leads to a loss of the ability to form new memories and a tendency to confabulate to fill the gaps (Korsakoff's syndrome).

Temporal lobes

Fortunately, unilateral damage to the hippocampal circuit causes little memory deficit, a fact which enables the operation of temporal lobectomy to be carried out safely on unfortunate sufferers of temporal lobe epilepsy. This condition is only too common and is very often resistant to drug treatment.

One very famous patient ('H.M.') who suffered from temporal lobe epilepsy had both his temporal lobes removed by an enthusiastic surgeon. He has not been able to remember anything from the day of his operation (though he now no longer has temporal lobe epilepsy!) and has been able since then to make a living from the fact that he is an ideal subject for studies of human memory. With constant rehearsal he can remember bits of information he has set his mind to, but if he is distracted at all, the memory is lost.

One big problem with the view that the main function of the hippocampus is in the selection and consolidation of memories is that this only seems to be true in humans. In other animals, hippocampal ablations seem to make very little difference to the ability to learn. The explanation seems to be that humans do much of their memorizing by *verbal encoding*, and it is this which is particularly affected by hippocampal damage. Other animals, of course, do not talk, and so hippocampal encoding does not play such an overwhelmingly important part in their memory storage. It has recently been shown that humans with hippocampal damage or presenting Korsakoff's syndrome can in fact memorize non-verbal material quite well, so long as the stimulus for retrieval is non-verbal and similar to the sought-after memory. As they cannot verbalize their storage of the item, they cannot retrieve it verbally. For instance, H.M. was trained in a non-verbal discrimination task, being rewarded with a penny for correct manual responses. No verbal instructions at all were given. Although he was quite unable to say how he had done it, he very quickly achieved 100% correct responses, showing that he had managed to remember this non-verbal task completely.

Chapter 26
Historical Epilogue

The early history of neurology, as of most scientific endeavours, was the result of two human interests which converged at times, and diverged at others. The first was simple curiosity. How do we see? How do our limbs move? It was heightened in this case by the most fundamental and fascinating questions of all. How do we think? What is consciousness? What is our Will? The second interest was dictated by practical problems presented when things go wrong with the nervous system. Why is this man paralysed down one side following a blow on his head, and what can we do about it? Why does this patient have fits beginning with a twitching at the corner of his mouth and progressing to generalized convulsions and unconsciousness? Happily, satisfactory answers to the first type of question, stemming from simple curiosity, often help to solve practical problems. Similarly, 'experiments of nature' which disturb the smooth running of the nervous system often reveal much about its normal functioning.

These two threads can be seen in the very earliest recorded attempts to make sense of the brain. In most ancient cultures dissection of human corpses was not allowed, either because they were thought to be Unclean (Ancient Hebrews), or they were needed by their previous owners (Babylonians), or were vengefully guarded by their spirits (Ancient Greeks). Thus knowledge of neuroanatomy was, of necessity, rudimentary and without this essential foundation neurology remained entirely speculative.

The Babylonians

The practical aim of Babylonian anatomy, such as it was, was not to understand sickness (the Babylonians took a very pessimistic view of their chances of defeating the demons they believed responsible for illness), but rather they hoped that by a minute and intricate survey of the entrails of sacrificial animals they could at least predict the course of a disease. They relied for cure on the supernatural powers of possessors of an 'oculus fascinus' to outface the 'evil eye' which was believed to cause disease.

The Egyptians

The Ancient Egyptians, on the other hand, seem to have had a much more highly developed knowledge of anatomy, because of the expertise which was required for their practice of embalming the dead. This was probably carried out by physicians, which helps to explain why the quality of Egyptian medicine around 1550 BC was so high. Such standards were not achieved again for 1700 years, until the time of Galen (*c.* 150 AD).

The Greeks

Basic neuroanatomical knowledge was lacking until the seventeenth century AD. What was missing in the way of empirical data was, however, substituted by a profusion of speculation. Alcmaen (*c.* 600 BC), who was the first Greek to recognize that the brain is the seat of consciousness and perception, nevertheless suggested that the brain secretes thought 'as the salivary glands secrete saliva and the lachrymal glands bring forth tears'. He also thought that some animals breathe through their ears and that the brain was cooled through the nostrils! Even Hippocrates (*c.* 400 BC), who was so *avant garde* in urging accurate clinical observation, deduction and correlation, believed that the brain was a gland which secreted the four cardinal humours: blood, phlegm, yellow bile (choli) and black bile (melancholi), and that it received its major input from the liver (Fig. 26.1). Aristotle (*c.* 350 BC), despite his manifold contributions to biology, doubted that the brain had anything to do with consciousness; he noted that it is the heart which thumps obtrusively at moments of high emotion, not the brain.

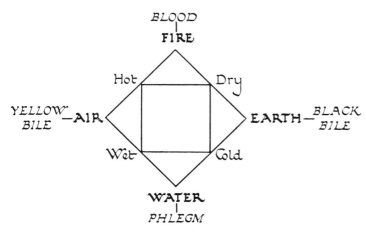

Fig. 26.1. Hippocrates' four cardinal humours. (From Singer C. (1928) *A Short History of Medicine.* Clarendon Press, Oxford. With permission.)

Galen (130–200 AD)

Galen was the foremost medical thinker of the Roman era. He based his physiology on Hippocratic and Vitalist ideas. For instance, he speculated that vision involved the transformation of visual images into visual spirits by the '*divinum oculi*', since when he looked into a person's eye, he saw a tiny image there reflected, as we now know, from the lens. These visual spirits were supposed to traverse the hollow optic nerve to reach the third ventricle, Galen's seat of consciousness and the abode of the soul.

We should not jeer too much at these naive ideas. Neither neuro-anatomy nor the science of optics existed then. Who knows with what amusement future generations will view our quaint conceptions in even 50 years time? It is worth remembering that after the fall of Rome, medical learning was kept alive only in the Arab world. In about 1000 AD, Avicenna of Persia wrote a textbook based on the teachings of Galen, which endured for longer than any other medical textbook. It was still in standard use, having been translated from Arabic by the Jews in the University of Montpelier, 650 years later. That is most unlikely to be the fate of this book.

The Renaissance

Real progress could not take place until advances in anatomy, physics and chemistry could come together to illuminate the functions of the nervous system. In Europe, anatomy was more or less proscribed until the seventeenth century by papal edicts which forbade dissection of the human body. Nevertheless, the liberal Holy Roman Emperor Frederick II (*stupor mundi*) allowed dissection at Salerno in the fifteenth century. The school at Montpellier was also fortunate in having free access to the bodies of executed criminals.

Vesalius

The modern era of physiology, as well as of anatomy, may be said to have started when Vesalius of Padua completed *De Humanis Corporis Fabrica* (Fig. 26.2). This book contained, in addition to beautiful illustrations of his painstaking dissections, many speculations about function. In the last chapter, Vesalius introduced experimental evidence derived from vivisection that the brain controlled the spinal cord, which in turn controlled muscles and limbs. Interestingly, although his experiments must have been somewhat bloody, he forbears to mention that arteries and veins actually do contain blood, rather than the spirituous air required by Catholic dogma. This may have been prudent self-censorship, designed to avoid the sort of trouble into which his contemporaries Galileo and Servetus propelled themselves.

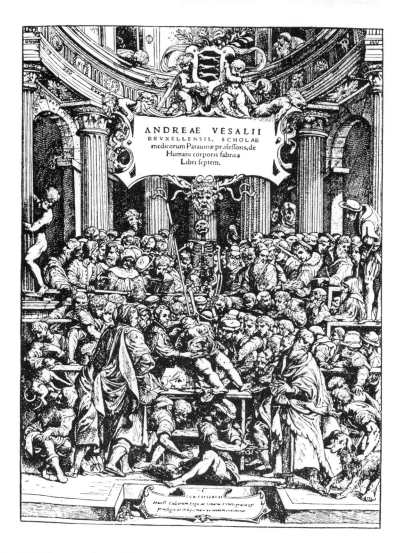

ANDREAE VESALII
BRVXELLENSIS, SCHOLAE
medicorum Patauinæ profeſſoris,de
Humani corporis fabrica
Libri ſeptem.

Fig. 26.2. Frontiscpiece of Vesalius' *De Humanis Corporis Fabrica* (from Singer (1928), with permission).

Paracelsus

Another contemporary, Paracelsus Theophrastus Bombastus, was much more outspoken. Even so he managed to avoid the Inquisition's fires. His writings were largely metaphysical, but because he spoke and wrote in vernacular German rather than scholarly Latin his ideas had a huge impact. His splendidly irreverent belief that the views of scholarly authorities were of no account, that only experience mattered, did much to hasten the modern era of scientific medicine.

Descartes

In 1662, Rene Descartes, a French mathematician and philosopher, published *De Homine*. This was not based on any experimental work at all, but nevertheless it has a reasonable claim to be the first proper textbook of physiology. Fernel's *De Homine* published 100 years earlier used the word 'physiology' for the first time but was very much rooted in the tradition of Vitalism—the idea that all living things are imbued with a life force independent of the material laws of physics and chemistry. However, Descartes offered the first thoroughly mechanistic approach to the workings of the body.

De Homine is particularly interesting to neurophysiologists, since Descartes placed the brain and central nervous system fairly and squarely in control of everything else. In this and in many other ways, his views have a very modern air about them. *De Homine* contains the first clear account of reflex action. Descartes believed all motor acts to be the consequence of sensory energy 'reflected' from the CNS (Fig. 26.3). He also saw clearly the importance of the concept of topographical mapping within the CNS. He believed that there must be a correspondence between the spatial arrangement of points in the outside world and the spatial arrangement of points within the brain representing, for example, the visual world, and speculates about the rules for 'mapping' one set onto the other by nervous connections.

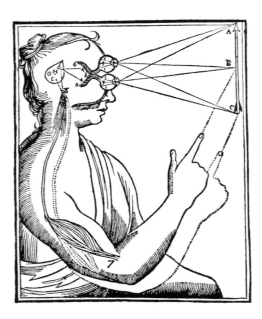

Fig. 26.3. Descartes' idea of the 'reflection' of visual energy into the pointing arm, and of topographical mapping in the cerebrum and pineal gland (from Singer (1928), with permission).

The mechanisms which he postulated for these operations were of course quite wrong. He conceived the nervous system according to the physics of his time, in terms of pipes, pulleys and levers. He revived the idea of Epistratus that nerves were hollow pipes conducting an unknown active principle from place to place. Thus, nerves were supposed to activate muscles by infusing them with this agent, causing them to swell up rather like bicycle tyres, and thus exert their actions. This theory was neatly refuted by Swammerdam (*c.* 1670) who simply immersed a forearm in water and showed that when muscles contracted there was no displacement of water, therefore they could not have swelled. This observation has only become explicable in our own day with the *sliding filament* theory of muscle contraction.

Galvani and bioelectricity

Descartes' speculations lacked experimental bases. Nobody had any inkling of the way in which nerves transmit signals, until Galvani's wife noticed that the frogs legs she was preparing for her husband's dinner twitched when they touched her copper and iron pans (Fig. 26.4). This serendipitous discovery of electricity proved immensely

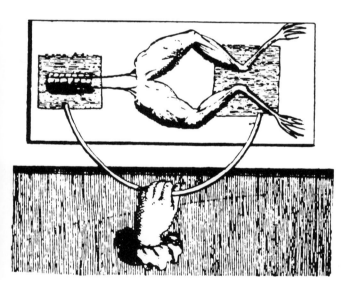

Fig. 26.4. Galvani found that completing the circuit between damaged spinal cord and frog leg muscles causes muscle to twitch (from Singer (1928), with permission).

important. It led to her husband's discovery of bioelectricity, to Volta's discovery of electrochemistry and, indirectly, to Faraday's discovery of electromagnetism (which led in turn to the modern electrical industry).

Electrophysiology

Following the discovery of the electrical nature of nervous transmission, a divergence between theory and practice in neurology began to take place. On the one hand were pure scientists such as: du Bois Raymond (1848) who finally observed the electrical potential change which occurs during a nervous impulse; Helmholtz (1850) who first managed to measure the velocity of conduction in human nerves; Caton (1875) who first recorded electrical waves from the cerebral cortex; Keith Lucas (1917) to whom credit for the all-or-none law of neuronal signalling should really go; Erlanger and Gasser (1924) who introduced the cathode ray oscilloscope to electrophysiology, and with it 'dissected' the compound action potential of whole nerves; and Adrian and Zotterman (1926) who first managed to record from single sensory nerve fibres. On the other hand there stood the clinical neurologists, who were unable to make much use of electrophysiology; it did not contribute significantly to attempts to alleviate sickness until well into the twentieth century.

Mesmer

The discoveries of Galvani and Faraday initially led in rather a different clinical direction, to the wild theories of Anton Mesmer about animal magnetism and its healing powers. Mesmer gave us the word 'mesmerize', but despite his immense financial success he became disillusioned and grew sceptical of magnetic healing entirely. James Braid took up his ideas, however, and came to the conclusion that mesmeric sleep was due to nervous fatigue, which he called 'neurohypnotism'. Sigmund Freud journeyed to visit the great neurologist Charcot who worked at the Salpêtrière hospital in Paris, to see this technique at first hand. Freud went on to use hypnotism in his initial probes into the mysteries of the Unconscious.

Clinical neurology and cerebral localization of function

The discoveries about nervous function made by the great clinical neurologists, such as Hughlings Jackson, Charcot, Head and Holmes, owed little to electricity, but much to the old-fashioned Hippocratic method of careful observation of symptoms and signs, later correlating them with post-mortem revelations about the location of pathological processes causing cerebral lesions. This classical technique led to perhaps the most important neurological concept of all, namely the general principle of *localization of function* within the nervous system.

Though the intellectual origins of the idea of cerebral localization
were respectable (Hippocrates, Galen, Descartes), its progress certainly was not. In the hands of the 'phrenologists', Gall and particularly Spurzheim, every real or imaginary bump in the skull was
supposed to reveal the degree of development of different cerebral
attributes in an individual (Fig. 26.5). Great skill and much money
was expended on meticulous measurement of people's heads in
vain attempts to detect abnormalities of the underlying brain, which
were alleged to be the clue to genius, mania or melancholy. The
excesses of the phrenologists brought them well-earned disrepute
and it was left to prodigiously respectable neurologists to rescue the
all-important idea of cerebral localization, using clinicopathological
correlation supplemented by experiment.

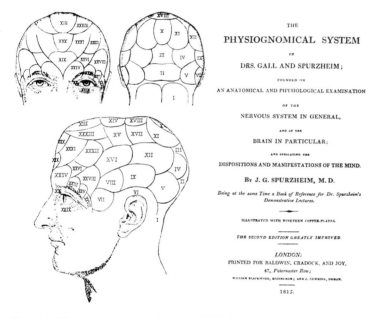

Fig. 26.5. The phrenological schemata of J.G. Spurzheim.

Robert Boyle (1649) had observed that pressure on the left side of
the brain caused right-sided paralysis and loss of speech, which
could be reversed by alleviating the pressure. Two hundred years
later, Fritz and Hitzig stimulated the exposed cerebral cortex and
showed that movements of the opposite side of the body could be
obtained from a restricted region in front of the Rolandic fissure.
David Ferrier further discovered that these movements were 'mapped' in the motor cortex in an orderly fashion with the face lateral,
the arm next, and the leg closest to the mid-line.

Hughlings Jackson

This 'movement map' had in fact been partially predicted some years earlier by Hughlings Jackson, who deduced it from the march of convulsions in certain types of epilepsy—first twitching of the face, then of the arm and then the leg. Jackson took the whole concept of localization of function much further, however. He introduced the idea of a hierarchy of functional centres in the brain which normally kept each other under control, but which could be released by disease, the 'highest' (i.e. those developed most recently in evolution and lying above the others anatomically) were the ones which, in general, suffered first. Some cerebral functions, such as memory, have not turned out to be localized in quite this way, and great tracts of the cerebral cortex have not yet been allocated a clearly defined function. (These facts have led some even now to deny the existence of any localization of function within the cortex whatever.) Nevertheless, this concept remains central to our present understanding of the nervous system.

CONCLUSIONS

This very short survey of some aspects of the history of neurophysiology was not intended to poke fun at our forefathers, but rather to trace the development of some of the important concepts in neurophysiology, such as nervous conduction, localization of function and mapping; to see how neurophysiological thought was very much conditioned by the thinking in other sciences at the time; and to deduce from their interests what past generations of neuroscientists conceived their aims to be. You will have noticed that the really fascinating basic questions mentioned at the beginning of the chapter, such as the nature of thought, of consciousness and of Free Will, become much less prominent after the Renaissance and the advent of the Scientific Method. Whilst these questions undoubtedly exercise the imagination of all thoughtful people, their answers are now seen to fall outside the province of neurophysiology, and in the domain of philosophers and theologians. It is perhaps no accident that, in the past, neurophysiologists tended to be either physicians or philosophers as well. Only in the twentieth century can we trace neurophysiology as a separate discipline. Today neurophysiologists confine themselves to trying to answer questions about the way in which the nervous system works in terms of anatomy, physics and chemistry, i.e. in terms of mechanisms whose operations can actually be measured. Questions about Consciousness, Free Will and the Soul, are for the most part of a completely different type (you cannot measure the Soul!), they are amenable to *a-priori* reasoning, introspection, speculation and faith.

The dualist position is that mental processes and their underlying physical correlates are two ways of describing the same thing, rather as a high-level computer language, such as Fortran, and the machine's own language, a series of 'noughts' and 'ones', both describe the same processes, but in totally different ways. Although at present the simple dualist position is not philosophically fashionable, it is nevertheless the one which the neurophysiologist must adopt if he is not to fall into the temptation of explaining away all difficult or awkward phenomena by recourse to vital spirits, etc.

The present aims of neurophysiology are therefore not to explain what thought or consciousness are, or the nature of Free Will, but to explain *how* we perceive, think and act. We attempt to understand the mechanisms underlying the way in which the nervous system acquires information about the outside world and the state of our own bodies by means of sensory receptors, how the CNS routes and re-routes coded signals to the particular parts of the body where they may be relevant, how it transforms these signals along the way, how information relevant to future survival is stored in our memories, and how the CNS effects movements.

Glossary

Anatomical terms

Afferent Pathways or signals passing towards a structure (usually sensory inputs).

Anterior Towards the front of a structure.

Ascending Running to higher (more rostral) levels of the nervous system.

Caudal Towards the tail end.

Centrifugal Flow of signals away from higher centres.

Centripetal Flow of signals towards higher centres.

Coronal section A section through the neuraxis cut at right angles to the long axis as if bends were straightened out. Thus in humans a coronal section of the forebrain (sometimes called frontal) is at right angles to a coronal section through the spinal cord (also called transverse), but this is not so in quadrupeds.

Descending Running to lower (more caudal) levels of the nervous system.

Dorsal Towards the top of a structure. In quadrupeds this also means towards the back surface of spinal cord and brainstem.

Dorsal horn of grey matter in spinal cord. Receives sensory signals from dorsal roots and descending control from brain. Projects sensory signals to higher centres and into ventral horn for reflex actions.

Efferent Pathways or signals passing away from structure (usually motor output).

Grey matter Regions of CNS that contain mostly nerve cell bodies, dendrites and axon terminals, but little white myelin. On surface of cerebral cortex but at core of spinal cord (dorsal and ventral horns).

Horizontal A section which is strictly horizontal, i.e. cut at right angles to vertical (applies to both bipeds and quadrupeds).

Lateral Further from mid-line.

Medial Towards mid-line.

Nucleus Distinguishable aggregation of nerve cell bodies, usually sharing common inputs and outputs, situated within the substance of the cerebral hemispheres (basal ganglia), cerebellum (cerebellar nuclei), brainstem (cranial nerve nuclei, etc.) and spinal cord.

Posterior Towards the back of a structure.

Projection neurone A neurone that sends an axon to a different level of the CNS (cf. cortico-cortical (association), commissural and local neurones, and interneurones whose axons remain at the same level).

Rostral Towards the top and front of the neuraxis.

Sagittal section A vertical anteroposterior section through the brain, cut along the long axis.

Sulcus Cerebral cortex is extensively folded to increase its surface area. Many of the fissures (sulci) produced by the infolding are the same in brains of the same species and are named. Each of these gives its name to the neighbouring outfolding (or gyrus).

Ventral Towards the bottom of a structure. In quadrupeds this also means towards the front surface of spinal cord and brainstem.

Ventral horn of grey matter in spinal cord contains ventral horn cells; these are the motoneurones whose axons, passing via the ventral roots, control all muscle activity. Hence they are called the final common pathway for action. Receives descending motor pathways and local (segmental) sensory and interneuronal signals for reflex action.

White matter Regions of CNS that contain mostly myelinated axon bundles. Lie deep in cerebral cortex, but on surface of spinal cord (dorsal, lateral and ventral columns).

Physiological terms

Accommodation The rise in threshold depolarization required to initiate a spike if application of depolarization is very slow. Also used of the decline in reflex responsiveness if stimuli applied slowly. Also used of the adjustment of curvature of the lens to focus eyes at different distances.

Adaptation Decline with time in response of sensory receptor, neurone or system of neurones despite maintained stimulation.

After potential Deviation of membrane potential from normal resting level after a spike or train of spikes.

Antidromic Propogation of impulse in the opposite direction to normal.

Collateral Important side branch of an axon, given off well before its termination and having a diameter as large as its parent.

Corollary discharge Neural signals accompanying a movement which pass to sensory centres in order to enable them to evaluate correctly the sensory input which was caused by the movement itself.

Electrotonus Local current spread causing deviation of membrane potential, decreasing with distance and with time, dependent only upon the passive electrical properties of the membrane.

Evoked potential Gross potential change recorded from a whole region following electrical or natural stimulation of its inputs.

Facilitation Subliminal effect of a first stimulus to cause additional excitation following a second stimulus, so that final effect is more than twice that of first stimulus applied alone.

Fatigue Decline in response of neurones or muscles due to protracted or excess activity. Therefore requires appreciable recovery time (cf. accommodation, adaptation, habituation).

Habituation Reduction in responsiveness of neurone or reflex if stimulus is repeated persistently.

Intrafusal Within the capsule of a muscle spindle (cf. extrafusal—the main muscle fibres).

Lamina A layer of neuropil and nerve cell bodies distinctive to those above and below it. Cerebral cortex, hippocampus, cerebellar cortex and spinal cord are laminated.

Modality A class of sensation (vision, touch, hearing, etc.). Also used of qualities, such as touch versus pressure, within one class.

Neurohormone Hormone released from nerve cells which acts on target structures at a distance (cf. neurotransmitter).

Neuromodulator Substance which modulates the chemical and electrical activity of neurones without itself being a transmitter.

Neuropil Tangle of dendrites and fine axon terminals with few cell bodies.

Neurosecretion Release of substances from neurones, triggered electrically or chemically, and usually mediated by the intracellular appearance of free Ca^{2+}.

Neurotransmitter Substance released by nerve cell axon terminals or dendrites, mediating normal chemical transmission from one neurone to the next.

Occlusion Where the sum of two reflex effects occurring simultaneously is less than the sum of their separate effects because some of the neurones employed are saturated by the first reflex and therefore cannot also be utilized by the second.

Orthodromic Flow of impulses in dendrites or axons in their normal direction of propagation.

Phasic A transient state.

Reafference Sensory input which is entirely a result of the animal's own movements (mostly supplied by proprioceptors).

Tonic A maintained, sustained or static state.

Further Reading

Chapter 1: Basic structure of the CNS

Bowsher D. (1979) *Introduction to the Anatomy and Physiology of the Nervous System,* 4th Edn. Blackwell Scientific Publications, Oxford.

Brodal A. (1981) *Neurological Anatomy in Relation to Clinical Medicine,* 3rd Edn. Oxford University Press, Oxford.

Gray's Anatomy (1973), 35th Edn. Longman, London.

Handbook of Physiology, Section 1: Neurophysiology. American Physiological Society. Williams & Wilkins, New York.

Hubel D. (ed.) (1979) *The Brain.* Scientific American Publications, W.H. Freeman, San Francisco.

Truex R.C. & Carpenter M.B. (1969) *Strong & Elwyn's Human Neuroanatomy,* 6th Edn. Williams & Wilkins, New York.

Chapter 2: Physiological techniques

Brazier M. (1975) *The Electrical Activity of the Nervous System.* Pitman Medical, London.

Hodgkin A.L. (1976) Chance and design in electrophysiology. *J. Physiol.,* 263, 1–21.

Hubbard J.L., Linas R. & Quastell D.M.J. (1969) *Electrophysiological Analysis of Synaptic Transmission.* Physiological Society Monograph No. 19. Edward Arnold, London.

Nastuk W.L. (ed.) (1964) *Electrophysiological Methods. Physical Techniques in Biological Research,* Vol. V. Academic Press, New York.

Chapter 3: The electrical properties of neurones

Aidley D.J. (1978) *The Physiology of Excitable Cells,* 2nd Edn. Cambridge University Press, Cambridge.

Armstrong C.M. (1981) Sodium channels and gating currents. *Physiol. Rev.,* 61, 644–683.

Eccles J.C. (1957) *The Physiology of Nerve Cells.* Oxford University Press, Oxford.

Hille B. (1978) Ionic channels in excitable membranes. *Biophys. J.,* 22, 283–294.

Hodgkin A.L. (1971) *The Conduction of the Nervous Impulse.* Liverpool University Press, Liverpool.

Hodgkin A.L. & Huxley A.F. (1952) A quantitative description of membrane current and its application. *J. Physiol.,* 117, 500–544.

Jack J.J.B., Noble D. & Tsien R.W. (1975) *Electric Current Flow in Excitable Cells.* Oxford University Press, Oxford.

Chapter 4: Synaptic transmission

Katz B. (1966) *Nerve, Muscle and Synapse.* McGraw-Hill, Maidenhead.

Shepherd G.M. (1979) *The Synaptic Organisation of the Brain.* Oxford University Press, Oxford.

Chapter 5: Introduction to sensory physiology

Adrian E.D. (1947) *The Physical Background of Perception.* Oxford University Press, Oxford.

Granit R. (1955) *Receptors and Sensory Perception.* Yale University Press, New Haven.

Handbook of Sensory Physiology (10 vols). Springer-Verlag, Berlin.
Mountcastle V.B. (1967) The problem of sensing and the neural codins of sensory events. In: *The Neurosciences*, Vol. I (ed. Schmitt F.O.), p. 393. Rockefeller University Press, New York.

Chapter 6: Visual system

Blakemore C.B. & Cambell F. (1969) On the existence of channels in the human visual system selectively sensitive to the orientation and size of retinal images. *J. Physiol.*, **203,** 237–260.
Cowey A. & Gross C. (1970) Effects of foveal prestriate and inferocortical lesions on visual discrimination. *Expl. Br. Res.*, **11,** 128–144.
Dowling F.E. (1979) Information processing by local circuits in the retina. In: *Neurosciences: Fourth Study Program* (ed. Schmitt F.O. & Worder F.G.), p. 163. M.I.T. Press, Cambridge, Massachusetts.
Hubel D.H. & Wiesel T.N. (1977) Functional architecture of monkey visual cortex. *Proc. Roy. Soc. Lond. B*, **198,** 1–59.
Kaneko A. (1979) Physiology of the retina. *Ann. Rev. Neurosci.*, **2,** 169–191.
Lennie P. (1980) Parallel visual pathways. *Vis. Res.*, **20,** 561–594.
Rodieck R.W. (1973) *The Vertebrate Retina.* W.H. Freeman, San Francisco.
Rushton W.H.H. (1972) Colour vision. *J. Physiol.*, **220,** 1–31.
The Psychology of Vision. (1980) *Phil. Trans. Roy. Soc. B*, **290,** 379–553.
Van Essen D.C. (1979) Visual areas of mammalian cerebral cortex. *Ann. Rev. Neurosci.*, **2,** 227–263.
Wald G. (1968) The chemistry of vision. *Science*, **162,** 230–239.
Zeki S.M. (1975) Functional organisation of projections from striate to prestriate cortex. *Cold Spring Harbor Symposium*, **40,** 591–600.

Chapter 7: Auditory system

Kay R. & Matthews D. (1972) On the existence in human auditory pathways of channels selectively tuned to the modulation present in frequency modulated tones. *J. Physiol.*, **225,** 657–677.
Merzenich M.M. & Brugge J.T. (1973) Representation of the cochlea in the superior temporal plane of the monkey. *Brain Res.*, **50,** 275–296.
Moller A.R. (1973) *Basic Mechanisms of Hearing.* Macmillan, London.
Syka J. & Aitken L. (1981) *Neuronal Mechanisms of Hearing.* Plenum, New York.
Von Bekesy G. (1960) *Experiments in Hearing.* McGraw-Hill, New York.
Whitfield I.C. (1967) *The Auditory Pathway.* Physiological Society Monograph No. 17. Edward Arnold, London.
Wilson J.P. & Evans E.F. (1977) *Physiology and Psychology of Hearing.* Academic Press, New York.

Chapter 8: Cutaneous sensations

Gordon G. (ed.) (1977) Somatic and visceral sensory mechanisms. *Br. med. Bull.*, **33**(2).
Gordon G. (1978) *Active Touch.* Pergamon, Oxford.
Rexed B. (1952) The cytoarchitectonic organisation of the cat spinal cord. *J. comp. Neurol.*, **96,** 415–466.
Vallbo A.B. (1979) Somaesthetic, proprioceptive sympathetic activity in human peripheral nerves. *Physiol. Rev.*, **59,** 919–958.
Wall P.D. (1970) Sensory and motor role of dorsal columns. *Brain*, **93,** 505–524.
Zotterman Y. (1976) *Sensory Functions of the Skin in Primates.* Wenner Gren Symposium. Pergamon, Oxford.

Chapter 9: Pain

Bonica J.J. (ed.) (1977) *Pain.* Raven Press, New York.

Melzack R. (1973) *The Puzzle of Pain*. Penguin, Harmondsworth.
Snyder S.H. (1976) Internal opiates and opiate receptors. *Sci. Am.*, **236**(3), 44–56.
Wall P.D. (1978) The gate control revisited. *Brain*, **101**, 1–18.
Willis W.D. & Coggeshall R.E. (1978) *Sensory Mechanisms of the Spinal Cord*. Plenum, New York.

Chapter 10: Position sense and kinaesthesia

Goodwin G.M., McCloskey D.I. & Matthews P.B.C. The contribution of muscle afferents to kinesthesia. *Brain*, **95**, 705–748.
McCloskey D.I. (1978) Mechanisms of kinaesthesia. *Physiol. Rev.*, **58**, 763–820.
Roland P.E. (1978) Sensory feedback to the cerebral cortex during voluntary movement in man. *Behav. and Brain Sciences*, **1**, 129–171.

Chapter 11: Vestibular system

Lamb J.F., Ingram C.G., Johnston I.A. & Pitman R.M. (1980) *Essentials of Physiology*. Blackwell Scientific Publications, Oxford.
Wilson V.J. & Melville-Jones G. *Mammalian Vestibular Physiology*. Plenum, New York.

Chapter 12: Smell and taste

Moulton D.G. (1976) Spatial patterning of response to odours in the peripheral olfactory system. *Physiol. Rev.*, **56**, 578–593.
Pfaffman C. (1979) Neural mechanisms and behavioural aspects of taste. *Ann. Rev. Psychol.*, **30**, 283–325.
Shepherd G.M. (1979) *Synaptic Organisation of the Brain*. Oxford University Press, Oxford.

Chapter 13: Introduction to motor control

Miles F. & Evarts E.V. (1979) Concepts of motor control. *Ann. Rev. Psychol*, **30**, 327–362.
Talbot R.E. & Humphrey D.R. (1979) *Posture and Movement*. Raven Press, New York.
The Control of Movement (1980) *Trends in Neuroscience*, **3** (11).
Thompson R.F. (ed.) (1976) *Brain Mechanisms in Movement*. Scientific American Publications. W.H. Freeman, San Francisco.
Towe A.L. & Luschei E.S. (1981) *Motor Coordination. Handbook of Behavioural Neurobiology*, Vol. 5. Plenum, New York.

Chapter 14: Spinal cord, muscle receptors and spinal reflexes

Lundberg A. (1975) Control of spinal mechanisms from the brain. In: *The Basic Neurosciences*, Vol. 1 (ed. Tower D.B.), p. 253. Raven Press, New York.
Matthews P.B.C. (1972) *Mammalian Muscle Receptors and their Central Actions*. Physiological Society Monograph No. 23. Edward Arnold, London.
Merton P.R. (1953) Speculations on the servocontrol of movement. In: *The Spinal Cord* (ed. Wolstenholm G.). Churchill, London.
Taylor A. & Prochazwka V. (1981) *The Muscle Spindle*. Macmillan, London.

Chapter 15: Motor cortex

Asanuma H. (1975) Columnar arrangement of neurones in motor cortex. *Physiol. Rev.*, **55**, 143–157.
Desmedt J.E. (1978) *Long Loop Mechanisms. Progress in Clinical Neurophysiology*, Vol. 4. Karger, Basel.
Evarts E.V. (1974) Sensorimotor cortex activity associated with movements triggered by visual as compared to somesthetic inputs. In: *Neurosciences Third Study Program* (ed. Schmitt F.O.), p. 327. M.I.T. Press, Cambridge, Massachusetts.

Penfield W. & Rasmussen T. (1950) *The Cerebral Cortex of Man*. Macmillan, New York.
Phillips C.G. & Porter R.W. (1977) *Corticospinal Neurones—their Role in Movement*. Physiological Society Monograph No. 34. Academic Press, London.

Chapter 16: Extrapyramidal system

Brazier M. (1978) The reticular formation revisited. IBRO Monograph 6. Raven Press, New York.
Denny-Brown S.D. (1966) *The Cerebral Control of Movement*. Liverpool University Press, Liverpool.
Kuypers H.G.M. (1973) Anatomical organisation of descending motor pathways. In: *New Developments in Clinical Neurophysiology*, Vol. 3 (ed. Desmedt !.), p. 38. Karger, Basel.
Massion J. (1967) The red nucleus. *Physiol. Rev.*, **47**, 383–436.

Chapter 17: Cerebellum

Blomfield D. & Marr D. (1970) How the cerebellum may be used. *Nature (London)*, **227**, 1224–1228.
Eccles J.C. (1973) *The Understanding of the Brain*. Springer-Verlag, Berlin.
Eccles J.C., Ito M. & Szentasothai J. (1967) *The Cerebellum as a Neuronal Machine*. Springer-Verlag, Berlin.
Holmes G. (1939) The cerebellum of man. *Brain*, **62**, 1–30.
Ito M. (1982) Cerebellar control of vestibulo-ocular reflex. *Ann. Rev. Neurosci.*, **5**, 275–298.
Kornhuber H.H. (1974) Cerebral cortex, cerebellum and basal ganglia. In: *Neurosciences Third Study Program* (ed. Schmitt, F.O.), p. 267. M.I.T. Press, Cambridge, Massachusetts.

Chapter 18: Basal ganglia

Cooper J.R., Bloom F.E. & Roth R.H. (1978) *The Biochemical Basis of Neuropharmacology*, 3rd Edn. Oxford University Press, Oxford.
Divac I., Gurilla R. & Öberg E. (1978) *The Neostriatum*. Pergamon, Oxford.
Marks J. (1977) Physiology of abnormal movements. *Postgrad. med. J.*, **53**, 713.
Martin J.P. (1967) *The Basal Ganglia and Posture*. Pitman Medical, London.
Poirier L. (ed.) (1979) *The Extrapyramidal System and its Disorders*. Raven Press, New York.

Chapter 19: Posture and locomotion

Grillner S. (1975) Locomotion. *Physiol Rev.*, **55**, 247–304.
Pearson K. (1976) The control of walking. *Sci. Am.*, **235**, 72–86.

Chapter 20: Eye movements

Carpenter R.H.S. (1976) *Movements of the Eyes*. Pion, London.
Miles F. & Lisberger D. (1981) Vestibulo-ocular reflex. *Ann. Rev. Neurosci.*, **4**, 273–299.
Robinson D.A. (1981) Neurophysiology of eye movements. *Ann. Rev. Neurosci.*, **4**, 463–503.

Chapter 21: Sleep, EEG, reticular system

Cartwright R.D. (1978) *A Primer on Sleep and Dreaming*. Addison-Wesley, Reading, Maryland.

Chapter 22: Autonomic nervous system

Cohen M.I. (1979) Neurogenesis of respiratory rhythm. *Physiol. Rev.*, **59,** 1105–1173.
Merrill E.G. (1974) Medullary respiratory neurones. In: *Essays on the Nervous System* (ed. Bellairs R. & Gray E.G.), p. 451. Oxford University Press, Oxford.

Chapter 23: Control of body weight, fluid balance and temperature

Anderssohn B. (1978) Regulation of water intake. *Physiol. Rev.*, **58,** 582–603.
Bligh J. (1973) *Temperature Regulation.* North Holland, Amsterdam.
Fitzsimmons F.T. (1979) *The Physiology of Thirst and Sodium Appetite.* Physiological Society Monograph No. 35. Cambridge University Press, Cambridge.
Friedman M.J. & Stricker E.M. (1976) Physiology of hunger. *Psychol. Rev.,* **83,** 409–431.

Chapter 24: Hemispheric specialization

Geschwind N. (1974) *Language and the Brain.* D. Reidel, Doordrecht, Netherlands.
Milner B. (1974) Hemispheric specialisation, scope and limits. In: *Neurosciences Third Study Program* (ed. Schmitt F.O.), p. 75. M.I.T. Press, Cambridge, Massachusetts.
Springer S.P. & Deutsch G. (1981) *Left Brain, Right Brain.* W.H. Freeman, San Francisco.

Chapter 25: Reward, learning and memory

Hilgard E.R. & Bower G.H. (1975) *Theories of Learning.* Prentice Hall, New Jersey.
Rolls E.T. (1975) *The Brain and Reward.* Pergamon, Oxford.
Snyder S.H. (1974) *Madness and the Brain.* McGraw-Hill, New York.

Chapter 26: Historical epilogue

Singer C. (1928) *A Short History of Medicine.* Clarendon Press, Oxford.

Index